W9-AGN-356

DISORDERS OF THE AUDITORY SYSTEM

DISORDERS OF THE AUDITORY SYSTEM

Frank E. Musiek
Jane A. Baran
Jennifer B. Shinn
Raleigh O. Jones

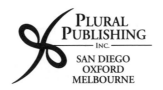

PLURAL
PUBLISHING
INC.

SAN DIEGO
OXFORD
MELBOURNE

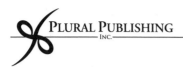

5521 Ruffin Road
San Diego, CA 92123

e-mail: info@pluralpublishing.com
Web site: http://www.pluralpublishing.com

49 Bath Street
Abingdon, Oxfordshire OX14 1EA
United Kingdom

Typeset in 10.5/13 Palatino by Flanagan's Publishing Services, Inc.
Printed in the United States of America by McNaughton & Gunn.

Library of Congress Cataloging-in-Publication Data

Disorders of the auditory system / Frank E. Musiek . . . [et al.].
    p. ; cm.
  Includes bibliographical references and index.
  ISBN-13: 978-1-59756-350-5 (alk. paper)
  ISBN-10: 1-59756-350-1 (alk. paper)
  I. Musiek, Frank E.
  [DNLM: 1. Hearing Disorders. 2. Auditory Diseases, Central. WV 270]
  LC-classification not assigned
  617.8—dc23
                         2011031036

Contents

Foreword

Writing a book on auditory disorders is a daunting task. Few individuals have the depth and breadth of knowledge to accomplish it effectively. But the authors of this volume, Drs. Frank E. Musiek, Jane A. Baran, Jennifer B. Shinn, and Raleigh O. Jones, are among a very small number of teams truly able to meet the challenge. This team has dealt with the issues and problems surrounding the evaluation of auditory disorders for many years, has devised a number of the tools in current use for clinical evaluation, and has applied them successfully in a variety of settings. They have been in the trenches. This team also reflects a fine working relationship between audiology, otology, and neurology critical to understanding the complex issues related to auditory disorders.

From a historical perspective, this volume might be viewed as the culmination of a steady march toward greater sophistication in the evaluation of auditory disorders. The 19th-century otologists, mostly in Germany, certainly differentiated conductive loss from what was then called "perceptive" loss; however, the modern era of diagnostic auditory evaluation began in 1948 with the historic paper by the British team of M. R. Dix, C. S. Hallpike, and J. D. Hood in the *Proceedings of the Royal Society of Medicine*, which demonstrated that unilateral perceptive loss (what we now call sensorineural loss) could be further differentiated into its cochlear and auditory nerve components by means of the alternate binaural loudness balance (ABLB) test.

This seminal observation stimulated international interest throughout the decades of the 1950s and 1960s in the development of a variety of methods for differentiating cochlear from eighth nerve disorders, based variously on the intensity difference limen (DL), Békésy audiometric threshold tracings, nonlinear distortion of tonal stimuli, the acoustic reflex, and variations on speech audiometry. The discovery of the auditory brainstem response (ABR) in the early 1970s, however, radically altered the search. It may be difficult for young audiologists today to appreciate how this single test altered the landscape of auditory diagnostic evaluation. In addition to its value in differentiating cochlear from auditory nerve sites, it has become the sine qua non of infant hearing screening, pediatric assessment of hearing loss, and evaluation of auditory neuropathy/auditory dyssynchrony disorder. Just a few years later the discovery of otoacoustic emissions (OAE) added another powerful tool to the audiologist's differential diagnostic armamentarium.

Today the combination of ABR and OAE is perhaps our most powerful set of diagnostic tools.

Interest in disorders central to the auditory periphery was advanced by many audiologists, especially in the United States, following the pioneering observations of the Italian investigators led by Ettore Bocca who, in the mid-1950s, demonstrated that "sensitized" speech audiometric measures could be used to reflect disorders at the level of the temporal lobes. Early in the next decade, Canadians Brenda Milner and Doreen Kimura demonstrated the right ear advantage/left ear disadvantage in dichotic listening. These two sets of observations suggested to many audiologists that speech audiometric tests, especially the dichotic variety, might identify children and adults with "central" auditory processing disorders. Later, frequency pattern, temporal pattern, and temporal resolution tests supplemented these measures. The authors of the present volume have been particularly active in this arena. Herein they bring us very nicely up to date on the present status of what has become, over the last five decades, a broad array of auditory disorders.

I would particularly recommend this book as an excellent text for an advanced undergraduate or graduate course on auditory disorders and their evaluation.

James Jerger
Richardson, TX
December 2011

Acknowledgments

Writing a book such as this one, which covers a wide range of difficult topics, is no easy task. Fortunately, I had three other authors who are also great friends who worked diligently to see this book to its finish. Longtime colleague and friend, Jane Baran, worked tirelessly in editing this text. Her extreme efforts need to be recognized, as without her numerous contributions this work could not have been completed. Jennifer Shinn, former student and friend, did an outstanding job of researching content and contributing many of the case studies. Jenn kept us going and provided much appreciated leadership and motivation—many, many thanks. Much appreciation to Raleigh Jones, our hardworking neurotologist, whose fine contributions regarding the medical and surgical aspects of hearing disorders are the underpinnings of this book. I am honored to work with these professionals.

We are thankful to Gary Jacobson and Devin McCaslin for their excellent contribution to the vestibular anatomy and physiology section of Chapter 2, and to Matthew Bush, who helped us out of so many difficult situations with his hard work and knowledge of otologic disorders. He was always there to lend a helping hand no matter what the task. We would also like to thank Curtis Given II, Michael Hoffer, Eric Smouha, Abbas Younes, Kathleen Arnos, Erik Musiek, and George Mencher for their thoughtful contributions to various chapters in the book.

Thanks to the patient, helpful, and kind people at Plural. We would especially like to recognize the late Sandy Doyle, who worked so courageously as the copy editor, to Caitlin Mahon for her expert editing, and to Angie Singh who never gave up on us and guided us to the completion of this text.

Finally, we have some personal acknowledgments, as this book would not have been completed without strong support from those close to us.

A heartfelt thanks to my wife Sheila, sons Erik and Justin, daughter-in-law Amy, and granddaughters Emma and Anna Kate for their love and encouragement. —FM

A special thanks goes out to my husband, David Hoffman, my daughter, Sarah Jane, and my loving parents, who continually offered their encouragement, love, and support throughout this endeavor. —JB

To my amazing family and loving husband. I am forever grateful for your unwavering love and support. —JS

To my wife, Dr. Jeannie Jones, whose professional and personal sacrifices and unwavering support have been the underpinning of my academic career. —RJ

1

Introduction

RATIONALE FOR THIS BOOK

The study of auditory disorders is the essence of a multidisciplinary approach for learning in the content areas of audiology and otology. It has been known for some time that, in order to create the optimal learning format for auditory disorders, both disciplines need to contribute to the knowledge base. More recently, however, other disciplines, such as neurology, pathology, and hearing science also have made important contributions to this area of study. One of the goals in writing this book was to include insights into auditory disorders from the perspectives of all of these disciplines.

When the idea for writing a book on auditory disorders was conceptualized, it had been a long time since such a book had been published. It was felt that an updated publication on auditory disorders directed toward AuD students, audiologists, and other professionals in related fields was needed. In addition, based on our own personal experiences, as well as considerable input from others in audiology and related disciplines,

there appeared to be a general lack of a comprehensive and full understanding of auditory disorders on the part of many graduate students and newly trained audiologists. This appeared to be especially true for disorders that affected the central auditory nervous system (CANS). This seemed perplexing because clinical audiologists are involved in the diagnosis and treatment of individuals with various disorders of the auditory system. As audiologists and health care professionals, we play an important role in guiding patients with hearing loss through the maze of professionals who sometimes need to be seen for optimal treatment. As a result, knowledge of disorders affecting the auditory system is critical. Clinical decisions regarding whether or not to refer, to whom to refer, the timing of the referral, and why the referral is needed depend on the audiologist's knowledge of hearing and vestibular disorders, associated medical conditions, and etiological bases.

This book covers the most common and/or significant disorders of the peripheral and central auditory systems. Not all auditory disorders are reviewed in this publication. To stay within the scope of the book, decisions had to be made as to which disorders to include and which disorders not to include in this text. Also, it was not our intent to provide a comprehensive review of vestibular disorders, although the reader will note that some vestibular disorders are discussed. These discussions are limited to disorders where the vestibular deficits are part of an auditory/vestibular disorder complex.

The references in this text are not always the original or first articles describing the disorders covered, but rather references that we believe will provide documentation on the disorders being discussed and lead the reader to more information, when desired. In many cases, recent review articles provided a framework that could be highly useful to the readers for whom this book was intended.

The coverage of auditory disorders in this book includes a review of disorders that can compromise the central auditory system, as well as the peripheral auditory system. In the authors' view, the topic of central auditory system disorders frequently has been overlooked or not covered to the degree that was warranted in past publications. In this text, disorders related to the central auditory system are a key area of coverage for a number of reasons. First, there is a considerable amount of new pathological information from the areas of neurology, neurotology, and neuroaudiology that impacts the diagnosis and treatment of central auditory disorders, which needs to be organized and made readily available. For example, relatively new findings have established the role of the central auditory system in tinnitus, which is a hearing loss symptom that was previously believed primarily to be a manifestation of inner ear pathology. In addition, it is now known that

noise-induced hearing loss, as well other peripheral disorders, may have significant effects on central auditory system function and long-term integrity. An understanding of the role of the central auditory system in hearing disorders and their related symptoms, as well as the potential for central auditory system compromise secondary to peripheral system compromise, is important for clinicians. Second, there is both increased knowledge of and interest in central auditory disorders as documented by the sharp increase in recent publications in this area and the demand for clinical services. Therefore, it is important for audiologists and related health care professionals to have access to information about central auditory disorders to effectively serve both patients who are being seen for central auditory assessments, as well as patients who may present with symptoms and preliminary audiologic findings that would result in a diagnosis of peripheral hearing loss, but who may also be at risk for central auditory compromise (e.g., as in the examples noted above).

OVERVIEW

Chapter 2, Structure and Function of the Auditory and Vestibular Systems, is critical as an early chapter in this book. Serious discussion of auditory and vestibular disorders, both peripheral and central, requires a working knowledge of the structure and function of the auditory and vestibular systems. This chapter focuses on the human auditory and vestibular systems to provide a reference and framework for the presentation of the hearing disorders and their sites of lesion included in subsequent chapters. Points of interest include both peripheral and central auditory aspects of auditory biology (see Musiek & Baran, 2007). For example, one point is the role of melanin, which is produced by the second layer of cells in the stria vascularis. If melanin is decreased, hearing sensitivity may suffer. This relationship is observed in albino animals, which often have hearing loss or are completely deaf when melanin levels are found to be reduced. Another highlight is information on traveling wave velocity. The velocity at the basal end of the cochlea is near 100 meters per second and slows to about 2 meters per second at the apical end. This information has much to do with greater neural synchronicity at the basal compared to the apical end of the cochlea. The implications of traveling wave velocity, in our view, has not been fully appreciated in either basic or applied research. In addition, new information on traveling wave velocity related to cochlear hydrops has emerged and resulted in the development of a potential clinical test for this particular inner ear condition, as discussed in the chapter on inner ear disorders. In the central auditory system one of the long-standing concepts remains one of the most revealing, that is, the concept of neural arborization. Within the CANS, there is a significant increase in the number of neurons available for processing as one moves through the CANS in a caudal to rostral direction. This increase in the number of neurons as one moves up the CANS assumes a greater capacity for complex functions in the higher CANS than the lower CANS or the auditory periphery. Although many advances in understanding the CANS have developed recently from molecular and microanatomic approaches, gross anatomic research has re-emerged as interest in functional imaging techniques has grown and its use as a tool to study the CANS has increased in popularity. Anatomic variances and asymmetries in both the normal and disordered human brain can be identified through the use of functional imaging techniques. Classic findings that the planum temporale and Heschl's gyrus are larger for the left hemisphere than the right still have relevant functional implications across several disciplines.

Chapter 3 addresses the auditory, vestibular, and radiologic test procedures discussed in this book. Although much of the audiologic information presented may be familiar information for audiologists, it may be useful to the student or the nonaudiologist reading this text. Throughout this book there has been a serious attempt to use similar forms, symbols, and terminology. A large number of case studies are included and consistency in the use of forms, symbols, and terminology should help reading efficiency. This becomes more evident when case studies utilizing vestibular, central auditory, and evoked potential assessments are reported. Chapter 3 provides an overview of the tests discussed in this text, as well as an introduction to the symbols, abbreviations, and terminology used. Whenever possible "classic" as well as "nonclassic" findings on the tests overviewed are reported for many of the auditory disorders discussed in subsequent chapters (as appropriate to the case or disorder being presented).

This chapter also includes an overview on contemporary radiology. Radiologic interpretation, of course, is based on anatomy. Therefore, we include radiologic information after the chapter on anatomy.

The two most common radiologic procedures, computed tomography (CT) and magnetic resonance imaging (MRI), are reviewed. Understanding elemental radiology on the part of the audiologist is one area that can markedly increase relevant communication with key medical personnel. Radiology can also provide insight as to the nature of a disorder and offer an excellent cross-check of audiologic test efficiency. Comparing audiologic evaluation results with radiologic evidence is one of the foundations of diagnostic audiology. Chapter 3 provides discussion of the basics of CT and MRI in a relevant, yet understandable manner. This is followed by a comparison of the two techniques revealing the advantages and limitations of each. Illustrations emphasizing the high utility of CT for osseous material, such as the temporal bone, ossicles, the bony cochlea, and the internal auditory canal, are provided. Other radiologic images revealing the application of MRI in viewing soft tissue structures, such as cranial nerves, brainstem, and cerebral substrate, are included. The case examples of both normal and abnormal radiologic images in subsequent chapters provide a highly relevant learning experience for the audiologist, student, or health care professional who has limited knowledge of or experience in interpreting the results of radiologic testing procedures.

Chapter 4 on the external and middle ear is the first that illustrates the book's organizational scheme for the four chapters that focus on a specific site of lesion (e.g., disorders of the outer and middle ear, the inner ear, the auditory nerve, and the CANS). Each of these chapters includes an anatomic review of the relevant anatomy, an introduction to each of the disorders discussed in the chapter, and information on the symptoms, incidence/prevalence, etiology/pathology, site-of-lesion, audiology, medical examination, audiologic management, and medical management for the disorders included. In a few instances, the disorders do not receive a full complement of information in each of the areas listed above. This occurred because of a paucity of information available, the rareness of the disorder, and/or the scope of the chapter. Typically, but not exclusively, these disorders were designated under "other disorders" at the ends of the chapters.

Chapter 4 covers the classic disorders affecting the outer and/or middle structures, such as atresia, Eustachian tube dysfunction, otitis media, cholesteatoma, glomus tumors, otosclerosis, and trauma. Mentioned briefly are external otitis, exostoses, osteomas, tympanic membrane perforations, tympanosclerosis, and ossicular chain disarticulation. Also, an audiologic mechanism that has been around for some time, but which is often not understood by many is highlighted. It is well known that, in early otitis media, there is a low-frequency tilt to the puretone audiogram. This is related to negative pressure increasing the stiffness of the ossicular chain. Later in the disease process, effusion may evolve, resulting in a significant "mass effect" that results in a high-frequency loss and an overall flat audiometric configuration (Jerger & Jerger, 1981).

Chapter 5 discusses disorders of the inner ear. These include trauma, noise-induced hearing loss, ototoxicity, Ménière's disease, autoimmune inner ear disease, presbycusis, superior semicircular canal dehiscence, and sudden idiopathic sensorineural hearing loss. Also overviewed are diabetes and perilymph fistula. Recently, there have been innovations in the study of a number of cochlear disorders; specifically mentioned are noise-induced hearing loss (NIHL) and Ménière's disease. A better understanding of the pathologic mechanisms underlying NIHL has emerged by the discovery of free radicals and their role in NIHL (as well as other diseases) (Kopke, Coleman, Liu, Campbell, & Riffenburgh, 2002). High-intensity sound results in overstimulation of the inner ear structures, which leads to the production of toxic, metabolic by-products, termed reactive oxygen species and free radicals. These free radicals result in oxidative stress on the hair cells and their related structures, and often result in damage to these inner ear structures. This new knowledge has created the potential for new approaches to the prevention and treatment of NIHL. Chemical agents that can resist the actions of free radicals have been shown to reduce the effects of NIHL. Although to date most of the research in this exciting area has been on animals, approaches to reduce the effects of free radicals are close to utilization with humans.

In disorders that affect the homeostasis of fluids within the inner ear (e.g., Ménière's disease), it has been postulated that the increase in endolymph in the scala media can result in stretching of the basilar membrane. This action in turn increases the stiffness gradient of the basilar membrane, especially in the more apical portions, which in turn causes the traveling wave to move faster. This increased velocity of the traveling wave can be captured in humans using the auditory brainstem response test (ABR) and high bandpass masking. Hence, for low frequencies, the resultant ABR latencies are shorter in patients with Ménière's disease when compared to individuals without the disease. This action is also related to an undermasking effect that occurs with this technique. This is an important physiologic correlate with genuine clinical impact on the diagnosis of Ménière's disease (Don, Kwong, & Tanaka, 2005).

Superior semicircular canal dehiscence syndrome is a vestibular disorder that recently has received much attention in otology and audiology. This often is a congenital condition that may reveal itself early on or after many years. Vestibular evoked myogenic potentials, also a relatively new technique, can help considerably in the diagnosis of this disorder. Given the mounting interest in this disorder and its impact in otology and audiology, its inclusion in this chapter was warranted.

Determining exactly what to include in Chapter 6 on the auditory nerve was somewhat difficult. Clearly, tumors of the eighth nerve traditionally are the key disorder to be covered. Decisions relative to what other disorders to include presented more of a challenge. Given the general awareness of auditory neuropathy/auditory dys-synchrony, it seemed reasonable to include it. Several other topics were considered, but most were extremely rare or little was known about them. The final topic included was one of interest to all the authors; hence, it was selected for inclusion in this chapter. This disorder is commonly referred to as vascular loop syndrome.

Chapter 6 reveals some new trends in the assessment and management of patients with eighth nerve tumors that are worth mentioning here. One is the evolution of a more conservative approach to the management of eighth nerve tumors. Small tumors in older individuals are now more commonly watched and monitored rather than immediately being surgically removed. This is because some small tumors simply do not grow or grow at a very slow rate; hence, surgery may not be necessary in some cases. Another trend that is emerging, although not without some controversy, is the by-passing of ABR testing, with the immediate and direct referral for MRI testing based primarily on a consideration of the patient's history and the audiogram. The final chapter on this controversial trend has not yet been written. By skipping the ABR and proceeding immediately to MRI testing, the total cost for MRI testing for patients who are considered to be at risk for eighth nerve tumors becomes exorbitant. This is because the overwhelming majority of people with unilateral sensorineural hearing loss, which is a primary consideration for referral for MRI testing, do not have tumors. Utilization of the ABR (a much less expensive diagnostic procedure) prior to referral for radiologic assessment would markedly reduce this overreferral for MRI testing. Each of these "trends" is discussed in greater detail in the auditory nerve chapter.

Chapter 6 also relays another controversial topic, that of auditory neuropathy/auditory dys-synchrony. The neurologic definition of this condition may be different from the audiologic one and this may create some difficulties in categorization. Of concern, however, is the inclusion of such disorders as hyperbilirubinemia (kernicterus at its pathological end point) as auditory neuropathies. Because hyperbilirubinemia does not primarily affect the auditory nerve, but rather the central auditory system and other central nervous system structures, it is not truly a peripheral neuropathy, but rather a CANS disorder. Further discussion of this controversy is included in Chapter 7, Disorders Affecting the CANS.

Chapter 7 is the largest chapter and addresses disorders that can affect the central auditory system. These disorders are driven more by their location than by the nature of the disease. That is, many disorders may affect the CANS if they are located within that system. On the other hand, some diseases that often can affect the central auditory system may not if their pathologic action is not in the right location (i.e., within the central auditory system). This chapter highlights vascular disorders, such as stroke involving the middle cerebral artery (MCA) and/or its branches. This vascular complex provides blood to most of the key auditory areas of the cerebrum. It is clear that disruption of the MCA complex will result in direct damage to cortical auditory structures. This in turn creates problems in higher level hearing processes. Despite this well-known link between anatomic damage and dysfunction, stroke patients seldom are evaluated audiologically.

Chapter 7 also brings attention to a prominent neurologic problem that also has an association with audiology, that is, Alzheimer's disease. Individuals with Alzheimer's disease often suffer from both peripheral and central auditory problems. Understanding the auditory factors in Alzheimer's and other degenerative disorders can be highly useful to patients suffering from these maladies. The use of standard audiologic tests, as well as central auditory procedures including both behavioral and electrophysiologic approaches, can provide considerable information that can help guide and counsel patients with Alzheimer's disease and their families. Indeed, it can be difficult to determine the degree of peripheral versus central auditory involvement in the patient with Alzheimer's disease, and for some patients (e.g., those with advanced stages of the disease), it may not be possible to obtain valid and reliable measures of auditory function. However, for many patients, some auditory testing can be completed and the use of both objective as well as subjective measures can lead to accurate diagnosis and subsequent management of the patient's auditory deficits. Deficits on the pure-tone audiogram can and should be corroborated with otoacoustic emissions (OAEs). If these individuals have valid sensitivity deficits, amplification can be a major help. Central auditory testing should rely heavily on auditory evoked potentials and laterality trends on behavioral test indices.

Special attention in this chapter focuses on surgical procedures that may disrupt the CANS. Epilepsy and other neurologic disorders at times may require surgery, which can involve compromise of higher auditory processes that can affect everyday communication. These patients should be evaluated prior to and after surgery to determine overall audiologic status and to inform optimal rehabilitative planning. This is a clinical population that all too often is overlooked by audiology in general.

Chapter 8 on tinnitus, hyperacusis, and auditory hallucinations could easily have been included in the context of other chapters. However, with the abundance of new information in these areas, it was decided to discuss these disorders in a section of their own. Tinnitus remains somewhat of a mystery in terms of a cure. However, advances in our understanding of tinnitus have changed. As mentioned above, greater acceptance of the role of the central nervous system in tinnitus has evolved due in part to the functional imaging work of Lockwood, Salvi, and Burkard (2002). This work (as well as similar studies by others) showed acti-

vation of the auditory cortex in patients experiencing tinnitus and has provided the basis for a new approach to the study of tinnitus. Although central tinnitus has long been entertained as a possibility, this concept now has gained support from many researchers who are investigating this bothersome malady.

Hyperacusis is a disorder that presents as exaggerated or inappropriate responses to sounds that are not uncomfortably loud to a typical person. It is a symptom that is often reported by patients who also report experiencing tinnitus, which has raised speculation that there may be a shared mechanism underlying the etiology and pathology of these two disorders. However, the exact mechanisms underlying hyperacusis remain unknown, but many theories abound. These theories, as well as some of the common peripheral and central conditions that may be associated with hyperacusis, are reviewed.

Perhaps for the first time in a book such as this, the disorder of auditory hallucinations is discussed. This topic was included for several reasons. One was that the prevalence of this disorder is much greater than most people suspect. Another was that auditory hallucinations are not a problem relegated only to those with psychiatric illnesses. In many instances, auditory hallucinations may have an auditory problem (peripheral or central) as their basis. Interestingly, there is much interest on the part of our European colleagues in this disorder. Perhaps one of the attractive reasons for the inclusion of this topic was the recent documentation of CANS involvement as revealed by functional imaging in patients experiencing auditory hallucinations (Shergill et al., 2004). As in the case of tinnitus, imaging studies have changed our thinking about auditory hallucinations. These studies implicate the auditory cortex as a possible physiologic basis for the perceptual experience of auditory hallucinations, and allow a refocusing of this disorder in more of an auditory context, at least for patients without comorbid psychiatric diagnoses. This relatively new information along with the historical view that auditory hallucinations often were linked to long-term and relatively severe hearing loss has served to create a logical interest from hearing professionals, and rightly so. In the same regard, some of the current treatments for auditory hallucinations are auditory in nature (Collins, Cull, & Sireling, 1989).

Chapter 9 on hereditary and congenital hearing loss provides background and foundational information on genetics and inherited hearing loss. Genetics is an area that recently has become of great interest to audiologists and hearing health care professionals. For example, the genetic protein, connexin 26, has become well known as playing an integral role in hearing and hearing loss in the past decade. Given this interest in genetics it seemed logical to include information on inherited hearing loss, highlighting basic information on chromosomes and genes. The chromosomes contain genetic material made up of deoxyribonucleic acid (DNA) arranged in units on the chromosomes, called genes. Genes carry the elements needed to form specific proteins that are critical for normal growth and development of the organism. There can be alterations in the DNA, which are termed mutations. These mutations eventually can result in incomplete or abnormal development and/or the degeneration of critical structures (Bayazit & Yilmaz, 2006). If genes coded for the development and/or maintenance

of structures that compose the auditory system undergo mutations due to DNA alterations, the result may be abnormal structure and function of this system and typically a hearing loss. This structural and functional alteration can be specific to the auditory system or it may involve the auditory and other systems. This has led to the categorization of genetically based hearing disorders as either nonsyndromic or syndromic. The former is where the mutation primarily affects the hearing structures. The latter is a more pervasive condition, with multiple systems often involved. This final chapter reviews the various syndromic and nonsyndromic hearing disorders utilizing an anatomic categorization. Categories include external and middle ear, cochlear, eighth nerve, and the CANS. In addition, this chapter discusses types of hearing loss usually noted in the various syndromes and the important roles of genetic evaluation and counseling in working with patients with potential genetic bases for their hearing losses.

SUMMARY

This text provides comprehensive information on a number of auditory disorders, but many disorders that affect or potentially could affect hearing function were not included as these were hearing disorders of extremely low incidence and felt to be beyond the scope of this book. However, we hope that this book provides sufficient pertinent information on disorders of hearing that readers will appreciate and value it, and will have the foundation needed to explore additional resources for information regarding disorders not covered in this text.

REFERENCES

Bayazit, Y. A., & Yilmaz, M. (2006). An overview of hereditary hearing loss. *ORL: Journal for Oto-Rhino-Laryngology and Related Specialties, 68*(2), 57–63.

Collins, M. N., Cull, C. A., & Sireling, L. (1989). Pilot study of treatment of persistent auditory hallucinations by modified auditory input. *British Medical Journal, 299*(6696), 431–432.

Don, M., Kwong, B., & Tanaka, C. (2005). A diagnostic test for Ménière's disease and cochlear hydrops: Impaired high-pass noise masking of auditory brainstem responses. *Otology and Neurotology, 26*(4), 711–722.

Jerger, S., & Jerger, J. (1981). *Auditory disorders.* Boston, MA: Little, Brown.

Kopke, R. D., Coleman, J. K., Liu, J., Campbell, K. C., & Riffenburgh, R. H. (2002). Candidate's thesis: Enhancing intrinsic cochlear stress defenses to reduce noise-induced hearing loss. *Laryngoscope, 112*(9), 1515–1532.

Lockwood, A. H., Salvi, R. J., & Burkard, R. F. (2002). Tinnitus. *New England Journal of Medicine, 347*(12), 904–910.

Musiek, F. E., & Baran, J. A. (2007). *The auditory system: Anatomy, physiology, and clinical correlates.* Boston, MA: Allyn & Bacon.

Shergill, S. S., Brammer, M. J., Amaro, E., Williams, S. C., Murray, R. M., & McGuire, P. K. (2004). Temporal course of auditory hallucinations. *British Journal of Psychiatry, 185,* 516–517.

2

Structure and Function of the Auditory and Vestibular Systems

INTRODUCTION

Hearing is a complex process that is critical to our everyday well-being. As humans we can hear an extremely wide range of frequencies and intensities. We can also discriminate small changes in intensity (on the order of 1 dB) and frequency (on the order of a few hertz). Even more amazing is the fact that the normal human auditory system can pick out sounds embedded in noise and understand what someone is saying across the room at large social gatherings (i.e., the cocktail party effect). These hearing skills, which we all take for granted, are a result of the ear (peripheral system) and the brain (central system) working together with great precision.

The vestibular system, which shares some anatomic structures with the auditory system, is responsible for our ability to perceive changes in head movements (acceleration and deceleration) and the orientation of the head with respect to gravity. Similar to the auditory system, the vestibular system has both peripheral as well as central components that work together to help us maintain our sense of balance.

Understanding the structure and function of the peripheral and central components of these two systems is the goal of much current research. It also is critical for advances in the diagnosis and treatment of disorders of the auditory system and any comorbid or related vestibular problems. An appreciation and understanding of the anatomy and physiology of these systems allows one to identify the location of the disordered region within the auditory and vestibular systems. This in turn provides insight as to the nature of the disorder that can lead to effective treatment. Therefore, it is safe to say that understanding disorders of the auditory and vestibular systems is an essential skill for the audiologist and hearing care professional that is dependent on a substantial knowledge of the structure and function of these two interrelated systems.

Although the topic of auditory and vestibular anatomy and physiology can only be overviewed in this chapter, it is hoped that the reader will be oriented well enough to fully grasp the essence of dysfunction of the auditory system. The anatomy and physiology of the auditory system is discussed first, followed by a brief overview of the vestibular system.

THE PERIPHERAL AUDITORY SYSTEM

The Temporal Bone

The temporal bone either houses or supports most of the structures of the auditory periphery. It is an integral part of the skull base and is composed of four fairly distinct segments. The squamous portion is part of the lateral cranium immediately superior to the ear canal. The bony ear canal is another segment of the temporal bone and constitutes the tympanic portion. Directly posterior to the tympanic portion is the mastoid segment, which is characterized by numerous air cells. The final segment is the petrous portion that houses the middle ear, the cochlea, and the vestibular apparatus. It is a wedge-shaped structure that courses medially in the base of the skull and divides the posterior cranial fossa from the middle cranial fossa (Figure 2–1).

On the posterior side of the petrous portion of the temporal bone there are a

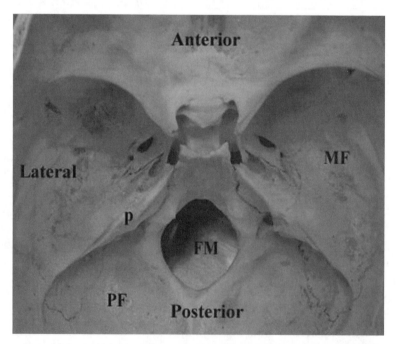

Figure 2–1. *A photograph of the base of the cranium with anterior, posterior, and lateral aspects depicted. Key: PF = posterior fossa, MF = middle fossa, FM = foramen magnum, p = petrous portion of the temporal bone which houses the middle and inner ears as well as the internal auditory meatus. (Reproduced with permission from Musiek and Baran, 2007.)*

number of key structures. The opening to the internal auditory meatus (IAM), also termed the porous acousticus, is located about two-thirds of the way along this structure and courses in a lateral to medial direction. Through this opening in the temporal bone exits the auditory, vestibular, and facial nerves that project to their respective nuclei in the brainstem (lateral, caudal pons). Also located on the posterior aspect of the petrous bone just lateral to the IAM opening is the opening for the vestibular and cochlear aqueducts. These openings are identified by small recesses in the posterior side of the petrous bone (Anson & Donaldson, 1981).

One of the main functions of the temporal bone is to provide a framework of support for the outer, middle, and inner ears as well as the seventh and eighth cranial nerves. In addition to support and stabilization of these structures, the temporal bone provides protection for most of the anatomic structures within the auditory periphery that support hearing.

The Outer Ear

Structure

The outer or external ear includes the pinna or auricle and the external auditory meatus (EAM), or ear canal. The pinna is "C"-shaped and is composed of a foundation of cartilage that is covered with skin. The structure of the pinna takes on a shape that conforms to the underlying cartilage, which results in its distinct appearance as a structure with numerous folds and recesses. These folds and recesses constitute specific anatomic sites or areas within the pinna for which particular terms are used (Figure 2–2). Referring back to the "C"-shaped structure of the pinna, the outer circular part of the "C" is termed the helix and just inside of

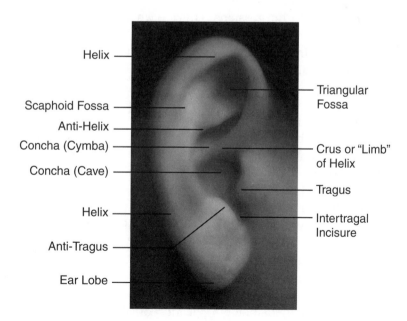

Figure 2–2. A photo of a human right pinna. (Reproduced with permission from Musiek and Baran, 2007.)

the helix is the antihelix. Located superiorly between the helix and antihelix is a groove called the scaphoid fossa, which lies next to the triangular fossa. Immediately inferior to the antihelix is a ridge, termed the crus of the helix. This ridge is responsible for much of the rigidity of the pinna. The deepest recess of the pinna is the concha, which leads to the opening to the ear canal. Anterior to the concha is a protective flap called the tragus, which can be pressed into the opening of the ear canal to serve as protection. Inferior and posterior to the tragus is a prominence termed the antitragus. At the most inferior aspect of the pinna is the ear lobe—probably the softest and most flexible of the pinna's structures. Between the ear lobe and the tragus is the intertragal incisure (Clark & Ohlemiller, 2008; Musiek & Baran, 2007). The various structures of the pinna are innervated by the fifth (trigeminal) and seventh (facial) cranial nerves (Musiek & Baran, 2007; Zemlin, 1998).

The anatomy of the pinna becomes useful when taking earmold impressions and when fabricating earmolds. Variances in the pinna's fine structure can be well-defined using the anatomy discussed above. This in turn can allow better and more precise communication between the audiologist or hearing instrument specialist and the earmold manufacturer concerning the need for attention to a particular area or areas of the earmold to be created or modified, which should result in a better fit, and ultimately, a more satisfactory hearing aid experience for the patient.

The second structure in the external ear is the EAM. This outer ear structure is shaped like a tube and averages 2.5 to 3.0 cm in length and 0.75 cm in diameter in the adult human. It originates at the con-

cha (an opening in the pinna) and ends at the tympanic membrane (Figure 2–3). The EAM is not straight, but rather curves like an elongated letter "S" that is lying on its side. However, it is important to note that there is great variation in the shape of the EAM in humans. Visual inspection of this structure will reveal some EAMs that are relatively straight, whereas in other instances the EAM will be observed to be curvier. Pulling on the posterior aspect of the pinna can help straighten the ear canal for visual inspection with otoscopy. This procedure can prove to be especially helpful when one is visually inspecting an ear canal that is quite curvy in nature.

The foundation of the outer third of the ear canal is cartilaginous, whereas the foundation of the medial two-thirds is bony. The entire length of the ear canal is covered by an epidermal lining and the outer third contains hair follicles and glands that secrete a waxy substance (i.e., cerumen). Innervation of the EAM comes from the fifth (trigeminal), seventh (facial), and ninth (glossopharyngeal) cranial nerves, making the EAM sensitive to tactile stimulation (Møller, 2000; Musiek & Baran, 2007; Zemlin, 1998).

Function

The pinna's main function is to help funnel sounds from the environment into the smaller diameter EAM. Because of its unique structure and size, the pinna tends to result in a slight enhancement of sounds in the vicinity of 5000 Hz (Shaw & Teranishi, 1968). This enhancement occurs because the unique configuration of the pinna in terms of its ridges and recesses results in a more efficient collection of sound in the higher frequency range and the wavelengths of lower fre-

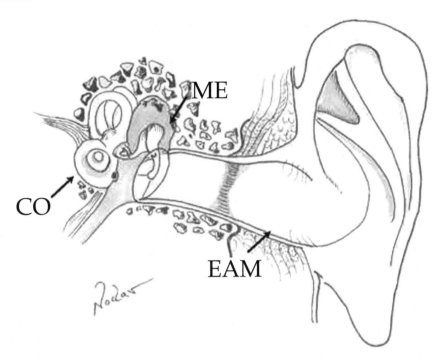

Figure 2–3. *A drawing of the outer, middle, and inner ears showing the location and configuration of the EAM. Key: EAM = external auditory meatus, ME = middle ear, CO = cochlea. (Adapted with permission from Musiek and Baran, 2007.)*

quency sounds are essentially larger than the pinna and can pass around this structure more readily than those of higher frequency sounds (Musiek & Baran, 2007). The pinna also helps with sound localization by creating complex resonances that change as the location of the sound source changes (Blauert, 1983).

The EAM helps to protect the ear with its debris-catching cilia and cerumen and it also serves as an acoustic resonator. The EAM peak resonance is around 3000 to 4000 Hz in the adult. At these frequencies, there is a gain of 10 to 15 dB in the acoustic signal with little or no gain at the frequencies below 1000 Hz (Dallos, 1973).

It also should be mentioned that, in addition to the pinna and the EAM, the head, and even the torso can exert differential effects on the sounds reaching the ear. The combination of these effects provides valuable auditory information that the normal auditory system uses to help identify the source of a sound (i.e., directional hearing). Most notable of the directional hearing effects is the head shadow effect, which can have a significant effect on the sound reaching the ear when the sound is originating from a source located on one side of the head versus the other. Take for example the situation where one has a sound being presented in a sound field to the right side of the head. In this case, the sound would have almost direct access to the right ear, but the head would interfere with the sound that is traveling to the left ear. The end result would be that the sound reaching the left ear would be of a lower intensity (especially at high frequencies) than the sound arriving at the right ear. The central auditory system is capable of detecting and analyzing these types of intensity differences, as well as "small" time of arrival differences that occur as a result of the further distance that the signal has to travel to reach one ear versus the other, to identify the source of a sound (see Musiek & Baran, 2007, for additional discussion).

The Middle Ear

Structure

The tympanic membrane (TM) marks the beginning of the middle ear and is oval-shaped and concave in its appearance (Figure 2–4). In the adult human, it averages 8 to 10 mm in diameter, with a slightly larger diameter along the vertical axis than along the horizontal axis. The membrane has three layers and measures about 0.1 mm in thickness (Gelfand, 1997;

Zemlin, 1998). These three layers include the epidermal (outer), the fibrous (middle), and the membranous (mucosal lining) layers. The fibrous layer is thicker in the center portion of the TM and thinner in the superior portion of this membrane. This "thinner" area is called the pars flaccida, which is the most elastic portion of the TM. For the most part, the remainder of the TM is stiffer (containing more fibers) and is referred to as the pars tensa (see Yost, 2000).

The TM has several important anatomic landmarks in addition to the pars flaccida and the pars tensa. The annular ligament is the rim around the TM, which anchors the membrane to the wall of the ear canal. The manubrium of the malleus attaches to the TM in its upper center portion, and the umbo is located in the center of the TM and marks the point of attachment for the most lateral aspect of the malleus. Coursing inferiorly and

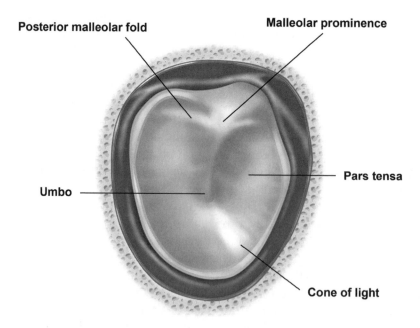

Figure 2–4. A drawing of a human right tympanic membrane.

in a slightly lateral direction is the cone of light, which simply is the otoscopic light that is reflected off the TM during otoscopy. With good observation skills, it is possible to visualize the long process of the incus through the TM. If observed, the location of the long process would be viewed in the superior-posterior quadrant of the TM.

The middle ear is identified, in part, by a cavity within the temporal bone that is bordered by the bony capsule of the cochlea medially and aspects of the temporal bone superiorly (attic), anteriorly, and posteriorly. The medial wall of the cochlea has two openings, the oval window (superior) and the round window (inferior), which are separated by the promontory. The ossicular chain, perhaps the most obvious structure in the middle ear, is composed of three bones, the malleus, the incus, and the stapes. Each of these bones has a detailed anatomy (see Musiek & Baran, 2007, for review). The stapes, the final bone in the ossicular chain, covers the oval window, and the round window is covered by a flexible membrane (also known as a secondary tympanic membrane) (Musiek & Baran, 2007; Zemlin, 1998).

In the anterior, inferior middle ear cavity is the opening to the Eustachian tube. This tube connects the middle ear cavity with the posterior aspect of the nasopharynx. Also located in the middle ear are the stapedius muscle tendon, which arises from the posterior wall of the middle ear and connects to the head of the stapes, and the tendon of the tensor tympani muscle, which courses through the middle ear cavity to connect to the malleus. In addition, a branch of the facial nerve that innervates the stapedius muscle (the smallest muscle in the body) transverses the middle ear space.

Function

Due to its concave structure, the TM has a rather complex displacement pattern that accommodates a wide range of frequencies and intensities (see Zemlin, 1998, for more in-depth explanation). Maximum displacement of the TM occurs in different areas and is dependent on the frequency of the sound stimulus. At high frequencies, the TM tends to vibrate in segments, whereas at low frequencies, there is less segmental vibration and the TM tends to vibrate more as a single unit (Gelfand, 1998).

A variety of functions are associated with the middle ear. The middle ear is an air-filled cavity. The volume of air within this cavity acts as a filter that limits or alters the transmission of some low-frequency sounds through the system. The structure also contributes to some complex resonance interactions with the ear canal and pinna resonances, altering the transmission of sound across the frequency range. The end result is primarily an increase in the intensity of the high-frequency components reaching the cochlea when these are compared to the levels represented in the original signal arriving at the outer ear.

The ossicular chain transmits vibrations from the eardrum to the cochlea. The stapes, the final bone in the ossicular chain, transmits these vibrations to the cochlea by horizontally rotating around an axis (a rocking-like movement) at high intensities, whereas a more piston-like movement of the stapes occurs for low intensities. The former type of movement may be related to stapedius muscle contraction, which occurs at high intensities (see Musiek & Baran, 2007, and Gelfand, 1998, for details). The ossicular chain also serves to stabilize movements related to the vibrations that are transmitted (Musiek & Baran, 2007).

The Eustachian tube's primary function is to allow fresh air into the middle ear cavity and balance the air pressure in the middle ear to that of the atmosphere. This is done when one opens the mouth or swallows. These actions result in contractions of the tensor veli palatini and levator veli palatini muscles, which function to open the Eustachian tube (Zemlin, 1998).

Transformer Action. Sound travels through air which is a low impedance medium. However, in hearing, sound (changes in air pressure) must be directed to a fluid-filled system, the cochlea, where the impedance is quite high. Therefore, without some help from the transformer action of the middle ear, most of the acoustic energy reaching the cochlea would be reflected back out of the ear. Three mechanisms contribute to the middle ear transformer effects: (1) an area ratio advantage between the TM and the stapes' footplate, (2) a lever advantage created by the middle ear bones, and (3) a "buckling" advantage due to the concave structure of the TM. The area ratio advantage relates to the fact that the TM has a much greater area than the stapes, which is the point of energy transfer to the inner ear. The area ratio of TM to stapes footplate is about 22:1, but the pars flaccida of the TM likely contributes little to this area ratio; hence, the effective ratio is estimated to be about 17:1. This area ratio focuses energy at the stapes, thus increasing the input greatly at this point in the auditory system (Gelfand, 1998; von Békésy, 1960). The lever advantage is created by the way the malleus and incus interact. The gain in force is related to the longer handle of the malleus (manubrium) moving the shorter handle of the incus (long process)

for about a 1.3:1 ratio advantage. Finally, the buckling action relates to the inward curvature of the TM, which on vibration imparts energy to the malleus. When this happens the TM moves proportionately more than the malleus (i.e., a "buckling effect"). The smaller displacement at the malleus in reference to the TM creates a greater or gain in force (Musiek & Baran, 2007). These three transformer mechanisms allow greater energy to be directed to the fluid-filled cochlea than would be the case if these mechanisms did not exist or did not function appropriately. If these mechanisms are compromised individually or collectively, a conductive hearing loss is expected.

The Acoustic Reflex. Stapedius muscle contraction is the end point of the acoustic reflex (AR). Because the stapedius muscle is located in the middle ear, it is reasonable to discuss this important reflex in this section of this chapter. However, it is important to highlight that the AR involves both peripheral and central mechanisms (Figure 2–5).

The AR pathway starts with sound entering the external ear and passing through the middle ear to the cochlea. The auditory nerve (see Figure 2–5) picks up the impulses from the cochlea and directs them to the ventral segment of the cochlear nucleus. The ventral cochlear nucleus then sends a fiber tract directly to the ipsilateral facial nerve nuclei and another branch to the contralateral superior olivary complex. The cochlear nucleus also sends fibers to the ipsilateral superior olivary complex, which then connects to its contralateral counterpart. The ipsilateral superior olivary complex connects to the facial nerve nuclei on both sides and the contralateral superior olive has input to the facial nerve nuclei.

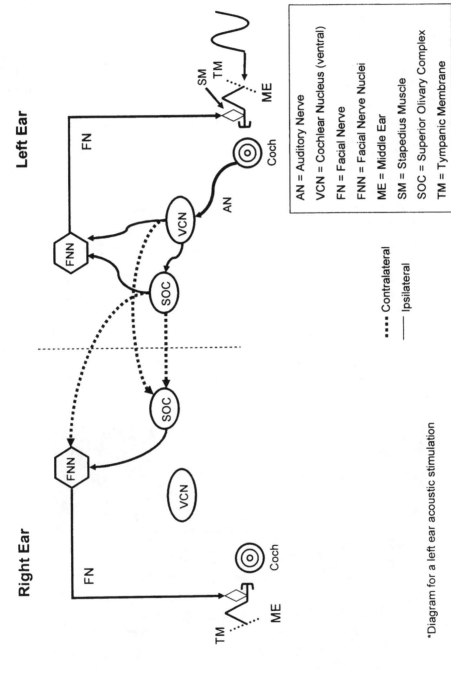

Acoustic Reflex

Right Ear

Left Ear

AN = Auditory Nerve
VCN = Cochlear Nucleus (ventral)
FN = Facial Nerve
FNN = Facial Nerve Nuclei
ME = Middle Ear
SM = Stapedius Muscle
SOC = Superior Olivary Complex
TM = Tympanic Membrane

••••• Contralateral
——— Ipsilateral

*Diagram for a left ear acoustic stimulation

Figure 2–5. A schematic of the acoustic reflex with the acoustic stimulus presented to the left ear. The vertical dotted line in the middle of the drawing represents the midline at the brainstem level. (Reproduced with permission from Musiek and Baran, 2007.)

Hence, there is bilateral input to the facial nerve nuclei resulting in bilateral acoustic reflexes even if there is only monaural stimulation. From the facial nerve nuclei the AR follows an efferent course back to the stapedius muscle in the middle ear (Borg, 1973).

Møller (2000) and Borg (1973) provide excellent accounts of the nature and physiology of the acoustic reflex. Probably the most popular explanation offered for the purpose of the acoustic reflex is that it serves to attenuate high intensity sounds and therefore may help to protect the inner ear. As has been documented by Møller (2000), the higher the intensity of an acoustic signal above the reflex threshold intensity, the greater the contraction of the AR, at least for individuals with normal auditory and facial nerve function. The action of the AR could be viewed as contributing to the nonlinearity of intensity coding within the auditory system as it results in a compression effect. In humans with normal auditory function, the AR is initiated at 70 to 90 dB HL for tonal stimuli and frequencies from 250 to 4000 Hz have little or no differential effects on the level of the threshold of the AR that is measured. The amplitude of the AR is largest for bilateral stimulation followed by ipsilateral and then contralateral stimulations (see Musiek & Baran, 2007). The latency of the AR also is variable and depends on a host of factors including stimulus type, intensity level, frequency, and how it is recorded.

The Cochlea

Structure: The Bony Cochlea

The cochlea is a bony shell similar in shape to a snail shell that is located within the petrous portion of the temporal bone (Figure 2–6). Inside this snail-like shell are fluids (endolymph and perilymph), special cells (hair and supporting cells), membranes (basilar, tectorial, Reissner's),

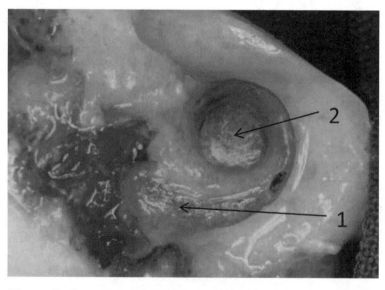

Figure 2–6. A photo of the bony cochlea situated in the temporal bone. Key: 1 = basal turn, 2 = helicotrema. (Courtesy of M. Pinheiro. Reproduced with permission from Musiek and Baran, 2007.)

nerve fibers, blood vessels, and special epithelium. The cochlea makes up part of the inner ear that also includes the vestibular apparatus. The latter structure has a highly identifiable external bony structure that includes the three semicircular canals and the less obvious areas for the utricle and saccule. The bony cochlea has two openings in the shell. The more superior is the oval window, which articulates with the stapes, and inferior to the oval window is the round window. As mentioned earlier, a bony eminence between the two openings is called the promontory (Zemlin, 1998).

Inside the bony cochlear shell is a spiral-shaped osseous structure called the osseous spiral lamina (OSL). The OSL is shaped like an evergreen tree with the basal part of the cochlea located where the lower branches would be and the apical part of the cochlea located toward the top of the tree (Figure 2–7). The bony cochlea is about 1 cm wide at the base and about 0.5 cm in length from base to apex. The "spiral" has from 2.2 to 2.9 turns in the human. The modiolus is the central part of the structure, which is composed of perforated bone that allows auditory nerve fibers to exit through small openings in the OSL and connect to the hair cells. The OSL has a shelf that spirals up the modiolus. This bony shelf is the supporting structure for the basilar membrane and the limbus. This shelf is wider at the base than at the apical end of the cochlea (Musiek & Baran, 2007; Zemlin, 1998).

Function: The Bony Cochlea

In general, the bony cochlea serves as a framework of support and protection for the membranous cochlea and the auditory nerve fibers. The oval and round windows supply access to the membranous inner ear and seal the inner ear fluids

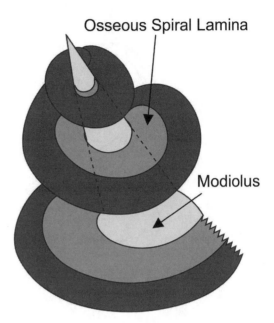

Figure 2–7. *A drawing of the osseous spiral lamina. The bony shelf spirals around the modiolus from base* (bottom of figure) *to apex* (top of figure). *(Reproduced with permission from Musiek and Baran, 2007.)*

with the stapes and the round window membrane serving these functions respectively. Because of its position, the promontory protects the round window. For example, if one were to perforate the lower segment of the TM with a probe, the probe would likely contact the promontory and not the round window. This is what happens when transtympanic electrocochleography is conducted. That is, a needle electrode after piercing the lower TM comes into contact with the promontory from where the recording takes place.

Structure: The Membranous Cochlea

The bony cochlea provides a spiral framework that is followed by the membranous cochlea (Figure 2–8). The membranous

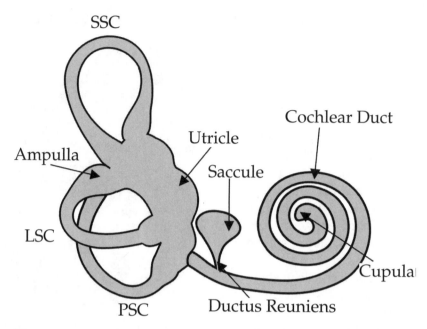

SSC

Cochlear Duct

Utricle

Ampulla

Saccule

LSC

Cupula

PSC   Ductus Reuniens

Figure 2–8. *A drawing of the membranous labyrinth. Key: SSC = superior semicircular canal, LSC = lateral semicircular canal, PSC = posterior semicircular canal. (Reproduced with permission from Musiek and Baran, 2007.)*

cochlea contains three ducts called scalae: the scala vestibuli (superior), the scala tympani (inferior), and the smallest scala that is situated between the other scalae, the scala media (often termed the cochlear duct) (Figure 2–9). The stapes' footplate articulates with the oval window, which opens into the vestibule and transfers energy down the scala vestibuli. The round window is located at the end of the scala tympani. Reissner's membrane and the basilar membrane (BM) divide the cochlea into the three ducts. Reissner's membrane separates the scala vestibuli from the scala media and the BM divides the scala media from the scala tympani. These ducts run the length of the cochlea except at the very end, termed the helicotrema, where the scala vestibuli and the scala tympani communicate. The scala media communicates with the vestibular system (specifically the saccule) via a narrowed channel called the ductus reuniens.

Two important fluid channels, the vestibular (VA) and cochlear (CA) aqueducts, play key roles in cochlear function. The VA is an endolymphatic channel that communicates from the posterior surface of the petrous bone to the saccule. The VA encompasses the endolymphatic duct and sac. The CA, which also opens to the petrous bone's posterior surface, courses to the scala tympani near the round window. This channel contains perilymph, a fluid highly similar to cerebral spinal fluid, which is found where it opens to the petrous bone surface (Figure 2–10).

The two main fluids in the cochlea are endolymph (in the scala media) and perilymph (in the scala vestibuli and

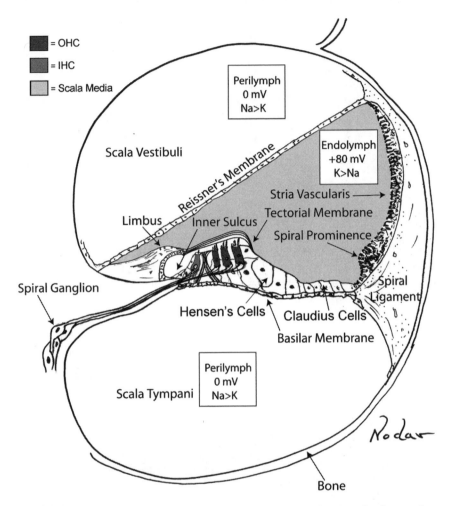

Figure 2–9. *A drawing of a cross-section of the cochlea showing the three scalae. Key: OHC = outer hair cells, IHC = inner hair cell. (Reproduced with permission from Musiek and Baran, 2007.)*

scala tympani). Endolymph is high in potassium and low in sodium and perilymph has just the opposite chemical concentrations.

The BM is composed of about 24,000 fibers and is 25 to 35 mm in length in the adult human. The BM supports the organ of Corti, the actual end organ for hearing. At its apex, the BM is wider than at its base (0.36 mm versus 0.04 mm). The BM is thicker at the base than the apex and it is also stiffer at the base than apex (Buser & Imbert, 1992; Musiek & Baran, 2007) (Figure 2–11).

Reissner's membrane is essentially avascular, has two layers of cells, and is permeable. From base to apex Reissner's membrane becomes wider like the BM; however, the scala media and the "shelf" of the spiral lamina become smaller and narrower, respectively, as one moves from the base to the apex.

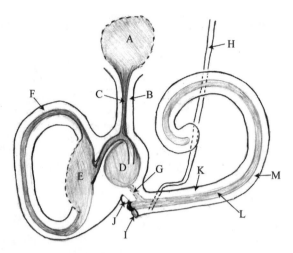

Figure 2–10. *A sketch of the membranous inner ear with a focus on the cochlear and vestibular aqueducts. Key: A = endolymphatic sac, B = vestibular aqueduct, C = endolymphatic duct, D = saccule, E = utricle, F = semicircular canals, G = ductus reunions, H = cochlear aqueduct, I = round window, J = stapes (oval window), K = scala vestibuli, L = scala media, M = scala tympani. (Reproduced with permission from Musiek and Baran, 2007.)*

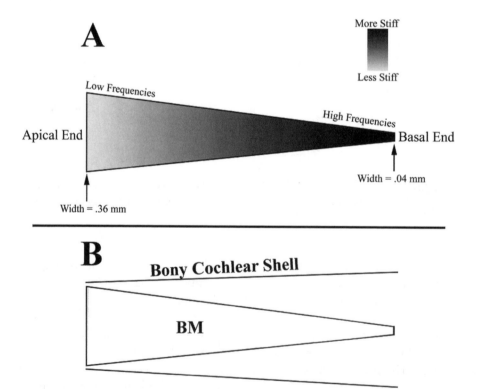

Figure 2–11. *A drawing looking done on the basilar membrane showing (A) the relative width and stiffness dimensions of the basilar membrane from its apical to basal end, and (B) the relationships between the basilar membrane and the bony shelf of the cochlea from apex to base. (Reproduced with permission from Musiek and Baran, 2007.)*

The organ of Corti is composed of supporting structures, sensory cells, membranes, and nerve fibers (Figure 2–12). This structure courses the length of the cochlea. Directly superior to the hair cells is the tectorial membrane, which interacts with the stereocilia of the outer hair cells and is anchored to the upper lip of the limbus. It appears that the tectorial membrane does not articulate with the stereocilia of the inner hair cells. On its underside and just above the inner hair cells' stereocilia is a bulge termed Hensen's stripe. This bulge in the membrane's underside reduces the distance between the tops of the stereocilia and the tectorial membrane, and may play a role in stimulation of the inner hair cells (see discussion later).

The reticular lamina is composed of tightly packed cells and forms a ceiling above the sensory and supporting cells of the organ of Corti. The stereocilia of the hair cells protrude through the lamina. The reticular lamina is composed of phalanges of Deiter's cells, inner and outer border cells, as well as the tops of the pillar cells (Figure 2–13). It keeps the endolymph from penetrating the internal structures of the organ of Corti. Hence, only the stereocilia and not the hair cells themselves are bathed in endolymph, which has a +80 mV charge.

The lateral wall of the cochlear duct is discussed next. The lateral wall is the location of the stria vascularis and the spiral ligament (see Figure 2–9). The stria vascularis is thought to play key roles in the production and absorption of endolymph. It is composed of three layers of cells. Marginal cells make up the

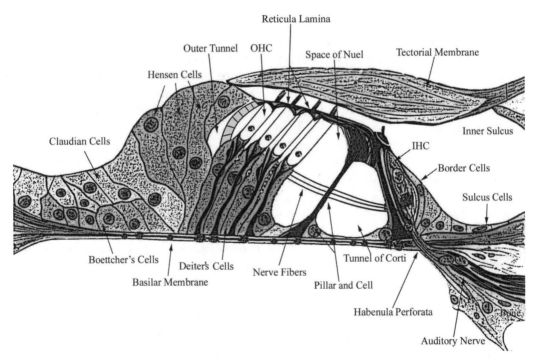

Figure 2–12. *A drawing showing the major structures within the organ of Corti. (Based on a drawing by Polyak, 1946. Reproduced with permission from Musiek and Baran, 2007.)*

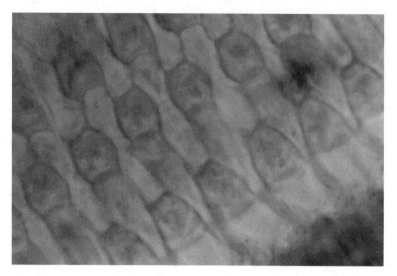

Figure 2–13. A micrograph from above the reticular lamina. (Courtesy of M. Pinheiro. Reproduced with permission from Musiek and Baran, 2007.)

first layer and are linked to ion channels and pumps. The intermediate cell layer is lateral to the marginal cells and contains melanin, and the basal cell layer is next to the spiral ligament. The cells in these three cell layers all are critical for the function of the cochlea. The stria vascularis also provides blood supply to the cochlea and maintains the metabolism of the inner ear (Slepecky, 1996).

The spiral ligament extends throughout the cochlea and covers the lateral wall of the scala media. It also extends inferiorly to the upper scala tympani. This structure supplies support to the lateral aspect of the BM as well as for Reissner's membrane.

Sensory Cells. There two types of sensory cells in the cochlea: inner and outer hair cells (IHCs, OHCs). The OHCs are organized in multiple rows (3–5) and the IHCs have only one row. These hair cells are located on the lateral and medial sides of the pillar cells respectively (Figure 2–14). There are about 3500 IHCs and 12,000 OHCs that course the length of the cochlea. Stereocilia are located at the top of both types of hair cells. The OHC's structure is different from that of the IHC (Figure 2–15). The OHCs are rather elongated tubelike structures that vary greatly in their length. The OHCs in the high-frequency regions of the cochlea are shorter than those located in the low-frequency regions (Geisler, 1998). Located within the OHCs are contractile proteins such as actin, myosin, prestin, and tubulin. There are also special structures along the outer walls of the OHCs called cisterns. These cisterns and chemicals allow for rapid expasion and contractile movements of the cells (discussed later). The OHCs usually have a −60 mV electrical charge and potassium ion channels. The OHCs have a cuticular plate on top that supports the stereocilia, which connect to the underside of the tectorial membrane.

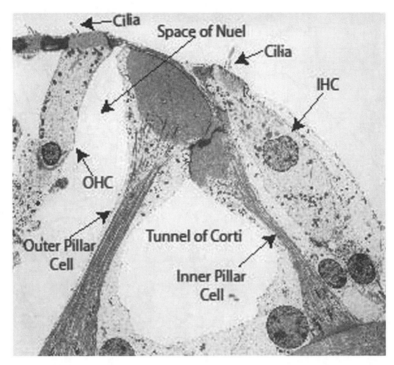

Figure 2–14. *A photo showing the tunnel of Corti. Key: IHC = inner hair cell, OHC = outer hair cell. (Courtesy of R. Mount, Hospital for Sick Children, Toronto. Reproduced with permission from Musiek and Baran, 2007.)*

Each OHC has three rows of stereocilia with a greater number of stereocilia at the base than the apex (about 150 to 50) of the cochlea. These stereocilia are stiff and form a "W" shape when looking down on the top of the hair cell.

The IHCs have a different structure than the OHCs. They have more mitochondria and both calcium and potassium channels and they do not have contractile proteins and cisterns. The IHCs have a −40 mV charge and about 50 to 70 stereocilia per cell, which are arranged in a "U" shape. The IHCs typically have three rows of stereocilia that are graded in length, and the stereocilia are longer at the apex of the organ of Corti than at its base.

Both the OHCs and IHCs have stereocilia that have pores that open when stimulated. This allows K^+ ions to pass into the cell resulting in depolarization. Tip-links are small filament bands that open the pores on movement in a certain direction. The tip-links are likely to be located toward the top of the stereocilia. Cross-links are similar in structure to tip-links, but they connect to the stereocilia closer to their midpoints. This allows the stereocilia to move in unison and also supplies some support for this movement (Geisler, 1998).

The hair cells are tuned so that cells located more basally respond to high-frequency sounds, whereas the more apically situated cells respond to lower fre-

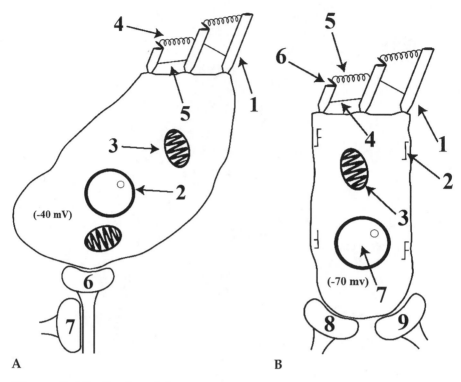

Figure 2–15. *Sketches of the inner (A) and outer (B) hair cells. Key for (A): 1 = stereocilia, 2 = nucleus, 3 = mitochondria, 4 = tip-links, 5 = cross-links, 6 = afferent nerve terminal, 7 = efferent nerve terminal; Key for (B): 1 = stereocilia, 2 = cisternae, 3 = mitochondria, 4 = cross-links, 5 = tip-links, 6 = pores, 7 = nucleus, 8 = efferent nerve terminal, 9= afferent nerve terminal. (Reproduced with permission from Musiek and Baran, 2007.)*

quency sounds. This arrangement of hair cells leads to the tonotopic representation of frequencies within the cochlea, with the higher frequency sounds being represented at the basal end of the cochlea and the lower frequency sounds at the apical end of the cochlea.

Supporting Cells. Supporting cells are located along the organ of Corti and include pillar cells, Deiter's cells, phalangeal cells, Hensen's cells, Claudian cells, border cells, and Bottcher's cells (Musiek & Baran, 2007; Slepecky, 1996). Next to the limbus are the border cells that divide the IHCs from the inner sulcus. The pha-

langeal cells support the IHCs and have stalks that separate these cells. These stalks or phalanges give rise to a flattened apical plate that contributes to the reticular lamina. A similar structure is observed in the case of the Deiter's cells, which support the OHCs. The inner and outer pillar cells enclose the tunnel of Corti and, because of their triangular structure, enhance the stiffness of this region where there is considerable movement of the BM. The space of Nuel is located next to the outer pillar cells. The lateral segment of the BM is where the Hensen's cells, the cells of Claudius, and Bottcher's cells are found. These all lend support to the lateral aspect of the BM. Between the most lateral OHCs and the Hensen's cells is a space called the outer tunnel.

Function: The Membranous Cochlea

The physiology of the cochlea can be separated into two major areas of study: cochlear mechanics and cochlear electrophysiology. Although these two areas of function will be presented separately, it is important to realize that cochlear mechanics and electrophysiology are interdependent and function smoothly as part of a larger continuum that helps make up the hearing experience. Some key broad-based functions of the cochlea are: (1) changing vibrotactile energy to electrical energy and (2) coding for intensity, frequency, and time. These functions require both mechanical and electrophysiologic processing.

Cochlear Mechanics. The ossicular chain's vibratory energy is imparted to the cochlea through the stapes' motion at the oval window. Key to starting mechanical functions of the cochlea is that, as the stapes pushes in (compression wave) or out (rarefaction wave) of the oval window, the round window membrane accommodates this movement. This interaction

between the oval and round windows cannot be compromised without affecting the cochlear hearing processes.

The input from the stapes displaces the fluid in the cochlea in a manner that creates a traveling wave (TW) that moves down the length of the cochlea. This TW causes an activation of subsequent mechanical and electrochemical processes in the cochlea. It has been estimated that the TW moves nearly 100 meters per second at the most basal segment but slows down to about 2 meters per second at the apical-most aspect of the cochlea (see Zwislocki, 2002). This velocity has implications for neural synchronization that are reflected in such measures as the auditory brainstem response (ABR). The ABR shows more synchronous activity derived from the basal end than the apical end of the BM.

Frequency can be coded in the cochlea in two ways, by place and by periodicity (temporally). The place theory, which was first described by von Békésy (1960), argued that sounds traveled down the BM and that frequency was coded by the point of maximum displacement of the BM by the traveling wave (TW), with high frequencies being represented more basally and low frequencies more apically (Figure 2–16). The TW reaches its maximum deflection at the place where the

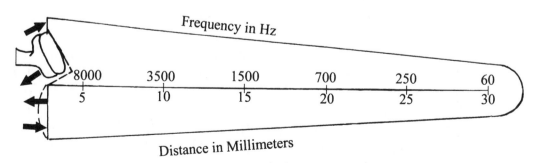

Figure 2–16. A drawing showing the relationship between frequency and its location on the human basilar membrane. (Reproduced with permission from Musiek and Baran, 2007.)

resonance of the BM matches that of the stimulating sound. This maximum deflection refers to the maximum amplitude point for the envelope (Figure 2–17). The difficulty with the place theory was that the tuning required for behavioral frequency discrimination was not consistent with the sharpness of the TW envelope; however, this problem was resolved with the discovery of the biological amplifier that will be discussed later.

Frequency also can be coded temporally. That is, the rapid movement of the BM (fine structure) is associated with the cycles of the acoustic stimulus that stimulate the hair cells and auditory nerve fibers accordingly. For example, if a 200-Hz tone were presented to the ear, the BM would move 200 times per second and the hair cells and auditory nerve would be stimulated and fire at the same rate. This kind of frequency coding may work feasibly for low-frequency tones, but not well for high-frequency stimuli as the firing rates needed to code high-frequency sounds are likely to exceed the physiologic capacities of the hair cells. Hence, common thinking is that temporal or periodicity processing and place of maximum displacement

work well for low frequencies but that, as the frequency of the stimulus increases, the place principle becomes more dominant (Geisler, 1998; Musiek & Baran, 2007; von Békésy, 1960; Yost, 2000).

Amplitude of the TW is how intensity is represented in the cochlea—the greater the intensity of the signal, the greater the amplitude of the TW envelope. However, with increases in intensity the displacement of the BM is not linear. The TW envelope has greater damping on the apical side; hence, the TW envelope has a sharper reduction in amplitude on the apical side than is reflected in the increase in amplitude on the basal side (see Figure 2–17). When intensity increases, not only does the vertical displacement increase, but so does the width of the envelope. This action results in more hair cells being stimulated, and in, turn more neural elements being activated. Because of the broader displacement of the envelope at high intensities, there is a decrease in the sharpness of the peak of the TW resulting in poorer frequency selectivity.

Nonlinearity associated with the BM is an important concept. As mentioned earlier, as intensity increases, so does BM displacement, but not in a linear fashion. At low intensities, there is proportionately more displacement of the BM than at high intensities (Figure 2–18). Like intensity, the representation of frequency on the BM is not linear. An octave change for a high-frequency sound on the basal part of the BM requires less space than an octave change at the low-frequency end of the BM. This nonlinearity can be viewed as a natural "compression" within the cochlea for both intensity and frequency (see Musiek & Baran, 2007; Yost, 2000).

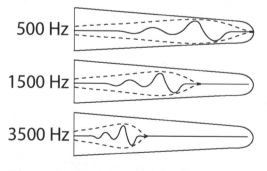

Figure 2–17. *A drawing of the location of the traveling wave on the basilar membrane for three frequencies. Note the envelopes* (dotted lines) *are not symmetric in their shapes. (Reproduced with permission from Musiek and Baran, 2007.)*

Hair Cell Mechanics. One of the hair cells' main functions is to convert vibra-

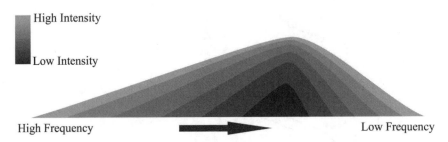

Figure 2–18. *A drawing showing basilar membrane displacements related to intensity increments of the stimulus. (Reproduced with permission from Musiek and Baran, 2007.)*

tory energy into electrical energy so that the nervous system can utilize these signals. This mechanical activity starts at the stereocilia. The OHC's stereocilia are imbedded in the underside of the tectorial membrane. If a TW is a compression wave, the BM will be deflected downward. Because the tectorial membrane and the BM are attached at different sites, a downward movement of the BM will result in the tectorial membrane pulling the stereocilia toward the limbus (or medial aspect of the organ of Corti). This movement at the stereocilia level results in the tip-links closing the pores of the stereocilia. As a result, no chemical transduction can evolve and the hair cell cannot depolarize. However, when the BM moves upward, such as is seen when the stimulus is a rarefaction wave, the tectorial membrane pulls the stereocilia in the opposite direction and the pores open up allowing K+ ions to enter the cell starting the depolarizing process (Figure 2–19). The stereocilia essentially move in unison because of the cross-link connections among the stereocilia (Geisler, 1998).

The IHCs are not embedded in the tectorial membrane; hence their stimulation related to the BM movement is somewhat different. The most popular theory is that there is fluid flow between the reticular lamina and Hensen's stripe on the underside of the tectorial membrane.

This fluid flow is increased in its effectiveness due to the restricted area created by Hensen's stripe. The fluid movement causes the defection of the stereocilia of the IHCs in the same direction for compression and rarefaction sounds waves as the OHCs, which starts the transduction process in the IHCs (Geisler, 1998; Musiek & Baran, 2007).

The hair cells, both inner and outer, are responsible for the transduction process. However, they do have different functions. As mentioned earlier, the OHCs have contractile proteins and cell wall structures that allow them to expand and contract. These cells will contract on upward defection of the BM and expand on downward movement. Because the OHCs are connected to the BM via their Deiter's cells, when they contract the result is the enhanced movement of the BM in an upward direction. Just the opposite happens when the BM moves downward. This creates an overall greater displacement of the BM and makes the incoming sound greater in intensity—a type of amplifier, hence, the name the "biological or cochlear amplifier." This biological amplifier is activated only for low-intensity sounds. Therefore, one might

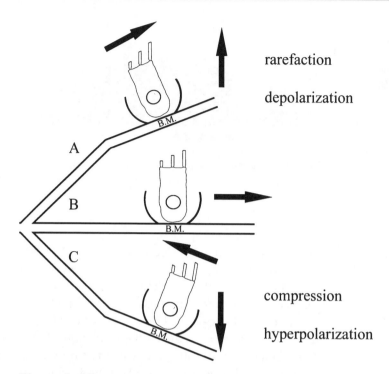

rarefaction

depolarization

A

B

B.M.

C

compression

hyperpolarization

Figure 2–19. *A schematic depicting basilar membrane movement and stereocilia deflection with changes in stimulus phase. A rarefaction stimulus causes an upward movement of the basilar membrane, which results in the stereocilia being deflecting away from the limbus and resulting in a depolarization of the hair cell (A). The resting phase of the basilar membrane shows no movement or deflection of the stereocilia (B). A compression stimulus results in basilar membrane movement in a downward direction, which results in the stereocilia being deflected toward the limbus and a hyperpolarization of the hair cell (C). (Reproduced with permission from Musiek and Baran, 2007.)*

say that it contributes to compression (of intensity) in the cochlea. As the area of the BM that is moved by OHC contraction/expansion is small, the BM response is sharpened. Hence, the biological amplifier not only amplifies sounds in the cochlea, it also sharpens the tuning of the BM for low-intensity sounds (Salvi, Clock Eddins, & Wang, 2007).

The expansion and contraction of OHCs results in another interesting phe-nomenon in hearing (Figure 2–20). The biological amplifier creates small acoustical signals that are sent back out of the cochlea in a reverse mechanical process, which vibrates the middle ear bones, which moves the tympanic membrane and results in subaudible sounds in the ear canal. These subaudible sounds can be picked up by a microphone and be recorded and displayed. We know these signals as otoacoustic emissions (OAEs).

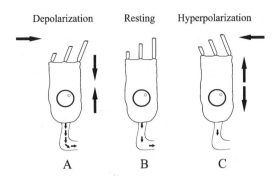

Depolarization　　Resting　　Hyperpolarization

A　　　　B　　　　C

Figure 2–20. *A drawing of depolarized (A), resting (B), and hyperpolarized (C) hair cells and the related electrical discharges to the auditory nerve. The vertical arrows show the contraction of the hair cell during depolarization (A) and expansion of the hair cell during hyperpolarization (C). (Reproduced with permission from Musiek and Baran, 2007.)*

Hence, OHC motility is linked to OAEs. If the OHCs are damaged, OAEs usually are absent and there is sensorineural hearing loss (Salvi et al., 2007).

Interestingly, the intensity range of OAEs is 30 to 40 dB about the same as the intensity range of the OHCs; that is, a hearing loss of 30 to 40 dB or more will result in absent OAEs. Furthermore, it is known that damage to IHCs, the auditory nerve, or the central mechanisms will not compromise OAEs (Geisler, 1998; Musiek & Baran, 2007).

The IHCs do not have motile properties like the OHCs, but they do play a major role in the transduction and coding of high-intensity acoustic signals. Perhaps too simply stated, the IHCs seem to take over where the OHCs leave off in terms of intensity coding. Although OHCs often are damaged by high-intensity sounds, IHCs often survive. The IHCs carry much of the information about sounds that reach the ear onto the central auditory

nervous system based on their reaction to high-intensity sounds and their rich neural supply.

Cochlear Electrophysiology. Cochlear mechanics initiate the transduction of vibratory energy to electrical energy. To recap, the BM moving upward as a result of a rarefaction sound wave results in shearing of the stereocilia of the hair cells by the tectorial membrane. This process results in the stereocilia being pushed away from the limbus and opens the pores of the stereocilia via increased tension on the tip-links. This pore opening allows K^+ ions to flow in and start the depolarization process (i.e., the hair cell fires). Downward deflection of the BM by a compression wave creates an opposite situation from what was just described and hyperpolarization takes place (i.e., the hair cell does not fire).

Three cochlear potentials are associated with hair cell depolarization. These include the endocochlear or resting potential, the cochlear microphonic (CM), and the summating potential (SP). The endocochlear potential is the electrical gradient that can be measured when the hair cell is not depolarizing, hyperpolarizing, or recovering from hyperpolarization. In this state, the hair cell is at about a −70 mV charge, whereas the scala media (endolymph) is at about a +80 mV charge (see Figure 2–9). This large differential in electrical charges, the endocochlear potential, is likely maintained by the intermediate cells of the stria vascularis. The endocochlear potential also is responsible for moving the K^+ ions through the channels of the stereocilia, which initiates the depolarization process. Hallowell Davis proposed a "battery model" many years ago that had as its main feature the stria vascularis as the energy source to maintain the intra- and extracellular charges in the cochlea (Davis, 1965; Wangemann, 2002a, 2002b).

The next cochlear potential to be discussed is the cochlear microphonic (CM), which was brought to prominence in auditory science by the classic experiment of Wever and Bray (1930). The CM is a summation of hair cell responses from along the BM to a sound stimulus (Salvi et al., 2007). As Wever and Bray demonstrated, the CM faithfully mimics the sound stimulus. This is one of the key characteristics in defining the nature of the CM. The CM occurs almost instantly and has little fatigability. Because the CM mimics the stimulus, positive and negative polarity stimuli will yield positive and negative polarity CMs. Therefore, if alternating polarity signals are averaged together, they essentially will cancel out this response. This is a procedure often used during electrocochleographic recordings to remove the CM from the resulting waveform in order to permit more accurate definition and identification of other potentials of interest within the waveform.

Salvi et al. (2007) nicely review some key characteristics of the CM. The CM is generated primarily by the OHCs; however, there is some contribution from the IHCs. The CM, depending on how it is recorded, can be obtained close to behavioral threshold—this is especially the case when using transtympanic electrocochleography. The CM amplitude generally increases monotically with intensity increases up to about 80 dB SPL, but then it "rolls over" slightly at higher intensities. This likely reflects the major role of the OHCs, which do not "handle" or code high intensities. The frequency of

the stimulus will influence the amplitude of the CM. The higher frequencies do not produce as large a response as the low frequencies. Low-frequency stimuli are capable of producing a CM at all three turns of the cochlea, whereas high-frequency stimuli precipitate responses only at the basal turn, a finding that is consistent with TW physiology.

The summating potential (SP) follows the CM in time (Figure 2–21). It is a DC potential that is generated by the OHCs and IHCs; however, the IHCs have a greater contribution to the SP than they do for the CM. The SP can be positive or negative depending if one is recording from the scala tympani or the scala vestibuli. This sometimes makes far-field recordings, such as is done with electrocochleography, difficult to understand and interpret. The SP can be recorded at low-intensity levels when the recording electrode is in or near the cochlea. However, in far-field recordings it is not often observed at low-intensity levels. At high intensities, the SP continues to increase in amplitude without the rollover effects noted for the CM. The SP cannot be cancelled out by an alternating polarity like the CM. It has been shown that, in disorders such as cochlear hydrops, the SP increases in amplitude (see Chapter 5, Disorders of the Inner Ear, and Clark & Ohlemiller, 2008; Dallos, 1973; Salvi et al., 2007).

The tuning curves of the IHCs and OHCs are sharp and highly similar to each other. These tuning curve responses are consistent with the vibration patterns and tuning of the BM (see Salvi et al., 2007).

The hair cells synapse with receptors on the auditory nerve. It appears that the hair cells' (afferent) neurotransmitter is glutamate (see Clark & Ohlemiller, 2008).

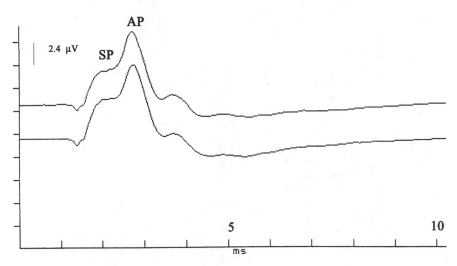

Figure 2–21. *A recording of a summating potential (SP) and action potential (AP) from a human during transtympanic electrocochleography. The components have been smoothed to better show the morphology. (Reproduced with permission from Musiek and Baran, 2007.)*

The Auditory Nerve

Once the cochlea has transduced the acoustic signal to electrical impulses and set up frequency and intensity codes, this information is passed on to the auditory nerve (AN). The AN, which preserves the cochlear codes, passes this information on to the brainstem, which is part of the central auditory system.

Structure

The AN connects the cochlea to the brainstem (Figure 2–22). The AN is part of the eighth cranial nerve, which also includes vestibular nerve fibers from the vestibular apparatus. In the adult human, the AN is approximately 22 to 26 mm long. The course of the afferent AN from the cochlea to the brainstem is not as simple as one may think. The AN fibers connect to the hair cells at the terminal buttons and from there course medially through the small openings in the shelf of the osseous spiral lamina called the habenula perforata. The AN continues medially to an enlarged cavity called Rosenthal's canal, which is where the spiral ganglion is located. The AN fibers proceed to form a trunk called the modiolus and then on into the internal auditory meatus (IAM) where they join the vestibular nerve (superior and inferior divisions) and facial nerve trunks (Figure 2–23). All these nerves course to the cerebellopontine angle (CPA) and then input to the cochlear nucleus in the brainstem (Møller, 2000).

There are two types of AN fibers, Types I and II. The Type I fibers connect to the IHCs and make up 90% of all AN fibers. The Type II fibers connect only to OHCs and constitute approximately 10% of the total AN population (Figure 2–24). The Type I AN fibers are myelinated, but the Type II fibers, for the most part, are not (Musiek & Baran, 2007; Spoendlin, 1972).

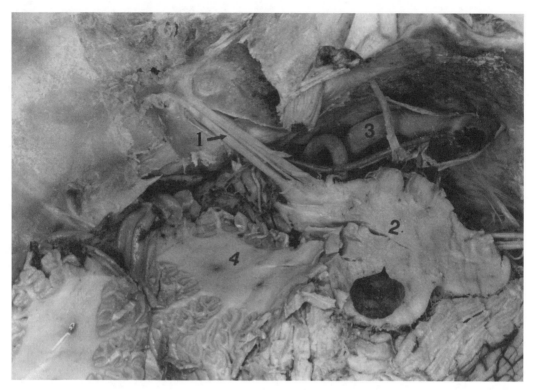

Figure 2–22. *A photo showing the base of the human brain. Key: 1 = the left seventh and eighth cranial nerves exiting the internal auditory meatus and connecting to the brainstem, 2 = the pons, 3 = basilar artery, 4 = the cerebellum. (Reproduced with permission from Musiek and Baran, 2007.)*

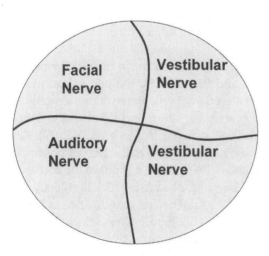

Figure 2–23. *A drawing of the internal auditory meatus as viewed when the nerves are exiting the internal auditory meatus and entering the brainstem at the cerebellopontine angle. (Reproduced with permission from Musiek and Baran, 2007.)*

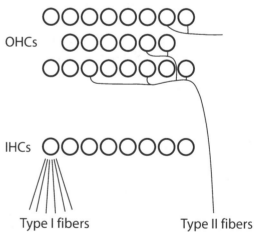

Figure 2–24. *A schematic showing Type I and Type II auditory nerve fibers and their connections to the inner and outer hair cells. Key: OHCs = outer hair cells, IHCs = inner hair cells. (Reproduced with permission from Musiek and Baran, 2007.)*

In a general sense, the tonotopic organization of the AN nerve reveals high frequencies on the outside of the nerve bundle and low frequencies in the core or middle (Figure 2–25). However, on closer inspection, the tonotopic organization is really more of a spiral following the spiral organization of the cochlea (Møller, 2000).

Function

If a tone burst is presented to the ear, the AN will respond by firing over the time period of the stimulus. The pattern that this firing rate over time yields is called a post-stimulus time histogram (PSTH). A PSTH for an AN fiber is shown in Figure 2–26. The latency of the compound action potential of the AN decreases with increases of intensity of the stimulus. Usually, the latency of the AN response is between 1 and 2 msec for a moderately intense click stimulus. The AN action potential probably is best known as wave I of the auditory brainstem response

or the "AP" of an electrocochleographic recording discussed earlier (Møller, 2000; Musiek & Baran, 2007).

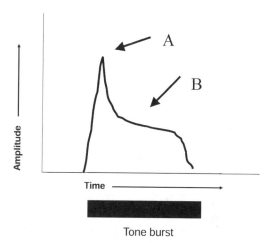

Figure 2–26. *A drawing of the firing rate over time known as a post-stimulus time histogram (PSTH) of an auditory nerve fiber to a tone burst. Key: A = initial abrupt strong response, B = the plateau portion of the neural response. (Reproduced with permission from Musiek and Baran, 2007.)*

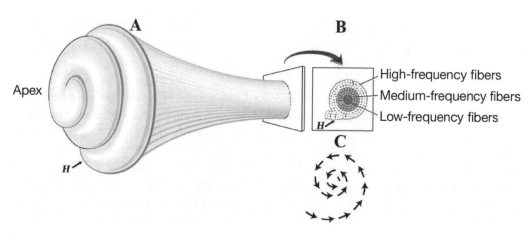

Figure 2–25. *A drawing showing the tonotopic arrangement of the auditory nerve. Key: A = auditory nerve core, B = cross-section of the auditory nerve depicting the tonotopic array of the nerve fibers, C = additional depiction of the tonotopic progression, H = hook area of the basal aspect of the cochlea. (Reproduced with permission from Musiek and Baran, 2007.)*

Frequency is coded in the AN by place (as earlier discussed) or firing rate (periodicity or temporal coding). Temporal coding is dependent on phase-locking, which means that the nerve fiber fires at the same point on the acoustic waveform. However, this does not mean that the nerve fiber fires on every cycle of the waveform. If the refractory period of the nerve fiber is too long, it may not be capable of firing on every cycle. In this case, the fiber may fire on every other or every third or fourth cycle. The cycles that are missed by one fiber are picked up by other available fibers of the AN. In aggregate, all cycles will be coded by AN fibers. This kind of frequency coding is commonly referred to as the volley principle (Musiek & Baran, 2007).

The characteristic frequency (CF) is the frequency to which the nerve fiber responds best, which usually is its lowest threshold. The farther away from the CF the stimulus, the greater the intensity is required for the nerve fiber to respond. Therefore, if one plots the intensity needed for the nerve fiber to fire as one moves gradually away from the CF (both on the low and high-frequency side), a physiologic tuning curve (TC) can be established (Figure 2–27). Tuning curves relate the frequency selectivity of the nerve fiber, that is, the sharper the TC, the better the frequency selectivity. Auditory nerve TCs are usually sharp at the high frequencies and broader at low frequencies unless there is damage to the OHCs of the cochlea or damage to the AN itself (Gelfand, 1998).

Intensity coding at the AN level is related to the spontaneous firing rate (SFR) of the neurons. Much of the work by Liberman (1978) as well as Kim and Parham (1991, 1997) have allowed a categorization of AN firing rates related to intensity

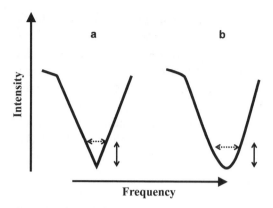

Figure 2–27. *A sketch of a sharp (a) and a rather broad (b) tuning curve similar to what may be recorded from auditory nerve fibers. (Reproduced with permission from Musiek and Baran, 2007.)*

coding. These authors relate that there is a range of SFRs with the lowest being less than 10 and the highest being about 100 spikes per second. Liberman (1978) divided AN SFRs into three categories: low = 0 to 0.5, medium = 0.5 to 18, and high ≥18 spikes per second. The high SFRs respond best to low-intensity sounds and the low SFRs respond best to high-intensity sounds. It is the combination of the low, medium, and high SFR neurons that allow the AN (in total) to have a relatively linear firing rate response to intensities from threshold to near 100 dB SPL. Hence, as intensities increase so do the firing rates of the individual neurons and more neurons respond (relating to the TW size).

One of the key phenomena of AN function is that of adaptation. Adaptation is the decrease in the amplitude of the AN action potential over time during stimulation without a change in the stimulus characteristics. Adaptation is a neural phenomenon, which is greater at high frequencies compared to low frequencies (Keidel, Kallert, & Korth, 1983). Damage to the AN increases adaptation. This was the basis for the clinical use of various tone decay tests to measure integrity of the AN.

THE CENTRAL AUDITORY SYSTEM

The central auditory system contains dramatically more auditory neurons than the AN. These neurons essentially increase in number and connections as one ascends the central auditory system (neural arborization). This marked increase in auditory neurons from thousands at the AN

level to practically millions in the auditory regions of the brain speaks to the high redundancy and complex functioning of the auditory brain (Figure 2–28).

The Cochlear Nucleus

Structure

The cochlear nucleus (CN) is the first structure of the central auditory system and is located on lateral aspect of the caudal-most pons in the brainstem. It is composed of three major nuclei groups: (1) the dorsal cochlear nucleus, DCN,

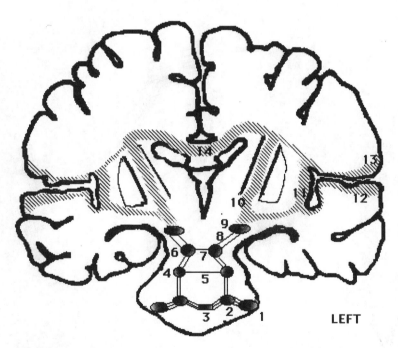

Figure 2–28. *A sketch of the brain showing a coronal view of the auditory pathways and areas. Key: 1 = cochlear nucleus, 2 = superior olivary complex, 3 = trapezoid body, 4 = nuclei of the lateral lemniscus, 5 = commissure of Prosbt, 6 = inferior colliculus, 7 = commissure of the inferior colliculus, 8 = brachium of the inferior colliculus, 9 = medial geniculate body, 10 = internal capsule, 11 = insula, 12 = Heschl's gyrus, 13 = inferior central gyri of the parietal lobe, 14 = corpus callosum. (Reproduced with permission from Musiek and Baran, 2007.)*

(2) the posterior ventral cochlear nucleus, PVCN, and (3) the anterior ventral cochlear nucleus, AVCN (Figure 2–29). The AN fibers project to the CN and enter between the AVCN and PVCN in an area termed the root entry zone. There are a variety of cell types in the CN (i.e., pyramidal, octopus, globular, multipolar, etc.), which are located in specific areas of this auditory structure. The CN has interneu-

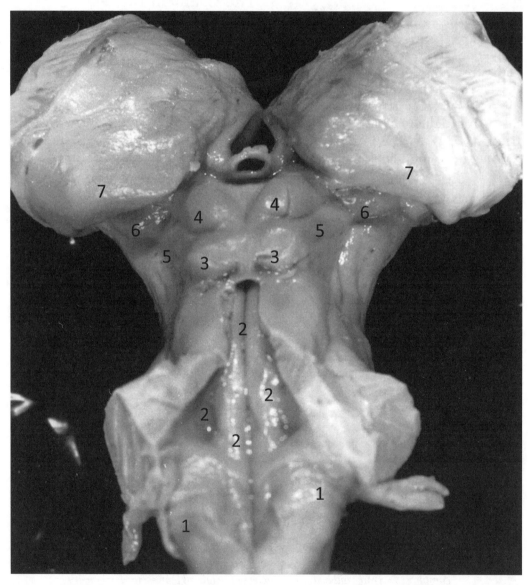

Figure 2–29. *A posterior view of the human pons, midbrain, and thalamus showing the ascending auditory pathway in these structures. Key: 1 = area of the cochlear nucleus, 2 = fourth ventricle, 3 = inferior colliculus, 4 = superior colliculus, 5 = brachium of the inferior colliculus, 6 = medial geniculate body, 7 = thalamus (numbers 1-2 pons, 2-4 midbrain, 6 thalamus). (Reproduced with permission from Musiek and Baran, 2007.)*

rons, such as the ventral tubercular tract, which provides neural communication among its nuclei. The neural outputs from the CN are both ipsilateral and contralateral with the latter being larger and more numerous. There are three major contralateral routes exiting the CN. The ventral and intermediate stria arising from the AVCN and PVCN project primarily to the opposite superior olivary complex (SOC), and to a lesser degree to the ipsilateral SOC. The dorsal stria, coming from the DCN projects mostly to the opposite lateral lemniscus (LL) tract (Pickles, 1998).

Function

The various cell types in the CN either modify or preserve the input firing pattern or PSTH from the AN. However, the PSTHs generated from the cells in the CN take on a variety of forms indicating sophisticated processing of the AN input. This kind of processing happens at each level of the auditory system. The CN has a tonotopic arrangement that is set up by the projections of the AN. In general, the low frequencies are in the lateral areas and the high frequencies are in the medial and dorsal regions of the DCN, PVCN, and AVCN. Therefore, each section of the CN has its own tonotopic arrangement (see Musiek & Baran, 2007; Romand & Avan, 1997). The TCs of the CN are similar to those of the AN. As intensity increases, the firing rate of CN neurons tends to increase rather linearly over a 30 to 40 dB range; however, some neurons do have a greater range of potential intensity changes. As was the case in the AN, the CN neurons can phase lock for tones up to the 3000 Hz to 4000 Hz range, indicating good temporal resolution. The CN is represented by wave III of the ABR, which occurs about 1.5 to 2.0 msec after wave I

(generated by the auditory nerve) in individuals with normal auditory function.

The Superior Olivary Complex

Structure

The superior olivary complex (SOC) is next in the ascending central auditory structures in the brainstem (Figure 2–30).

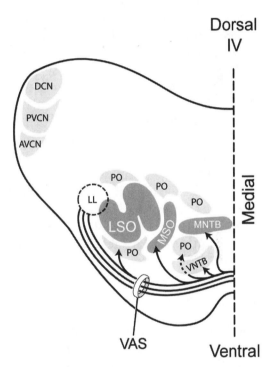

Figure 2–30. A drawing of a transverse section of the brainstem showing the superior olivary complex (based on the cat). Key: LSO = lateral superior olive, MSO = medial superior olive, MNTB = medial nucleus of the trapezoid body, VNTB = ventral nucleus of the trapezoid body, VAS = ventral acoustic stria, LL = lateral lemniscus, PO = periolivary nuclei, DCN = dorsal cochlear nucleus, AVCN = anterior ventral cochlear nucleus, PVCN = posterior ventral cochlear nucleus, IV = fourth ventricle. (Reproduced with permission from Musiek and Baran, 2007.)

It receives heavy input from the contralateral CN as mentioned earlier. Although the SOC is at the same level as the CN, it is located deep in the pons. The main structures in this complex are the lateral superior olive (LSO), the medial superior olive (MSO), the nuclei of the trapezoid body, and groups of periolivary nuclei surrounding the lateral and medial olive. For the most part, there are only three cell types in the SOC—much less than in the CN. In the LSO, high frequencies are located medially and low frequencies are represented laterally within this structure, whereas for the MSO the high frequencies are represented toward the ventral end and the low frequencies toward the dorsal end. The LSO is tuned higher than the MSO (based on animal data) (Møller, 2000; Moore, 2000; Musiek & Baran, 2007).

The output connections of the SOC are mostly crossed connections to the nuclei of the lateral lemniscus (NLL) and the inferior colliculus (IC). These crossing fibers make up what is termed the acoustic chiasm. The SOC also has ipsilateral connections to the NLL and IC (Musiek & Baran, 2007).

Function

The SOC is the prominent structure for bilateral representation of monaural acoustic input. This permits precise comparisons of ipsilateral and contralateral inputs along time, intensity, and to some degree, frequency domains. This sets up the cuing (for the rest of the central auditory system) of time and intensity differences that are essential for sound lateralization (within the head) and sound localization functions. The terms interaural timing (ITD) and intensity differences (IID) have become entrenched in describing localization and lateralization functions. Fusion is another function of the

SOC that can be defined as the combining and integration of information from the two ears. For example, if one ear could hear only high frequencies and the other ear only low frequencies, the SOC could combine these inputs allowing hearing along the entire frequency spectrum.

The TCs of the SOC are sharp and sensitive to change. Further frequency analysis has to do with place in the SOC as mentioned earlier. As one would expect, the SOC neurons have good phase locking—similar to the phase-locking capabilities of CN neurons. Intensity coding for the SOC also is similar to that of the CN. The SOC is represented in large part by wave IV of the ABR; however, this auditory structure also may contribute to other ABR waves. Finally, the SOC plays major role in the acoustic reflex (discussed earlier) and in masking level differences (Møller, 2000).

The Lateral Lemniscus

Structure

The lateral lemniscus (LL) and the nuclei of the LL (NLL) represent two anatomic entities (Figure 2–31). The LL refers to the major pathway on each side of the brainstem that courses from the caudal pons to the midbrain (inferior colliculus). This pathway carries the majority of all neural impulses from lower nuclei to more rostral nuclei. In the LL, the contralateral fibers are far greater in number than are the ipsilateral fibers. The NLL has two main parts: the ventral (VNLL) and dorsal (DNLL) divisions. The VNLL division receives projections from the AVCN and the trapezoid body contralaterally and the DNLL receives projections from the SOC and AVCN ipsilaterally. Neural projections from these nuclei are primarily

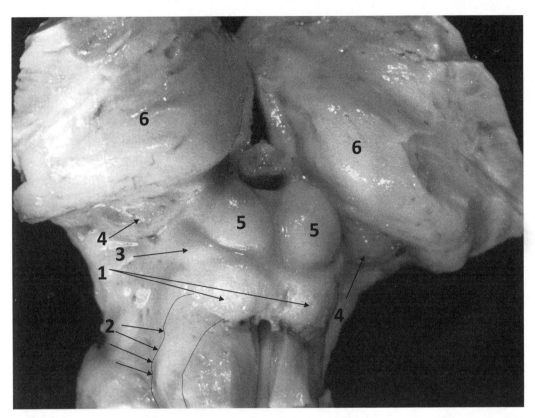

Figure 2–31. *A photo showing the upper pons, midbrain, and thalamus. Key: 1 = inferior colliculus, 2 = lateral lemniscus pathway (demarcated), 3 = brachium of the inferior colliculus, 4 = medial geniculate body, 5 = superior colliculus, 6 = thalamus. (Reproduced with permission from Musiek and Baran, 2007.)*

ipsilateral and course to the IC (Møller, 2000; Schwartz, 1992). It is worthwhile to note that many fibers from the CN and SOC bypass the NLL. Stellate, multipolar, globular, elongated, and ovoid cells are found in the NLL (Covey & Casseday, 1986).

Function

The tonotopic arrangement of the NLL is poorly understood with several different kinds of arrangements being hypothesized (see Musiek & Baran, 2007, for discussion). The NLL is known to be sensitive to interaural time differences, preserving this function from the SOC. Perhaps one of the most notable functions of the NLL

is the primary role that these nuclei play in the generation of wave V of the ABR. This is the largest and most consistent wave of the ABR (Møller, 2000).

Inferior Colliculus

Structure

The IC is situated within the midbrain and is the largest of the ascending brainstem auditory nuclei (see Figure 2–31). It has three divisions, including the central nucleus, the dorsal nucleus, and the lateral nucleus (Morest & Oliver, 1984). The central nucleus is the key auditory player, although the other divisions also contribute to the hearing anatomy. The IC essentially receives major inputs from all more caudal nuclei in the pons both ipsilaterally and contralaterally. The IC is on the receiving end of the acoustic chiasm earlier mentioned. Primarily disc-shaped and stellate cells are found in the IC's central nucleus. The projections from the IC primarily run ipsilaterally to the MGB in the thalamus via a large pathway — the brachium; however, there are also contralateral projections that often course through the commissure of the IC (Ehret, 1997; Musiek & Baran, 2007).

Function

The central nucleus of the IC has a tonotopic organization that runs dorsolaterally to ventromedially for low to high characteristic frequencies. The TCs of the IC are mostly sharp and some even double peaked, indicating complex frequency coding. There are both monotonic and nonmonotonic intensity functions found in the IC. Although most fibers increase firing rate with increases in intensity over a wide range, some fibers "roll over" at sensation levels of less than 10 dB (Popelár & Syka, 1982). This provides a large range of intensity functions for the IC — perhaps more than is seen for other auditory brainstem nuclei.

Most of the neurons in the IC are regarded as good temporal processors, but their phase-locking ability is not quite as sharp as that noted for more caudal auditory nuclei. The IC has a large population of neurons that are sensitive to tone modulations (as compared to steady-state tones). The IC also is sensitive to interaural time and intensity differences similar to the neurons of the SOC, hence, it also plays an important role in localization and binaural hearing (Ehret, 1997; Erulkar, 1959).

The Medial Geniculate Body

Structure

The medial geniculate body (MGB) is located on the dorsal-caudal aspect of the thalamus (see Morest, 1965, for classic descriptions) (see Figure 2–31). The MGB is divided into dorsal, ventral, and medial segments with the ventral being the "most" auditory. The dorsal and medial segments are multisensory, but both of these segments have large areas of auditory representations. The main projections from the IC are ipsilateral with the key input from the central nucleus coursing to the ventral portion of the MGB (Morest, 1965; Winer, 1992).

Output projections from the MGB are interesting. The ventral segment fibers lead to the primary auditory cortex, the medial segment fibers course to the insula, and the dorsal segment fibers project to the secondary auditory areas, insula, and even primary auditory cortex (Musiek & Baran, 2007; Streitfeld, 1980). There also are connections from the MGB to the amygdala, at least in some animals (LeDoux, 1986). Cells types in the ventral MGB are predominately large bushy cells and small stellate cells (Winer, 1992).

Function

The tonotopic organization of the ventral MGB reveals low frequencies laterally and high frequencies medially. The TCs are multiformed-broad, narrow, multipeaked, and some "unusual" (Musiek & Baran, 2007).

Intensity coding in the MGB features mostly nonmonotonic fibers. This differs somewhat from previously discussed intensity coding for lower nuclei. This could mean less activity for high intensities at this level within the auditory system.

There also is a decrease in phase locking (temporal processing) at the MGB compared to other nuclei, with the majority of MGB fibers locking onto low-frequency stimuli. However, the MGB (especially the ventral segment) is sensitive to interaural time and intensity differences similar to more caudal auditory nuclei. Excitatory and inhibitory interactions at the MGB for contralateral and ipsilateral stimulations, respectively, enhance localization processing (Musiek & Baran, 2007).

The MGB contributes to the middle latency response (MLR). However, other nuclei in the thalamic area and auditory cortex may also contribute to the MLR (McGee, Kraus, Littman, & Nicol, 1992).

Auditory Cortex and Subcortex

Structure

The subcortex for purposes of this chapter includes the brain structures between the MGB and the auditory cortex (Figure 2–32). The internal capsule is a pathway through

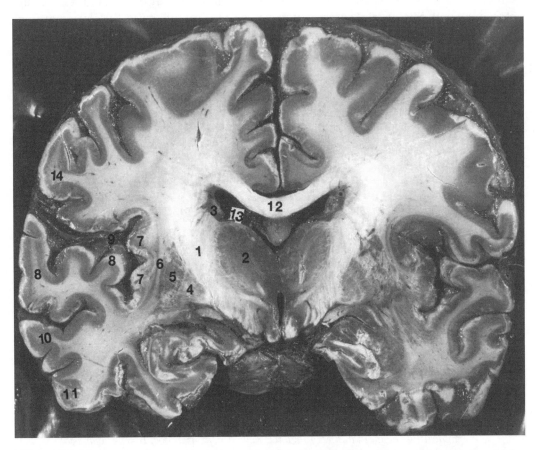

Figure 2–32. The human cerebrum (coronal view). Key: 1 = internal capsule, 2 = thalamus, 3 = caudate, 4 = globus pallidus, 5 = putamen, 6 = external capsule, 7 = insula, 8 = superior temporal gyrus, 9 = sylvian fissure, 10 = middle temporal gyrus, 11 = inferior temporal gyrus, 12 = corpus callosum, 13 = lateral ventricle, 14 = inferior parietal lobe. (Reproduced with permission from Musiek and Baran, 2007.)

which the auditory tracts project to the cortex and associated areas. The internal capsule is bordered medially by the caudate and lateral ventricle and laterally by the putamen and globus pallidus, which together are termed the lenticular process. Lateral to the lenticular process is the external capsule and the insula. In the external capsule is the claustrum, which is gray matter that is responsive to acoustic stimuli (Musiek, 1986).

Neurons from the ventral and dorsal portions of the MGB course through the internal capsule to the primary and secondary auditory areas and the medial segment of the MGB sends fibers that proceed beneath the internal capsule then turn laterally under the lenticular process to reach the external capsule and insula (Roullier, 1997).

The use of imaging studies in humans has changed the view of the auditory cortex. These authors feel it is difficult and somewhat arbitrary to define primary and secondary areas. Hence, areas of the cortex that have been shown to be highly responsive to acoustic stimuli are discussed here. A key structure is the lateral or Sylvian fissure (Figure 2–33) that separates the superior temporal lobe from the frontal and parietal lobes. Located deep in the posterior half of the Sylvian fissure are Heschl's gyrus and the planum temporale (Figure 2–34). Other structures that are considered auditory are the (central) gyri of the inferior parietal lobe, the inferior-posterior frontal lobule, the supramarginal gyrus, the angular gyrus, and portions of the superior temporal gyrus (posterior two-thirds) (see Figures 2–32 and 2–34).

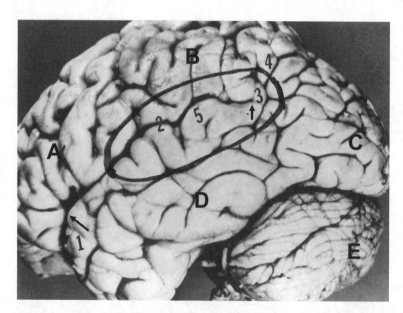

Figure 2–33. *A left lateral view of the human brain with the circled area indicating the main auditory regions. Key: A = frontal lobe, B = parietal lobe, C = occipital lobe, D = temporal lobe, E = cerebellum, 1 = temporal pole, 2 = Sylvian fissure (arrows marking the beginning and end of this fissure), 3 = supramarginal gyrus, 4 = angular gyrus, 5 = superior temporal gyrus. (Modified from Waddington, 1974, with permission.)*

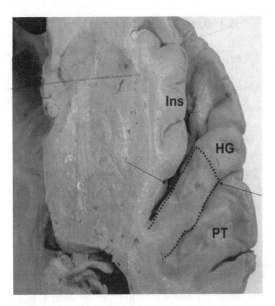

Figure 2–34. *A photo of the brain (horizontal section) of the human brain that defines the primary auditory cortex (within the dotted lines). Key: INS = insula, HG = Heschl's gryus, PT = planum temporale. [Note: the arrows are pointing to the temporal sulcus (anterior) and Heschl's sulcus (posterior)]. (Reproduced with permission from Musiek and Baran, 2007.)*

Also, the insula should be considered as an auditory area (see Figure 2–34). Further discussion of Heschl's, the planum temporale, and the insula follows.

Heschl's gyrus is often considered the primary auditory cortex in humans. There can from one to three gyri composing Heschl's gyrus in an individual brain. Generally, the left Heschl's gyrus is larger than the right (Campain & Minkler, 1976; Musiek & Reeves, 1990). The planum temporale is located immediately posterior to Heschl's gyrus and immediately anterior to the supramarginal gyrus. It also is larger on the left side than the right side (Geschwind & Levitsky, 1968). The insula is a cortex medial to the mesial temporal lobe. It has a series of long and short gyri with adjacent sulci. It is also larger on

the left than right side (Mesulam & Mufson, 1985). Recently the insula has been viewed as a key structure in auditory function (Bamiou, Musiek, & Luxon, 2003).

There is also a different view of the anatomy of the auditory cortex termed the core–belt arrangement (Kaas, Hackett, & Tramo, 1999). The core is the main auditory region, surrounded by a belt and parabelt. There is an outflow of fibers from the core to the belt and parabelt regions. Primarily, the connections to other parts of the brain are via the parabelt region (see Musiek & Baran, 2007).

There are intra- and interhemispheric connections involving the cerebral auditory areas. The interhemispheric connections are presented later. The main intrahemispheric connection is via the arcuate fasciculus, which is part of the longitudinal fasciculus. This tract courses from the area around the supramarginal gyrus (often referred to as Wernicke's area) to the frontal lobe picking up neural connections along the way. This is how Heschl's gyrus conveys impulses to the frontal lobe (Musiek, 1986).

Function

The tonotopic arrangement of Heschl's gyrus reveals the low frequencies in the lateral aspect and the high frequencies in the medial posterior aspect (Musiek & Baran, 2007). The core–belt organization, however, is different in this auditory structure when compared to the organization that has been seen in lower auditory structures (based on primates). The core has anterior, middle, and posterior segments with the anterior and posterior segments running from low to high in a lateral to medial manner. The middle segment runs low to high in a posterior to anterior manner (Hackett, Preuss, & Kaas,

2001). The TCs of the auditory cortex are sharp and multipeaked. In regard to intensity coding, the auditory cortex has both monotonic and nonmonotonic fibers. Generally, as intensity increases most fibers fire at a higher rate and more fibers respond. Some, however, do "roll over" with intensity increases. At the cortex, there also may be some interesting interactions for intensity increases with inhibitory fibers. In other words, inhibition may result in decreases rather than increases in firing rate and numbers of fibers activated (see Musiek & Baran, 2007).

The auditory cortex responds better to modulated tones than to steady-state tones (Evans & Whitfield, 1964). The cortical neurons also respond better to slow as opposed to fast modulation rates (<50 per sec). Most auditory cortex fibers can respond to periodicities (pure-tone cycles) only up to 100 Hz. However, individual abrupt stimuli like click stimuli yield faster responses (Phillips & Hall, 1990). The overall capacity of cortical neurons to temporally process sounds is not as fast as is observed for more caudal auditory structures.

The auditory cortices play an important role in localization. Time and intensity differences are utilized to trigger localization processes and there appears to be stronger cortical activity for contralaterally compared to ipsilaterally directed signals (see Musiek & Baran, 2007).

A number of evoked potentials are relevant to the function of the auditory cortex and subcortex. The MLR is generated from the thalmocortical pathway and auditory cortex. The late potentials N1,P2 also are generated by the auditory cortex. Although the event-related potentials (P300, MMN) likely have numerous generators, the auditory cortex certainly plays a role in these responses (McPherson, 1996; Musiek & Baran, 2007).

The Corpus Callosum

Structure

The corpus callosum (CC) is the largest commissure in the brain connecting the two hemispheres and is responsible for transferring information from one hemisphere to the other (Figure 2–35) (see Musiek & Baran, 2007). The CC is heavily myelinated and in adult humans is about 6.5 cm anterior to posterior and is about 1 cm in thickness. Its fibers run from cortex to cortex. Some connect to the same locus in the other hemisphere (homolateral fibers) and some connect to other regions (heterolateral fibers). The CC is organized to transfer information from every main area of the hemispheres; hence, it has different anatomical regions (see Figure 2–35). The posterior sixth of the CC is the splenium where visual fibers from the occipital lobes cross. Just anterior to the splenium is the isthmus or sulcus (a thinned region) where auditory fibers from the temporal lobe reside. Proceeding anteriorly is a division known as the trunk or body where somatosensory and motor fibers from the parietal lobe cross. Anterior to the trunk is the genu for frontal lobe and olfactory fibers. Beneath the genu is the anterior commissure for which there is much controversy regarding the fiber types, but they could be auditory or olfactory.

Function

The key function of the CC is the transfer of impulses between the two hemispheres. There are both excitatory and inhibitory fibers within the CC. The heavily myelinated fibers that are excitatory have an interhemispheric transfer time (ITT) of 3 to 6 msec and the inhibitory fibers may

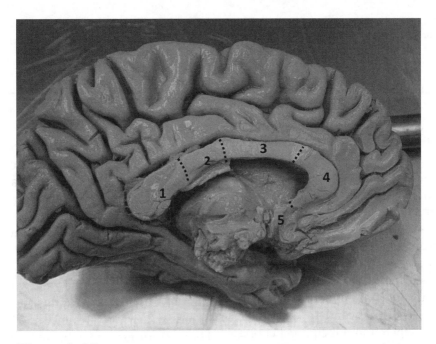

Figure 2–35. *A view of the human corpus callosum. Key: 1 = splenium, 2 = sulcus or isthmus, 3 = trunk or body, 4 = genu, 5 = anterior commissure. (Reproduced with permission from Musiek and Baran, 2007.)*

have an ITT of more than 100 msec. The ITT in humans changes with age. The best ITT is found in teenagers with individuals who are older and younger yielding increased ITTs (Salamy, 1978).

The transfer of information from one hemisphere to the other can be critical to our perception. Each hemisphere is dominant for certain processes and it is the timely exchange of these processes that allows the brain to work efficiently. A relevant example of this exchange of hemispheric information is dichotic listening for speech. When speech is presented in the dichotic mode, the right hemisphere receives input from the left ear and the left hemisphere receives input from the right ear. If a verbal response is required, the information in the right hemisphere must be transferred to the speech hemisphere, which is the left hemisphere. If this func-

tion is compromised, a left ear deficit in dichotic listening will result. This deficit takes place because the ipsilateral pathways to the cortex are suppressed during dichotic listening leaving only the contralateral system to function for speech perception (Kimura, 1961; Musiek, Kibbe, & Baran, 1984).

Recent research also has demonstrated that the CC may play a role in modulating the functions (inhibitory-excitatory) in each hemisphere. Although it is difficult at this time to theorize how this may influence various auditory processes, it indeed seems to be an exciting avenue for future research. Needless to say, the CC plays important roles in audition. It allows the efficient exchange of information across all sensory systems and therefore is critical to both auditory and speech perception processing.

THE EFFERENT SYSTEM

Structure

Coursing along a similar tract as the afferent auditory system is the descending or efferent auditory system (EAS). This system is smaller and less well understood than is the afferent system. The EAS starts at the auditory cortex where it likely has several areas of input including fibers from secondary auditory regions. It courses caudally through the internal capsule and on to the MGB where some reciprocal routes to the cortex are noted. The EAS fibers descend to the inferior colliculus where more reciprocal connections involving the MGB and cortex are present. It then descends farther along the LL and into the area around the SOC where it becomes known as the olivocochlear bundle (OCB).

The OCB can be divided into two main descending tracts, the lateral olivocochlear (LOC) and medial olivocochlear (MOC) systems. The LOC is primarily an ipsilateral route and the MOC a contralateral route to the cochlea. These ipsilateral and contralateral routes descend from the OCB area to the cochlear nucleus, exit the brainstem via the internal auditory meatus, and run along the vestibular tracts out to the cochlea. The LOC fibers finally connect to the afferent fibers leaving the IHCs and the MOC fibers connect directly to the OHCs (Sahley, Nodar, & Musiek, 1997).

Function

The function of the rostral portion of the EAS remains somewhat a mystery. The number of reciprocal connections as well as some available data indicates that both excitation and inhibition influences can be exerted on the incoming acoustic signal (Mitani, Shimokouchi, & Nomura, 1983). It also seems likely that the rostral and caudal portions of the EAS work together and that the rostral portion also has some influence on the OCB. More research on the rostral EAS is certainly indicated as it may play a subtle, but important, role in hearing that is yet to be discovered.

The caudal EAS, which we will refer to as the OCB, was first studied over 50 years ago by Galambos (1956). Galambos demonstrated that, if the OCB was stimulated electrically in animals, it resulted in reduced firing rates of the AN fibers. These findings have been interpreted to mean that the OCB may have inhibitory influences on the afferent auditory system. It was discovered that the OCB also could be stimulated and the same effect measured if an acoustic signal was presented to one ear and a noise was presented to the opposite ear (Folsom & Owsley, 1987). This has become known as the "suppression effect" and can be measured using otoacoustic emissions or evoked potentials in humans.

Activation of the OCB also has been shown to enhance hearing in noise (Kawase & Liberman, 1993). If the OCB is activated either electrically (as was done in the Galambos' study) or by contralateral noise when a listener is being asked to detect a signal in noise, the detection threshold will improve relative to the conditions in which the OCB is not stimulated. A number of experimental studies have shown similar effects, and this phenomenon is now considered to be one of the mechanisms that allows hearing in noisy situations to be enhanced (see Musiek & Baran, 2007; Sahley et al., 1997).

VASCULAR SUPPLY FOR THE AUDITORY SYSTEM

The Peripheral System

Functions of the peripheral and central auditory systems are highly dependent on blood supply. The external ear's blood supply comes from branches of the external carotid artery, whereas the middle ear receives its blood supply from branches of the internal carotid. The cochlea and AN's vascular supply comes from the vertebrobasilar system.

The pinna and external auditory meatus are supplied mostly, but not exclusively, by the superficial temporal artery and posterior auricular artery. There is some controversy regarding the tympanic membrane's blood supply, but playing key roles are branches of the deep auricular and maxillary arteries. The middle ear (soft tissue) receives vascular input from branches of the internal carotid, maxillary (tympanic branch), posterior auricular (mastoid branch), and middle meningeal (petrosal branch) arteries, as well as branches of the ascending pharyngeal and pterygoid arteries (Anson & Donaldson, 1981; Clark & Ohlemiller, 2008; Musiek & Baran, 2007).

The internal auditory or labyrinthine artery (IAA), which is a main branch of the basilar or anterior inferior cerebellar artery (AICA) (brainstem), is key for blood supply of the cochlea and AN. The IAA divides within the IAM into cochlear and vestibular branches, which supply the auditory and vestibular nerves before proceeding externally to the cochlea. The cochlear artery branches into the spiral modiolar artery (SMA) and the cochleovestibular artery (CVA). The SMA spirals around the modiolus giving off branches en route and the CVA coils following the cochlea. These two main vessels give off branches that make up the network of radiating arterioles that supplies much of the cochlea (Musiek & Baran, 2007; Smith, 1973). These arteries have as their counterparts veins and collecting venules in similar anatomic areas, which return the impure blood back to the main veins and onto the heart.

The Central System

The central auditory nervous system in terms of its vascular supply can be segmented into the brainstem and cortex. The brainstem auditory structures are supplied by the vertebrobasilar system and the cortex by the internal carotid system. In the brainstem, the vertebral arteries, which course rostrally on both sides of the spine, join together to form the basilar artery a few millimeters below the pontomedullary junction. The basilar artery is located on the ventral side of the brainstem. The basilar artery gives off the anterior inferior cerebellar artery (AICA), which with circumferential branches supplies blood to the cochlear nucleus. Smaller branches off the basilar artery called paramedial or pontine penetrating arteries, penetrate the pons to supply the SOC and some of the LL deep in the pons (Waddington, 1974).

Proceeding rostrally another main branch of the basilar artery is the superior cerebellar artery, which indirectly supplies the LL and the IC. The MGB is most likely supplied by the posterior thalamic group arteries, which are a multivessel complex arising from the posterior cerebral artery (Musiek & Baran, 2007; Waddington, 1974).

The auditory cortex and associated areas are supplied with blood primarily by the middle cerebral artery (MCA). The MCA has anterior, middle, and posterior temporal arteries that branch to cover the anterior, middle, and posterior temporal lobe. The MCA also has a central sulcus branch that supplies the parietal lobe. The angular artery feeds the angular gyrus and possibly the supramarginal gyrus. The insula's vascular supply is from the fronto-opercular artery (from the anterior MCA), which branches into a variety of insular arteries. The corpus callosum's anterior four-fifths has as its vascular supply the pericallosal artery, a branch of the MCA, and its posterior one-fifth is supplied by the posterior cerebral artery (Musiek & Baran, 2007; Waddington, 1974).

THE VESTIBULAR SYSTEM

Structure

The vestibular system serves to maintain static and dynamic balance by initiating a series of reflexes that are recruited when the head is moved during daily activities (e.g., walking or running). This system also provides information regarding spatial orientation and a subjective sense of movement. This elegant system consists of five end organs for each ear that act as integrating accelerometers, nerves that carry electrical signals to the brainstem, and diffuse projections that are routed throughout the central nervous system. The peripheral vestibular system is physically connected to the peripheral auditory system at the vestibule, which is located between the middle ear cavity and the internal auditory meatus. Because of this, it is not uncommon for disease to affect both the auditory and vestibular systems (e.g., Ménière's disease). The peripheral vestibular system is housed in a series of hollow tunnels called the bony labyrinth that are located within the very hard petrous portion of the temporal bone. The membranous labyrinth is suspended within the bony labyrinth by perilymph and supporting connective tissue. The membranous labyrinth is filled with endolymphatic fluid, which has an ionic composition that is higher in K^+ and lower in Na^+ than perilymph.[1]

The peripheral vestibular system is shown in Figure 2–36. The vestibular end organs consist of the horizontal (or lateral), anterior (or superior) and posterior semicircular canals, and the utricle and the saccule. Together, there are a total of five peripheral end organs, which act to transduce acceleration of the head or the head and body into an electrical code. The three semicircular canals convert angular acceleration and deceleration and the latter two end organs (i.e., the utricle and saccule) transduce linear acceleration and deceleration. The anatomic structures of the end organs are, at the same time, both similar and different. Each consists of a mass that sits atop stereocilia that project from hair cells. It is the effect of inertia on the mass that results in deflection of the stereocilia and electrical transduction at the base of the hair cells. Each of the semicircular canals is oriented in a different plane making this system sensitive to

---

[1]It is believed that the "dark cells" of the cristae (i.e., semicircular canal system) and maculae (utricle and saccule) are responsible for producing the endolymphatic fluid found in the vestibular apparatus (Kimura, 1969).

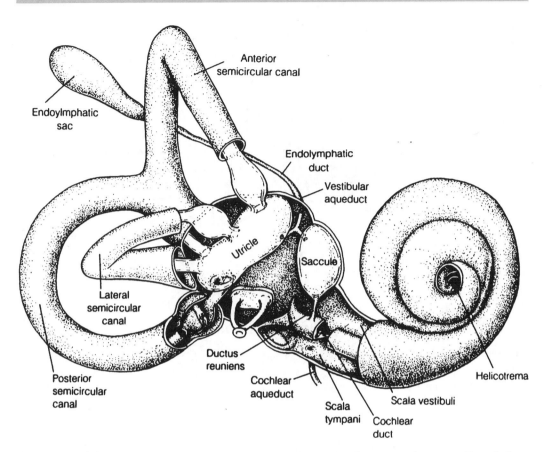

Figure 2–36. The anatomy of the membranous labyrinth. Illustration by Mary Dersch from Pender, 1992, with permission of Daniel Pender. This material is copyrighted and any further reproduction or distribution is prohibited without express permission of the author.

angular acceleration in nearly all directions. Specifically, the horizontal canal is tilted upward approximately 30° anteriorly in relationship to the horizontal plane and two vertical semicircular canals are oriented at 45° in the sagittal plane. The sense organ located at the ampullated end of each semicircular canal is called the cristae ampullaris. Each cristae consists of: (1) a gelatinous mass that fills the ampulla from the floor to the ceiling, called the cupula, (2) hair cell stereocilia, and (3) a single, taller, more rigid kinocilium that projects up from each hair cell into the cupula (Figure 2–37). The stereocilia project from hair cells and both afferent and efferent nerve fibers approximate the base of the hair cells. The cupula and the endolymph have the same specific gravity (i.e., 1.0; Money et al., 1971). When the head is not in motion, the cupula is suspended in the endolymph in a neutrally buoyant position and the primary afferent nerve fibers fire at a tonic resting rate. Acceleration of the head in the plane of a canal results in the endolymph lagging behind the canal walls and results in fluid motion. The cupula seals the ampullar cavity, and because the flow of endolymph is impeded, pressure

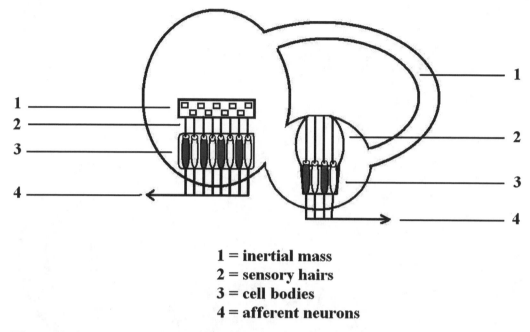

1 = **inertial mass**
2 = **sensory hairs**
3 = **cell bodies**
4 = **afferent neurons**

Figure 2–37. An illustration of the receptor mechanisms of the semicircular canals and otolith system. The stimulus of the otolith organs is provided by the inertia of the otolith crystals. The stimulus of the semicircular canals is provided by the inertia of the endolymph in the canal system.

is exerted on the cupula, thus bending it in the direction opposite that of the head movement. This distortion of the cupula results in shearing of the stereocilia and kinocilia that causes a change in the electrical discharge rate at the base of the hair cells. The end organs are polarized so that head movement in one direction results in depolarization of the end organ and an increase in the firing rate, whereas movement in the opposite direction results in hyperpolarizaton and a decrease in the discharge rate.

The saccule and the utricle are located in the vestibule and each has a sensory neuroepithelium called a macula. The macula of the saccule is oriented primarily in the vertical plane and the macula of the utricle is oriented in the horizontal plane. The mass in the macular organs (see Figure 2–37) are calcium carbonate crystals (i.e., 5–7 μm), referred to as "oto-

liths" or "otoconia" (Lindeman, 1969). These crystals reside on a sticky, reticulated "net" called the otolith membrane. The stereocilia and kinocilia project from hair cells up into the otolith membrane; however, the polarization pattern is more complex than in the cristae. Each macular organ has an anatomic line running through it called a striola. The hair cells are oriented in opposing directions around the striola. In the utricle, the hair cells are oriented toward the striola, whereas in the saccule, the hair cells are oriented away from the striola. This unique organization of hair cells allows the otolith organs to transduce linear head motion in nearly any direction. Here again, both afferent and efferent primary nerve fibers approach the base of the hair cells.

Electrical activity from the vestibular end organs is routed through either the superior or inferior division of the vestibular portion of the eighth cranial nerve. The superior vestibular nerve contains afferent fibers from the horizontal and anterior semicircular canals, the utricle, and part of the saccule, which provide electrical impulses to this pathway. The inferior vestibular nerve contains afferent fibers from the posterior semicircular canal and the majority of the saccule. In total, the vestibular branches of the eighth nerve consist of 18,000 single nerve fibers that discharge at a rate that varies between 10 and 100 spikes per second. This means that, at any moment, there can be well over 1 million spikes per second flowing from each of the two peripheral vestibular systems to the central vestibular system.

The origin of the second-order neuron in the vestibular system is the vestibular nuclei (i.e., the vestibular equivalent of the cochlear nuclei). There are four vestibular nuclei in the pons: the superior, medial, lateral, and inferior vestibular nuclei. The vestibular nuclei act as gating centers for electrical activity generated from the peripheral vestibular system (Figure 2–38). For example, electrical activity from the vestibular nuclei is routed to the eye movement pathways so that we can view a stationary object while walking or running in such a way that the target remains still on the center of clear vision of the retina. The cerebellum regulates vestibular responses. Specifically, the vestibulocerebellum (i.e., flocculus, nodulus, uvula, and vermis) receives input from the primary vestibular afferents and also sends projections to the vestibular nuclei (see Figure 2–38). In this regard, inhibitory connections between the flocculus and the vestibular nuclei

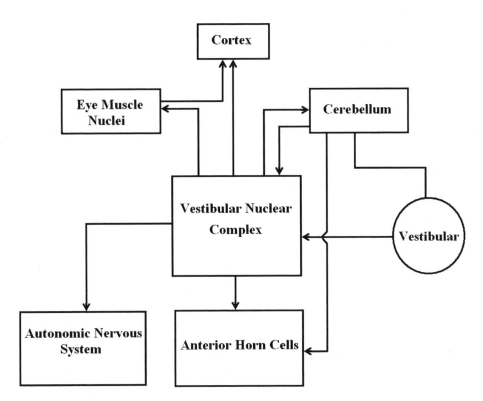

Figure 2–38. A block diagram illustrating the vestibular nuclei and their connections.

make it possible for patients to centrally compensate (i.e., improve the dynamic properties of the vestibulo-ocular reflex) after the loss of all or part of a single end organ system (Ito, 1993). Connections between the vestibular nuclei, the cerebellum, and the descending spinal cord pathways (e.g., the lateral and medial vestibulospinal pathways, and the reticulospinal pathway) also enable us to correct postural deviations so we do not fall (see Figure 2–38). Connections between the vestibular nuclei, the reticular activating system, and the autonomic nervous system are responsible for the generation of secondary reactions such as pallor, sweating, nausea, and vomiting that occur when function is lost either temporarily or permanently in one vestibular end organ (see Figure 2–38). Finally, connections between the vestibular nuclei and cortical centers located in the parietal and temporal lobes make it possible for the brain to interpret the pattern of electrical signals ascending from the brainstem as motion (see Figure 2–38).

Function

Three primary vestibular reflexes act to maintain our balance. The vestibulocolic reflex (VCR) acts on neck muscles to stabilize the head based on the signals received from the vestibular end organs. The vestibulospinal reflex (VSR) serves to stabilize the body, also based on signals received from the end organs. Finally, the purpose of the vestibulo-ocular reflex (VOR) is to maintain clear vision during head motion. It accomplishes this task by generating compensatory eye movements during head accelerations that act to keep the fovea of the retina on an object of interest. For example, the VOR is recruited to stabilize the environment

when a person is running on a treadmill. An intact VOR enables that person to either read a magazine or watch a monitor at the same time. For the sake of simplicity we describe changes that occur in the VOR when a person turns the head to the left. The horizontal VOR is shown in Figure 2–39.

When the head is turned to the left, endolymph lags behind and bends the stereocilia and kinocilia of the cristae ampullaris in both lateral semicircular canals. In this case, the left end organ is housed in the leading ear for the head movement and the endolymph moves in a clockwise fashion deflecting the stereocilia and kinocilia of the cristae toward the utricle. Because of the arrangement of the stereocilia in the lateral canals, this action results in an increasing firing rate in the superior portion of the vestibular nerve on the left side. The stereocilia and kinocilia of the cristae ampullaris in the right lateral canal, or the lagging ear, are deflected away from the utricle driving the firing rate in the right vestibular nerve below its tonic resting rate. The two medial vestibular nuclei (MVN) each receive input from the lateral semicircular canals via the superior vestibular nerves. In this case of a head turn to the left, the increased peripheral input from the left end organ is received by the left MVN and a corresponding decrease is received by the right MVN. The left MVN routes the increased activity to both ipsilateral and contralateral secondary vestibular neurons. Specifically, the left MVN sends projections to the ipsilateral oculomotor nucleus (III) and sends decussating projections to the contralateral abducens nucleus (VI). On the right side, a similar but opposite chain of events occurs. The right MVN relays the decrease in neural activity to the ipsilateral abducens nucleus and also across the midline to the

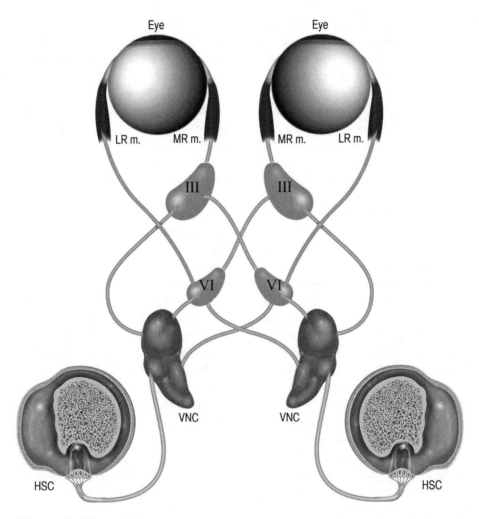

Figure 2–39. *Dorsal perspective of the horizontal vestibulo-ocular reflex (VOR) pathways. Key: HSC = horizontal semicircular canal, VNC = vestibular nuclear complex, VI = abducens nuclei, III = oculomotor nuclei, LRm = lateral rectus muscle, MRm = medial rectus muscle.*

left oculomotor nucleus. The abducens and oculomotor nuclei send motor projections to the effector organs of the horizontal VOR (i.e., extraocular muscles).

In our example of a head turn to the left, the right abducens nucleus and left oculomotor nucleus relay the increased neural input received from the vestibular nuclei through motor neurons to the left medial rectus and right lateral rectus muscles. This pattern of input to these two extraocular muscles causes them to contract, which results in a slow deviation of the eye to the right that is proportional to the head turn.

Facilitating this rightward deviation of the eyes is the corresponding decrease in neural drive to the antagonist extraocular muscles (i.e., left lateral rectus and right medial rectus). The decrease in activity that has been relayed from the vestibular nuclei of the lagging ear to the left abducens and right oculomotor nuclei decreases the neural drive to the oculomotor and abducens nerves and from there to the right medial rectus and left lateral rectus resulting in a relaxation of these muscles. The medial longitudinal fasciculus (MLF) is the brainstem pathway that coordinates the outputs of the vestibular nuclei to the oculomotor and abducens nuclei making it possible for these compensatory eye movements to be conjugate (i.e., for the visual axes to be parallel).

In the situation where there is sustained rotation (i.e., if the person was in a continuously rotating chair), this slow deviation of the eyes in the opposite direction of the head turn will drive the eyes to the lateral extremes in the orbits. Neurons in the paramedian pontine reticular formation (PPRF) interrupt the flow of electrical activity from the vestibular periphery, which results in the eyes returning quickly to midline. The neurons in the PPRF go through a refractory cycle and inputs from the vestibular system again drive the eyes in the direction opposite the head turn. This rhythmic, repetitive, sawtooth-shaped eye movement is referred to as "nystagmus" and it will continue as long as the asymmetry exists between the two vestibular end organs (it is the velocity of the slow eye deviation that is measured in quantitative assessments of vestibular system function).

Due to endolymph-cupular dynamics, the vestibular system is less sensitive to angular accelerations of less than 0.05 Hz and greater than 3 Hz (Baloh & Honrubia, 2001). For example, if rotation in the yaw plane (i.e., rotating about a superior-inferior axis) is sustained at a constant velocity, fluid motion will approximate the speed of the canals and the cupulae will drift back to their neutral position (Goldberg & Fernandez,

1971). In this case, it would seem intuitive that the subject being rotated would no longer perceive the sensation of rotary motion once the cupulae return to their static state. However, horizontal VOR responses to a sustained rotational stimulus persist approximately three times longer than the "drive" from the periphery. This prolongation of the VOR after cessation of the neural drive from the peripheral end organs has been termed "velocity storage" and is under the control of a neural integrator (NI) that is located in the brainstem and cerebellum. The NI acts to adjust the output of vestibular afferent activity allowing the VOR response to be extended one order of magnitude beyond what the canal responses produce, thereby enhancing the low-frequency response of the VOR. In order for the velocity storage mechanism to function, several anatomic structures must be intact. These include the peripheral end organs, the vestibular portions of the eighth cranial nerve, the vestibular nuclei, the commissural fibers connecting the vestibular nuclei (i.e., "direct" and "indirect" pathways), and the connections between vestibular nuclei and the cerebellum. The velocity storage mechanism manifests itself in many of the quantitative tests that are used clinically. Impairment in the velocity storage system has been shown to result in stereotyped abnormalities on quantitative tests of vestibular system function and may contribute to balance impairments in unsteady, falls-prone patients (Jacobson, McCaslin, Patel, Barin, & Ramadan, 2004).

Vascular Supply for the Vestibular System

The labyrinthine artery supplies the peripheral vestibular end organs and is known to have a variable origin (Baloh & Honrubia, 2001). It arises most commonly from a branch of the AICA, but occasionally can be a direct branch of the basilar artery or the superior cerebellar artery. Once the labyrinthine artery enters the inner ear it bifurcates into the common cochlear artery and the anterior vestibular artery. The common cochlear artery has two branches: the main cochlear artery and the vestibulocochlear artery, which turns into the posterior vestibular artery. The main cochlear artery nourishes structures within the cochlea (e.g., basilar membrane). The posterior vestibular artery supplies the ampulla of the posterior semicircular canal and the majority of the saccule (Schuknecht, 1993). The anterior vestibular artery supplies the vestibular portion of the eighth cranial nerve, the ampullae of the anterior and lateral semicircular canals, the macula of the utricle, and a small part of the saccule (Baloh & Honrubia, 2001). The different sources of blood supply to the different end organs can be a source of the varying findings often encountered during quantitative vestibular testing.

SUMMARY

This chapter presented an overview of some key aspects of the auditory and vestibular systems in regard to their structures and functions. The efferent pathways also were discussed as well as the vascular anatomy of the peripheral and central auditory systems and the vestibular system. This chapter serves as an orientation and reference for the subsequent chapters on disorders of hearing that, by their nature, require grounding in structure and function of the auditory system.

Acknowledgments. The vestibular portion of this chapter was written by Gary Jacobson, PhD and Devin McCaslin, PhD, Professor and Associate Professor, respectively, Department of Hearing and Speech Sciences, Vanderbilt University. The authors also gratefully acknowledge Allyn & Bacon for the extensive use of *The Auditory System: Anatomy, Physiology, and Clinical Correlates* by *Musiek and Baran*.

REFERENCES

Anson, B. J., & Donaldson, J. A. (1981). *The surgical anatomy of the temporal bone and ear* (3rd ed.). Philadelphia, PA: W. B. Saunders.

Baloh, R. W., & Honrubia, V. (2001). *Clinical neurophysiology of the vestibular system* (3rd ed.). New York, NY: Oxford University Press.

Bamiou, D. E., Musiek, F. E., & Luxon, L. M. (2003). The insula (Island of Reil) and its role in auditory processing: Literature review. *Brain Research Reviews, 42*(2), 143–154.

Blauert, J. (1983). *Spatial hearing. The psychophysics of human sound localization.* Cambridge, MA: MIT Press.

Borg, E. (1973). On the neuronal organization of the acoustic middle ear reflex. A physiological and anatomical study. *Brain Research, 49*(1), 101–123.

Buser, P. A., & Imbert, M. (1992). *Audition.* Cambridge, MA: MIT Press.

Campain, R., & Minckler, J. (1976). A note on the gross configurations of the human auditory cortex. *Brain and Language, 3*(2), 318–323.

Clark, W. W., & Ohlemiller, K. K. (2008). *Anatomy and physiology of hearing for audiologists.* Clifton Park, NY: Thomson Delmar Learning.

Covey, E., & Casseday, J. H. (1986). Connectional basis for frequency representation in the nuclei of the lateral lemniscus of the bat Eptesicus fuscus. *Journal of Neuroscience, 6*(10), 2926–2940.

Dallos, P. (1973). *The auditory periphery: Biophysics and physiology*. New York, NY: Academic Press.

Davis, H. (1965). A model for transducer action in the cochlea. *Cold Spring Harbor Symposia on Quantitative Biology, 30,* 181–190.

Ehret, G. (1997). The auditory midbrain, a "shunting-yard" of acoustical information processing. In G. Ehret & R. Romand (Eds.), *The central auditory system* (pp. 259–303). New York, NY: Oxford University Press.

Erulkar, S. D. (1959). The responses of single units of the inferior colliculus of the cat to acoustic stimulation. *Proceedings of the Royal Society of London B Biological Sciences, 150*(940), 336–355.

Evans, E. F., & Whitfield, I. C. (1964). Classification of unit responses in the auditory cortex of the unanaesthetized and unrestrained cat. *Journal of Physiology, 171,* 476–493.

Folsom, R. C., & Owsley, R. M. (1987). N1 action potentials in humans. Influence of simultaneous contralateral stimulation. *Acta Otolaryngologica, 103*(3–4), 262–265.

Galambos, R. (1956). Suppression of auditory nerve activity by stimulation of efferent fibers to the cochlea. *Journal of Neurophysiology, 19*(5), 424–437.

Geisler, C. D. (1998). *From sound to synapse: Physiology of the mammalian ear*. New York, NY: Oxford University Press.

Gelfand, S. A. (1997). *Essentials of audiology*. New York, NY: Thieme Medical.

Gelfand, S. A. (1998). *Hearing: An introduction to psychological and physiological acoustics* (3rd ed.). New York, NY: Marcel Dekker.

Geschwind, N., & Levitsky, W. (1968). Human brain: Left-right asymmetries in temporal speech region. *Science, 161*(837), 186–187.

Goldberg, J. M., & Fernandez, C. (1971). Physiology of the peripheral neurons innervating semi-circular canals of the squirrel monkey. I. Resting discharge and response to constant angular accelerations. *Journal of Neurophysiology, 34*(4), 635–660.

Hackett, T. A., Preuss, T. M., & Kaas, J. H. (2001). Architectonic identification of the core region in auditory cortex of macaques, chimpanzees, and humans. *Journal of Comparative Neurology, 441*(3), 197–222.

Ito, M. (1993). Neurophysiology of the nodulofloccular system. *Revue Neurologique (Paris), 149*(11), 692–697.

Jacobson, G. P., McCaslin, D. L., Patel, S., Barin, K., & Ramadan, N. M. (2004). Functional and anatomical correlates of impaired velocity storage. *Journal of the American Academy of Audiology, 15*(4), 324–333.

Kaas, J. H., Hackett, T. A., & Tramo, M. J. (1999). Auditory processing in primate cerebral cortex. *Current Opinion in Neurobiology, 9*(2), 164–170.

Kawase, T., & Liberman, M. C. (1993). Antimasking effects of the olivocochlear reflex. I. Enhancement of compound action potentials to masked tones. *Journal of Neurophysiology, 70*(6), 2519–2532.

Keidel, W. D., Kallert, S., & Korth, M. (1983). *The physiological bases of hearing* (pp. 82–108). New York, NY: Thieme-Stratton.

Kim, D. O., & Parham, K. (1991). Auditory nerve spatial encoding of high frequency pure tones: Population response profiles derived from d' measure associated with nearby places along the cochlea. *Hearing Research, 52*(1), 167–179.

Kim, D. O., & Parham, K. (1997). Physiology of the auditory nerve. In M. J. Crocker (Ed.), *Encyclopedia of acoustics* (pp. 1331–1378). New York, NY: John Wiley & Sons.

Kimura, D. (1961). Some effects of temporal lobe damage on auditory perception. *Canadian Journal of Psychology, 15,* 156–165.

Kimura, R. S. (1969). Distribution, structure, and function of dark cells in the vestibular labyrinth. *Annals of Otology, Rhinology, and Laryngology, 78*(3), 542–561.

LeDoux, J. E. (1986). The neurobiology of emotion. In J. E. LeDoux, & W. Hirst (Eds.), *Mind and brain: Dialogues in cognitive neuroscience* (pp. 342–346). Cambridge, UK: Cambridge University Press.

Liberman, M. C. (1978). Auditory-nerve response from cats raised in low-noise chamber. *Journal of the Acoustical Society of America, 63*(2), 442–455.

Lindeman, H. H . (1969). Studies on the morphology of the sensory regions of the vestibular apparatus with 45 figures. *Ergebnisse der Anatomie und Entwicklungsgeschichte, 42*(1), 1–113.

McGee, T., Kraus, N., Littman, T., & Nicol, T. (1992). Contributions of medial geniculate body subdivisions to the middle latency response. *Hearing Research, 61*(1–2), 147–154.

McPherson, D. L. (1996). *Late potentials of the auditory system.* San Diego, CA: Singular Publishing Group.

Mesulam, M., & Mufson, E. (1985). The insular of Reil in man and monkey architectonics, connectivity, and function. In E. G. Jones & A. Peters (Eds.), *Cerebral cortex* (Vol. 4, pp. 179–226). New York, NY: Plenum Press.

Mitani, A., Shimokouchi, M., & Nomura, S. (1983). Effects of stimulation of the primary auditory cortex upon colliculogeniculate neurons in the inferior colliculus of the cat. *Neuroscience Letters, 42*(2), 185–189.

Møller, A. R. (2000). *Hearing: Its physiology and pathophysiology.* New York, NY: Academic Press.

Money, K. E., Bonen, L., Beatty, J. D., Kuehn, L. A., Sokoloff, M., & Weaver, R. S. (1971). Physical properties of fluids and structures of vestibular apparatus of the pigeon. *American Journal of Physiology, 220*(1), 140–147.

Moore, J. K. (2000). Organization of the human superior olivary complex. *Microscopy Research and Technique, 51*(4), 403–412.

Morest, D. K. (1965). The laminar structure of the medial geniculate body of the cat. *Journal of Anatomy, 99,* 143–160.

Morest, D. K., & Oliver, D. L. (1984). The neuronal architecture of the inferior colliculus in the cat: Defining the functional anatomy of the auditory midbrain. *Journal of Comparative Neurology, 222*(2), 209–236.

Musiek, F. E. (1986). Neuroanatomy, neurophysiology, and central auditory assessment. Part II: The cerebrum. *Ear and Hearing, 7*(5), 283–294.

Musiek, F. E., & Baran, J. A. (2007). *The auditory system: Anatomy, physiology, and clinical correlates.* Boston, MA: Allyn & Bacon.

Musiek, F. E., Kibbe K., & Baran J. A. (1984). Neuroaudiological results from split-brain patients. *Seminars in Hearing, 5*(3), 219–229.

Musiek, F. E., & Reeves, A. G. (1990). Asymmetries of the auditory areas of the cerebrum. *Journal of the American Academy of Audiology, 1*(4), 240–245.

Pender, J. D. (1992). *Practical audiology.* Philadelphia, PA: JB Lippincott Company.

Phillips, D. P., & Hall, S. E. (1990). Response timing constraints on the cortical representation of sound time structure. *Journal of the Acoustical Society of America, 88*(3), 1403–1411.

Pickles, J. O. (1988). *An introduction to the physiology of hearing* (2nd ed.). London, UK: Academic Press.

Popelár, J., & Syka, J. (1982). Response properties of neurons in the inferior colliculus of the guinea-pig. *Acta Neurobiologiae Experimentalis, 42*(4–5), 299–310.

Romand, R., & Avan, P. (1997). Anatomical and functional aspects of the cochlear nucleus. In G. Ehret & R. Romand (Eds.), *The central auditory system* (pp. 97–192). New York, NY: Oxford University Press.

Roullier, E. (1997). Functional organization of the auditory pathways. In G. Ehret & R. Romand (Eds.), *The central auditory system* (pp. 3–65). New York, NY: Oxford University Press.

Sahley, T. L., Nodar, R. H., & Musiek, F. E. (1997). *Efferent auditory system.* San Diego, CA: Singular Publishing Group.

Salamy, A. (1978). Commissural transmission: Maturational changes in humans. *Science 200*(4348), 1409–1411.

Salvi, R.J., Clock Eddins, A. C., & Wang, J. (2007) Cochlear physiology II: Mostly electrophysiology. In F. E. Musiek & J. A. Baran, *The auditory system: Anatomy, physiology, and clinical correlates* (pp. 112–149). Boston, MA: Allyn & Bacon.

Schuknecht, H. (1993). *Pathology of the ear.* Philadelphia, PA: Lea & Febiger.

Schwartz, I. R. (1992). Superior olivary complex in the lateral lemniscal nuclei. In D. B. Webster, A. N. Popper, & R. R. Fey (Eds.), *The cochlea* (pp. 117–167). New York, NY: Springer-Verlag.

Shaw, E. A. G., & Teranishi, R. (1968). Sound pressure generated in an external ear replica and real human ears by a nearby point source. *Journal of the Acoustical Society of America, 44*(1), 240–249.

Slepecky, N. (1996). Cochlear structure. In P. Dallos, A. N. Popper, & R. R. Fay (Eds.), *The cochlea* (pp. 44–129). New York, NY: Springer-Verlag.

Smith, C. A. (1973). Vascular patterns of the membranous labyrinth. In A. J. D. De Lorenzo (Ed.), *Vascular disorders and hearing defects* (pp. 1–22). Baltimore, MD: University Park Press.

Spoendlin, H. (1972). Innervation densities of the cochlea. *Acta Otolaryngologica, 73*(2), 235–248.

Streitfeld, B. D. (1980). The fiber connections of the temporal lobe with emphasis on Rhesus monkey. *International Journal of Neuroscience, 11*(1), 51–71.

von Békésy, G. (1960). *Experiments in hearing.* New York, NY: McGraw-Hill.

Waddington, M. (1974). *The atlas of cerebral angiography with anatomic correlation.* Boston, MA: Little, Brown.

Wangemann, P. (2002a). K+ cycling and the endocochlear potential. *Hearing Research, 165*(1–2), 1–9.

Wangemann, P. (2002b). K(+) cycling and its regulation in the cochlea and the vestibular labyrinth. *Audiology and Neurotology, 7*(4), 199–205.

Wever, E. G., & Bray, C. W. (1930). Action currents in the auditory nerve in response to acoustical stimulation. *Proceedings of the National Academy of Sciences of the United States of America, 16*(5), 344–350.

Winer, J. A. (1992). The functional architecture of the medial geniculate body and primary auditory cortex. In D. B. Webster, A. N. Popper, & R. R. Fay (Eds.), *The mammalian auditory pathway: Neuroanatomy* (pp. 222–409). New York, NY: Springer-Verlag.

Yost, W. A. (2000). *Fundamentals of hearing: An introduction* (4th ed.). San Diego, CA: Academic Press.

Zemlin, W. R. (1998). *Speech and hearing science: Anatomy and physiology* (4th ed.). Boston, MA: Allyn & Bacon.

Zwislocki, J. J. (2002). *Auditory sound transmission: An autobiographical perspective.* Mahwah, NJ: Lawrence Erlbaum.

3

Audiologic, Vestibular, and Radiologic Procedures

Examination of Hearing Sensitivity

Although the examination of type of hearing impairment can be dated to the late 1700s by measures such as tuning fork tests, our more precise methods of audiologic assessment began in the 1920s with the advent of the Western Electric 1-A audiometer. Advances in technology have changed dramatically over the years but, many of the fundamental principles of assessment remain the same. Therefore, for readers who are not familiar with traditional audiologic assessment measures, a review of the fundamentals of peripheral assessment certainly deserves attention. It is beyond the scope of this chapter to provide all of the details necessary for a thorough understanding of audiologic test procedures; instead, this chapter provides a general overview of relevant evaluation measures.

The audiometer is the primary tool used by audiologists in the assessment of peripheral hearing sensitivity. It allows the audiologist to evaluate a patient's sensitivity for a variety of different sound stimuli such as pure tones and speech. When performing a hearing evaluation, results are plotted on a pure-tone audiogram (Figure 3–1). This is a graphic representation of hearing, which is plotted as thresholds (i.e., lowest intensity level at which a stimulus is audible) in decibels (dB hearing level; dB HL) as a function of frequency (Hz). The frequencies typically evaluated include the octave frequencies from 250 through 8000 Hz. The reason for this is that most of the sounds critical for the understanding of speech fall within this particular frequency range. In some cases, however, additional frequencies may be tested. Such cases would include the assessment of patients at risk for noise-induced hearing losses, where the interoctave frequencies of 3000 and 6000 Hz also are assessed, and the testing of patients who are being monitored for potential ototoxic effects of medications, where ultra-audiometric frequencies (i.e., frequencies above 8000 Hz) are tested.

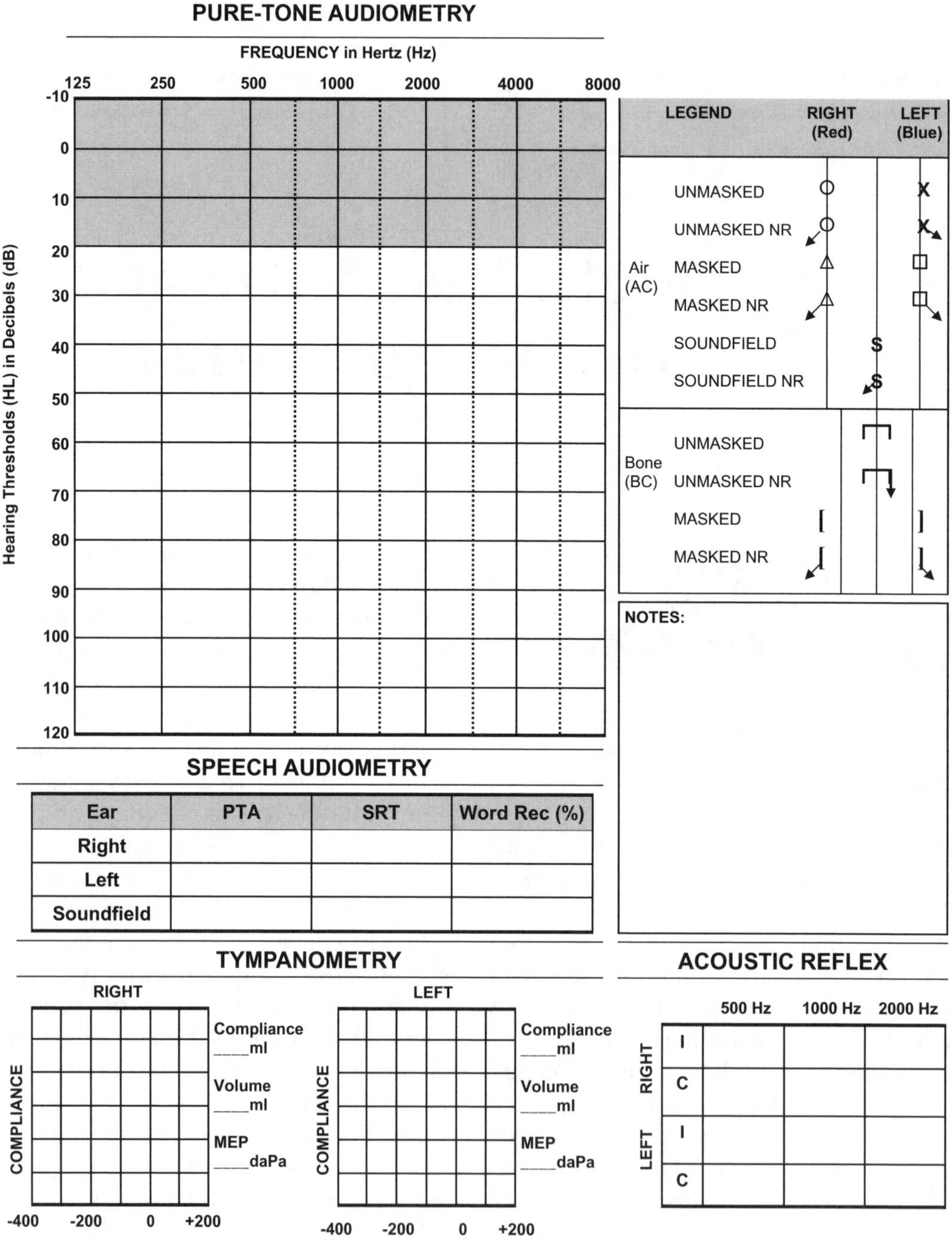

PURE-TONE AUDIOMETRY

FREQUENCY in Hertz (Hz)

Hearing Thresholds (HL) in Decibels (dB)

LEGEND		RIGHT (Red)	LEFT (Blue)
	UNMASKED	O	X
	UNMASKED NR	O	X
Air (AC)	MASKED	△	□
	MASKED NR	△	□
	SOUNDFIELD	S	
	SOUNDFIELD NR	S	
	UNMASKED		⌐
Bone (BC)	UNMASKED NR		⌐
	MASKED	[	]
	MASKED NR	[	]

NOTES:

SPEECH AUDIOMETRY

Ear	PTA	SRT	Word Rec (%)
Right			
Left			
Soundfield			

TYMPANOMETRY

RIGHT

COMPLIANCE

Compliance ____ml

Volume ____ml

MEP ____daPa

-400　-200　0　+200

LEFT

COMPLIANCE

Compliance ____ml

Volume ____ml

MEP ____daPa

-400　-200　0　+200

ACOUSTIC REFLEX

		500 Hz	1000 Hz	2000 Hz
RIGHT	I			
	C			
LEFT	I			
	C			

Figure 3–1. An example of the audiogram used for the case studies presented in this book.

Several different classification systems have been recommended for quantifying the degree of hearing loss, but perhaps the most widely used one is the Jerger classification system introduced in 1980 (see Jerger & Jerger, 1980) (Figure 3–2). In addition to quantifying the degree or severity of hearing loss, the audiologist will determine the type of hearing loss. It is generally accepted that there are three types of hearing loss: (1) conductive hearing loss, (2) sensorineural hearing loss, and (3) mixed hearing loss. Conductive hearing losses are hearing losses that occur because of a loss of sound conduction from the outer ear to the cochlea, whereas hearing losses that are sensorineural in nature are the result of cochlear or retrocochlear involvement. Mixed hear-

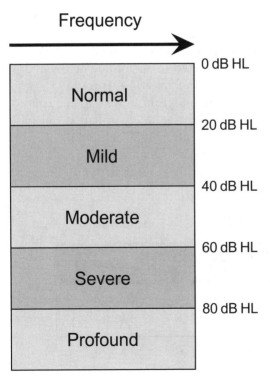

Figure 3–2. *Jerger's classification system used for defining degree of hearing loss.*

ing losses are exactly what the name would suggest, a combination of a conductive and sensorineural hearing loss.

The audiologist's role is to accurately measure a patient's behavioral hearing sensitivity, and in doing so, to determine if a hearing loss is present. If a hearing loss is present, the audiologist must ultimately determine the type, degree, and configuration of the hearing loss in order to implement appropriate referrals and rehabilitation. However, one must keep in mind that the pure-tone audiogram is only one method for the evaluation of hearing. Although the pure-tone audiogram is the cornerstone of audiologic assessment, its greatest limitation is that it provides limited information with respect to the processing and subsequent comprehension of auditory information (i.e., it is simply an auditory detection measure).

Speech audiometry is another critical component of traditional audiologic assessment. It provides additional information with respect to the functional performance of the auditory system. Typically, two speech measures are made during this assessment: (1) speech recognition threshold (SRT) or speech awareness (SAT) threshold, and (2) word recognition performance at suprathreshold levels. The SRT is determined by presenting a closed set of two-syllable words and determining one's threshold for speech. In this test procedure, the patient either repeats the stimuli presented or points to pictorial representations of the presented stimuli. For children and other difficult-to-test populations who are not able to complete the SRT test procedure, SATs are often employed. In this measure, the individual being tested does not have to recognize the stimulus being presented, but rather only has to detect that a signal is being presented (in this case the signal is a speech signal as opposed to a pure-tone signal). The SRT should be in good agreement ($\pm$7 dB) with the pure-tone average (i.e., either the average threshold intensity at 500, 1000, and 2000 Hz for patients with relatively flat hearing losses, or the better two frequency average for patients who have steeply sloping hearing losses). However, if an SAT measure is derived rather than an SRT, the SAT often is obtained at a lower intensity level than the SRT would be for reasons explained above. As a result, there is likely to be a greater difference between the SAT and the pure-tone average when this speech threshold measure is derived. Word recognition testing compliments SRT testing by evaluating the percentage of words that patients are able to identify correctly at suprathreshold levels. This provides information about the patient's speech recognition abilities, and helps significantly in determining the best rehabilitative approaches to patient care.

Tympanometry and Acoustic Reflexes

Immittance audiometry is an important tool in diagnostic audiology and otology. It provides information that can aid in the detection of a variety of outer and middle ear auditory disorders as well as in the documentation of normal/abnormal cochlear and lower brainstem function. For the purposes of this book, we briefly orient the reader to two primary measures of immittance audiometry: tympanometry and acoustic reflex thresholds.

Tympanometry allows clinicians to measure the amount of compliance of the middle ear system. Maximum compliance is achieved when the air pressure in the external ear is equal to the air pressure within the middle ear system. This measurement is accomplished by sealing the ear canal and varying the air pressure in the ear canal to measure the movement of the tympanic membrane. The results are displayed as a tracing called a tympanogram that plots compliance as a function of middle ear pressure. In addition, information about the peak pressure, maximum compliance, and equivalent ear canal volume (referred to as volume below and in subsequent chapters) are provided. A normal tympanogram will yield the following: peak pressure, compliance, and volume measurements (Table 3–1).

There have been several classification systems with respect to tympanometry,

Table 3–1. Normative Values for Tympanometry as a Function of Age

	Pressure (daPa)	Volume* (cc/ml)	Compliance (cc/ml)
Adults	−150 to +50	0.9 to 2.0	0.3 to 1.7
Children	−150 to +50	0.3 to 0.9	0.25 to 1.05

Note. An equivalent ear canal volume measurement of >2.0 cc/ml with a Type B tracing suggests a perforated TM or patent PE tube.

*Equivalent ear canal volume.

Sources: Based in part on normative data provided by Margolis & Hunter, 2000; see also ASHA, 1997.

but perhaps the most widely used is the Jerger classification system (Jerger, 1970) in which a number of tympanograms have been categorized based on their specific shapes and characteristics (Figure 3–3). Using this classical description scheme, clinicians have adopted the following universal tympanogram descriptors:

Type A: Type A curves demonstrate normal pressure, volume, and compliance values.

Type A_s: The "s" in A_s stands for "shallow." These tracings typically demonstrate a normal middle ear pressure measurement and a compliance peak that is significantly reduced, but there continues to be some mobility or compliance in the system.

Type A_d: The "d" in A_d stands for "discontinuous" or "deep" and represents the exact opposite of the A_s tracing. The A_d tracing typically demonstrates normal pressure; however, there is a very high compliance peak. This is typically associated with too much flaccidity of the tympanic membrane and can be secondary to ossicular disarticulation.

Type B: Type B tympanograms can occur under several conditions. The curves are sometimes referred to as "flat" because there is no observable compliance peak due to a lack of compliance in the system. An important measure to evaluate in these cases is the volume.

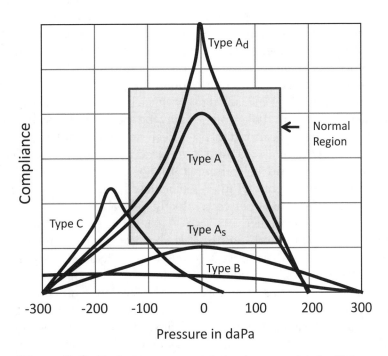

Figure 3–3. Typical tympanometric tracings associated with normal and abnormal middle ear function.

If the tracing reflects a normal volume, there likely is effusion in the middle ear causing the lack of mobility. However, if there is an abnormally small volume present, it may be that the probe tip has been occluded or blocked by cerumen, debris, or the ear canal wall. A tracing that reflects a large volume typically suggests a patent pressure equalization (PE) tube or a perforation of the tympanic membrane.

Type C: Type C tympanograms suggest some degree of Eustachian tube dysfunction. The tracing will demonstrate normal volume and compliance, but excessive negative pressure will be present.

In addition to peak pressure, compliance, and volume measurements, many clinicians also assess the tympanogram width or gradient as this can be another indicator of middle ear pathology. The tympanometric width is derived by measuring the tympanometric width (in daPa units) at a point that is half the peak admittance on the positive side of the tympanogram. Normative values for children range between 80 to 159 daPa (Margolis, Hunter, & Giebink, 1994) and for adults between 51 to 114 daPa (Margolis & Heller, 1987). Abnormally large tympanometric widths are indicative of middle ear dysfunction and can be observed in such middle ear conditions as otitis media; however, abnormally narrow tympanometric widths have not been confirmed to be a reliable indicator of middle ear dysfunction (see Margolis & Hunter, 2000, for discussion). Other methods have been introduced for measuring the tympanometric gradient that express the gradient as a ratio measure (see Nozza, 2003); however, the tympanometric width measurement described above is more often employed as it is the tympanogram measure provided on many commercial immittance audiometers.

Acoustic reflex testing is a direct measure of the acoustic stapedial reflex. It is defined as the lowest intensity level at which a reflex can be measured. Because the stapedial muscle contracts in response to loud sounds, a direct measure of the integrity of the stapedial reflex can be accomplished through this technique. Because there are both ipsilateral and contralateral inputs within the brainstem, the stapedial reflex can be recorded with either ipsilateral or contralateral stimulation. Depending on the pattern of responses observed, varying inferences regarding the site of lesion can be made. In most normal hearing individuals, this reflex can be observed around 70 to 90 dB HL. Reflexes are elevated or absent when insufficient intensity is delivered to the cochlea secondary to compromise of the outer and/or middle ears. In individuals with cochlear hearing losses, the reflexes may be present at normal or elevated threshold levels, but they typically are reduced in terms of their sensation levels (SL). For patients with profound sensory (cochlear hearing losses), the reflexes are likely to be absent.

Elevated or absent acoustic reflexes can be indicative of retrocochlear involvement (see Wilson & Margolis, 1999). The auditory nerve, the low pons, and the facial nerve must all be intact to provide a normal acoustic reflex. In the ipsilateral reflex, the neural response to the stimulus courses from the auditory nerve to the superior olivary complex and then to the facial nerve nuclei and back down the facial nerve to the stapedius muscle ipsilaterally. A lesion anywhere along this route can affect the ipsilateral reflex. The contralateral reflex pathway is similar to the ipsilateral, but its course crosses midline in the low pons connecting to the contralateral facial nerve nuclei and then the contralateral stapedius muscle. Therefore, the contralateral reflex can be affected by midline and contralateral brainstem lesions and dysfunction of the contralateral facial nerve (see Chapter 2: Structure and Function of the Auditory and Vestibular Systems).

Measurement of acoustic reflex decay can also be utilized clinically. This requires a presentation of 500- or 1000-Hz stimulus at 10 dB SL re: the pure-tone threshold over a 10 second time period. If the amplitude of the response decreases more than half of maximum over the 10-second time period, it may indicate retrocochlear involvement (Wilson & Margolis, 1999).

Auditory Processing Tests

Central auditory processing evaluations seek to determine how efficiently and effectively patients are able to process complex auditory stimuli. The pure-tone audiogram is extremely limiting in that it only provides information about hearing sensitivity. However, many patients with significant lesions of the central auditory nervous system (CANS) demonstrate normal hearing sensitivity, but are significantly impaired in the "processing" of auditory information. So the pure-tone audiogram usually is not helpful in documenting the auditory deficits experienced by these patients and additional behavioral and/or electrophysiologic testing will be needed to identify the patient's auditory processing disorder. The tests described below can be administered to patients who report concerns regarding hearing (particularly in background noise) yet demonstrate normal peripheral hearing sensitivity in an effort to determine if the presence of a central auditory processing deficit is the basis for the patient's auditory symptoms (Musiek & Chermak, 2007).

The assessment of central auditory processing generally takes on two forms: (1) behavioral assessment (Figure 3–4), and (2) electrophysiologic assessment. The behavioral assessment seeks to provide information regarding a patient's functional performance, whereas the electrophysiologic assessment provides information regarding the neural integrity of the CANS (see section below).

It is recommended that the evaluation of a patient's central auditory processing disorder (CAPD) include tests of temporal processing, dichotic listening, monaural low-redundancy speech perception, auditory discrimination tasks, and binaural interaction tests (American Academy of Audiology [AAA], 2010). Table 3–2 provides a listing of some of the clinically available tests within these areas of auditory processing.

Tests of temporal processing evaluate the ability of the auditory system to process small and rapid changes of sound over time (see Lister, Roberts, & Lister, 2011; Musiek et al., 2005). Although there are four subtypes of temporal processing (resolution, sequencing, integration, and masking), only the first two mentioned areas commonly are used in the assessment of patients being evaluated for central auditory processing deficits due to lack of available clinical measures for the latter two areas. Pattern perception tests (frequency and duration) assess among other things temporal sequencing ability.

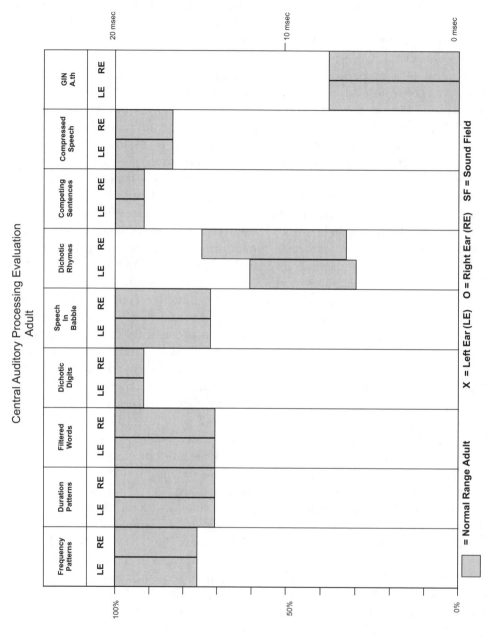

Figure 3–4. Summary form used to record behavioral central auditory processing test results. Note that this particular form reflects adult normative values.

Table 3–2. Some Clinically Available Tests of Central Auditory Function Categorized According to the Auditory Process Assessed

	Test Name	*Reference*
Temporal Processing	Gaps-In-Noise (Temporal Resolution)	Musiek et al., 2005 Shinn, Musiek & Chermak, 2009 Lister, Roberts, & Lister, 2011
	Random Gap Detection (Temporal Resolution/ Fusion)	Keith, 2000
	Frequency Pattern Test	Musiek & Pinheiro, 1987
	Duration Pattern Test (Temporal Sequencing)	Musiek, Baran, & Pinhiero, 1990
Dichotic Listening	Dichotic Digits	Musiek, 1983 Musiek, Gollegly, Kibbe, & Verkest-Lenz, 1991
	Staggered Spondaic Words	Katz, 1962
	Dichotic Sentences	Fifer, Jerger, Berlin, Toby, & Campbell, 1983
Monaural Low-Redundancy Speech Perception	Time Compressed Speech	Wilson, Preece, Salamon, Sperry, & Bornstein, 1994
	Filtered Words	Willeford, 1977
Binaural Function (interaction)	Masking Level Difference (MLD)	Lynn et al., 1981
	Listening in Spatialized Noise (LISN-S)	Cameron & Dillon, 2007 Cameron et al., 2009

The Gaps-in-Noise (GIN) and Random Gap Detection tests are clinical measures of temporal resolution. These tests have been found to be sensitive to cortical lesions (Musiek et al., 2005; Musiek & Pinheiro, 1987).

The dichotic listening tests evaluate the binaural integration and separation abilities of the CANS and are sensitive to cortical lesions, and to a lesser extent brainstem involvement (Baran & Musiek, 1999; Musiek & Pinheiro, 1985). Dichotic tasks are most useful in cases of deficient interhemispheric transfer where marked left ear deficits are the hallmark.

The monaural low-redundancy tests are among the least sensitive of the central measures, but they provide an ecological validity, which is beneficial to the test battery (Baran & Musiek, 1999). These tests are designed to degrade the auditory signal by filtering (filtered speech), increasing the rate (compressed speech), or placing the signal in competition (speech-in-noise or speech-in-speech).

Perhaps the most widely recognized binaural function test is the masking level difference (MLD) test. This measure, although not a direct assessment, provides insight into localization and lateralization abilities by creating a "release from masking" by changing the phase relationships at the two ears. This procedure has been shown to be highly sensitive to brainstem involvement (Lynn, Gilroy, Taylor, & Leiser, 1981). MLDs work best for low-frequency stimuli, such as 500-Hz tones and spondee word stimuli.

Electroacoustic and Electrophysiologic Assessment

Electroacoustic and electrophysiologic procedures are procedures that evaluate the acoustical and electrical cellular responses of the auditory system. Electroacoustic and electrophysiologic evaluations of hearing have a long-standing history. The use of electrophysiologic measures can be traced back to the early 1930s with routine clinical use beginning in the early 1980s (see Hall, 2007). Otoacoustic emissions (OAEs) relatively speaking are a more recent discovery. They were initially described by David Kemp in the 1970s (Kemp, 1978), but did not become clinically integrated until the mid to late 1990s. Traditionally, when one thinks of how hearing is assessed, it is through our oldest measure of hearing, behavioral pure-tone audiometry. However, electroacoustic and electrophysiologic assessments play a critical role with respect to differential diagnosis specifically in regard to the subspecialty of neuroaudiology. Both electroacoustic as well as electrophysiologic auditory assessments, like pure-tone testing, can provide measurements of hearing sensitivity. However, these assessment tools provide a means for the objective measurement of auditory function with respect to both sensitivity and integrity from the level of the cochlea through the auditory cortex (see Hall, 2007; Musiek & Lee, 1999; Robinette & Glattke, 2002, for detailed reviews).

Electroacoustic Measures

Electroacoustic evaluation as it relates to OAEs has significantly changed the face of diagnostic audiology. Otoacoustic emissions provide clinicians with objective information specifically regarding the integrity of the outer hair cells of the cochlea. They are unique in their ability to provide information regarding the active biological process at this level of the auditory system, which is not readily available by any other means of assessment. This active process is a result of an "echo" caused by stimulation of the hair cells. That is to say, the recorded response is shaped by, and similar to, the eliciting acoustic signal. In order for this process to occur and emissions to be present, the outer and middle ear systems must be functioning normally for the stimulating signal to travel through to the cochlea and the emission to travel back through the middle ear to be recorded by a probe microphone placed in the ear canal.

In general, OAEs are categorized as either spontaneous or evoked. For the purposes of this book, we focus on the evoked otoacoustic emissions, which include both distortion product otoacoustic emissions (DPOAEs) and transient evoked otoacoustic emissions (TEOAEs) as they are the most widely utilized in clinical assessment. Both DPOAEs and TEOAEs are elicited by placing a probe in the ear of the patient. The probe tip is placed securely within the external auditory meatus and the stimulus is delivered either as a pair of tones (DPOAEs) or as a click stimulus (TEOAEs).

Distortion product otoacoustic emissions are elicited by a nonlinear process within the cochlea. This process occurs when two tones that are close in frequency, are presented to the cochlea. The mechanics of the inner ear create a distortion of the signals. In a healthy ear with normal hearing or near-normal hearing sensitivity, a response is measured. The tones used to elicit this distortion are labeled as f_1 and f_2. The most robust response (the distortion product) for a particular frequency is observed by applying the formula, $2f_1-f_2$. Interpretation of DPOAEs is performed by measuring the level of the response (the emission) in reference to the noise floor or as an absolute scale (level of the DPOAE). The noise floor is the measurable noise recorded in the ear canal. The response is recorded as a function of amplitude above the noise floor for the particular frequency(s) of interest. If a response that meets clinical criterion for level above the noise floor is present, then the response is considered to be present (Figure 3–5).

Transient otoacoustic emissions are another means by which cochlear function can be measured. TEOAEs are elicited through the use of a transient signal such as a click stimulus. The emission onset occurs approximately 4 msec following stimulation. The TEOAE is a broad-spectrum response; however, it does provide frequency information as the response follows the tonotopic arrangement of the basilar membrane. Similar to DPOAEs, the TEOAE is determined to be present or

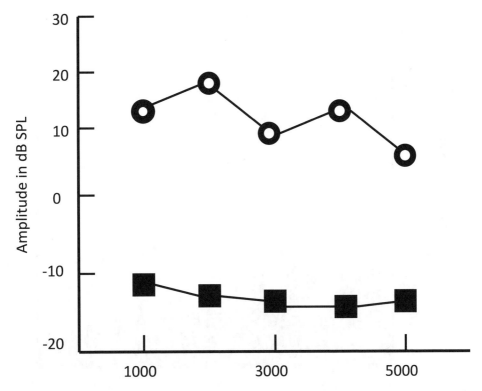

Figure 3–5. *An example of a normal DPOAE response (○ = dB SPL values for the right ear, filled boxes = noise floor in dB SPL).*

absent based on the relationship between the response and the noise floor. If the response is repeatable and exceeds the noise floor, then it is considered to be present. Like DPOAEs, TEOAEs are indicative of cochlear outer hair cell function. Figure 3–6 demonstrates an example of a present TEOAE response.

Although not a direct measure of hearing sensitivity, OAEs provide general information regarding outer hair cell function within the cochlea. There are many applications for OAEs. These include, but are not limited to, infant screening, pediatric assessment, ototoxicity monitoring, general monitoring, and differential diagnosis of cochlear versus retrocochlear involvement. Patients who present with normal hearing sensitivity

typically will demonstrate normal OAEs. The general clinical observation with respect to OAE interpretation is that in individuals with present OAEs, hearing is likely to be better than 30 dB HL (specifically for TEOAEs). However, those with absent OAEs will likely demonstrate hearing thresholds greater than 30 dB HL. It should be noted that, if there is involvement or pathology of the outer or middle ear systems, often no valid interpretation can be made regarding cochlear integrity as the absence or low amplitude of the response can be due to the presence of the outer or middle ear pathology rather than cochlear involvement.

Otoacoustic emissions are invaluable with respect to their role in the differential diagnosis of cochlear versus retrocochlear

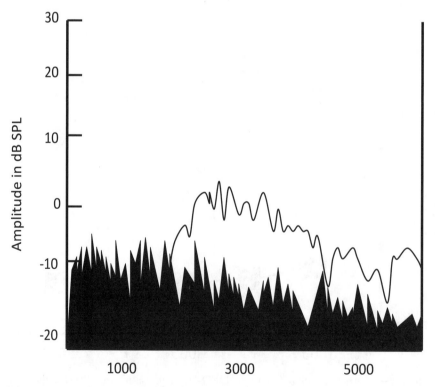

Figure 3–6. An example of a normal TEOAE response (white area is the TEOAE response, black area is the noise floor).

involvement. Individuals who have either eighth nerve or central auditory involvement, in the absence of comorbid cochlear conditions, will present with normal OAEs, but will likely demonstrate abnormalities on pure-tone audiometry and ABR testing in cases with eighth nerve involvement and on behavioral and electrophysiologic measures in patients with CANS compromise (see Robinette & Glattke, 2002).

Given the fact that the degree of hearing sensitivity cannot be directly determined, otoacoustic emissions are certainly limited in their diagnostic utility. That is to say, in individuals who present with absent OAEs, all that can be concluded is that they have at least a mild to moderate degree of hearing loss. Therefore, OAEs are a useful screening measure, but lack strength with respect to threshold determination. This is why objective measures of hearing through electrophysiologic assessment can and should be a critical component of a diagnostic battery for many patients.

Electrophysiologic Measures

Electrophysiologic assessment of the auditory system can be used for both the neurodiagnostic evaluation of the integrity of the auditory system as well as the evaluation of hearing sensitivity. This type of assessment measures neurobioelectrical activity arising from within the auditory nerve and the CANS. It has a long-standing history in clinical audiology spanning more than three decades and it continues to be an integral component of today's diagnostic evaluation.

Electrophysiology (also referred to as evoked potentials [EPs]), like pure-tone audiometry, can be used to assess hearing sensitivity. However, these procedures also provide a mechanism for the objective measurement of neural integrity within the auditory system. Therefore, evoked potentials can be useful tools in the differential diagnosis of a variety of auditory disorders as they allow for measurement of not only the auditory nerve, but the entire CANS through the level of the cortex (if a combination of EPs are used). The following discussion will provide an overview of the early, middle, and late evoked potentials that are used in audiologic assessment.

Electrocochleography (ECochG) was the first of the auditory evoked potentials to be discovered in the 1930s (Hall, 2007). Today, it has relatively widespread clinic use with respect to the neuroaudiological evaluation of Ménière's disease, as well as intraoperative monitoring. This potential is typically obtained by placing one of three types of electrodes (canal, tympanic membrane, or transtympanic) into the external auditory meati of both the involved and uninvolved ears with a disk electrode placed at Fpz (ground). Using an alternating click stimulus both a summating potential (SP, a direct current receptor potential reflecting cochlear electrical activity in response to acoustic stimulation) and an action potential (AP, a postsynaptic potential generated by the auditory nerve) are extracted (Figure 3–7). The ratio between these two potentials is calculated in order to determine if abnormalities are present. Abnormal results will vary depending upon the type of electrode utilized. Transtympanic electrodes yield less variance with a SP/AP ratio of greater than 30% falling outside the norm, whereas ear canal electrodes require a SP/AP ratio of 50% or greater to be considered abnormal by many investigators (see Ferraro, 2000, and Hall, 2007, for reviews). This test has proven to be useful in the diagnosis of Ménière's disease as patients with this disease typically present with abnormally large SP/AP ratios (Ferraro, 2000).

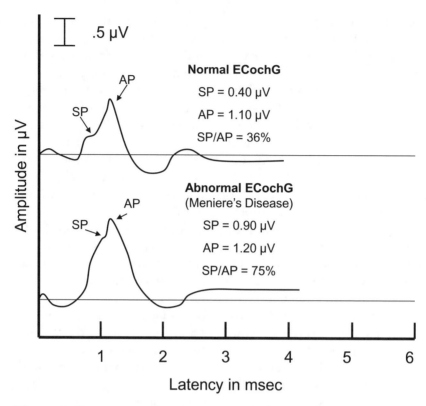

Figure 3–7. *A schematic representation of a normal* (upper tracing) *and abnormal* (lower tracing) *ECochG response.*

The auditory brainstem response (ABR) is an early auditory evoked response that is generated by neurobiological activity within the auditory nerve and the central auditory pathways (see Hall, 2007). The ABR (also referred to as the brainstem auditory evoked potential [BAER]) provides information regarding the integrity of the auditory system through the level of the brainstem (including the auditory nerve). The response usually occurs within the first 10 msec after stimulus presentation. For neurodiagnostic purposes, it is typically obtained using a 100 μsec click stimulus fed through insert earphones that is generally presented at 80 or 90 dB nHL (Figure 3–8); however, this intensity level may need to be increased depending on variables such as waveform morphology and/or degree of hearing sensitivity. Repetition rates vary depending on clinician preference; however, they generally range from 15 to 30 clicks per second with filter settings of 150 to 3000 Hz (or 30 to 3000 Hz for young children and newborns). For the ABR, neurobiological activity is recorded from a noninverting electrode that is typically attached at either the high forehead (F_z) or the vertex (C_z) while the inverting electrodes are either placed on the earlobes or mastoids (A_1 and A_2). The patient is normally grounded with an electrode at the mid-forehead or the contralateral ear. In order to obtain adequate recordings, it is critical that excellent contact with the

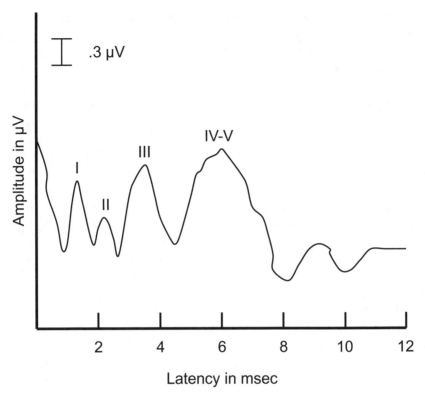

Figure 3–8. *An example of a normal auditory brainstem response.*

scalp be obtained, which is achieved by having low electrode impedances. It is recommended that individual electrode impedances fall below 5 kΩ and that the impedance be balanced to within 2 kΩ across the electrode array. For the purposes of determining threshold sensitivity, the same recording parameters as mentioned above may be used. When hearing sensitivity is being assessed, it is recommended that threshold measures be determined by decreasing the intensity level of the stimulus in 10 dB steps until the threshold is established. The threshold in ABR testing is defined as the lowest intensity level at which an identifiable and repeatable waveform (i.e., wave V) is observed.

There are several indices, which are used to evaluate the integrity of the audi-tory system, specifically with respect to suspicion of retrocochlear involvement (Musiek, Shinn, & Jirsa, 2007). Five primary peaks are typically analyzed with respect to the ABR. These includes waves I through V; however, primary emphasis is placed on analysis of waves I, III, and V. Presence of these waveforms is first established and then absolute, interwave, and interaural latencies are measured. These ABR measures include analysis of the absolute latencies of waves I, III, and V, interwave latency comparisons for I–III, III–V, and I–V, and an interaural comparison of the absolute latency difference of wave V (ILD). It is also recommended that a comparison between the behavioral threshold for the ABR stimulus and the EP threshold for the same stimulus be completed. If any of following common indices used in a neurodiagnostic evaluation fall outside the normal range, then retrocochlear involvement would be suspected: (1) absence of a full or any part of a response, (2) poor waveform replication, (3) increased absolute or interwave latencies, (4) an abnormal ILD, (5) an abnormal increase in latency with increase in stimulation rate (although not highly diagnostic), (6) a significant difference between the behavioral and electrophysiologic threshold, and (7) an abnormal wave I–V amplitude ratio (Musiek et al., 2007). These measures should be interpreted with the audiogram so that when necessary, hearing loss can be taken into account. Although it is recommended that each individual clinician obtain their own normative data, the following table (Table 3–3) provides the normative data used by the authors in their practices (Musiek, 1991; Musiek, Baran, & Pinheiro, 1994).

Although magnetic resonance imaging (MRI) with contrast has certainly become the gold standard for detection of retrocochlear lesions such as acoustic neu-romas, ABR as a screening tool demonstrates excellent sensitivity and specificity. Most authors report that for medium and large acoustic neuromas, sensitivity is on the order of more than 90%; however, the sensitivity decreases (50–80%) for small lesions when traditional ABR indices are used (Schmidt, Sataloff, Newman, Spiegel, & Myers, 2001; Zappia, O'Connor, Wiet, & Dinces, 1997). Recently, however, it has been demonstrated that the use of a novel index of comparing behavioral versus electrophysiologic thresholds yields almost 100% sensitivity for detecting small acoustic neuromas (Bush, Jones, & Shinn, 2008). This is a promising development in the identification of small acoustic tumors; however, additional confirmation of the efficacy of this procedure is needed.

Given some of the negative variables associated with MRI (cost, patient comfort, etc.), it can be argued that the ABR is an appropriate and viable alternative to imaging as a screening procedure for retrocochlear involvement. In addition, some could possibly argue that there are overreferrals for MRIs, especially given

Table 3–3. Cutoff Criteria for Abnormal ABR Measures for Adult Patients

Index	*Abnormal Cutoff Criterion**
Absolute Wave V Latency	>6.1 msec with less than 40 dB HL hearing loss
I–III Interwave Comparison	>2.3 msec
III–V Interwave Comparison	>2.4 msec
I–V Interwave Comparison	>4.4 msec
Interaural Wave V Latency Difference	>0.3 msec with symmetrical hearing loss
Wave V–I Amplitude Ratio	<0.75
Wave V High Rep Rate	shift of >0.1 msec in the latency of wave V for every 10 click rate increase +0.2 msec
Behavioral vs. EP Threshold	>30 dB nHL difference

*Utilizing an 80 dB nHL rarefaction click at a low repetition rate.

the low confirmation rate. Therefore, the application of the less costly ABR test may help reduce the number of overreferrals. Moreover, ABR provides a functional (physiological) measure that is not provided by MRI.

The middle latency response (MLR) was first reported in the 1950s, but it has gained more attention in recent years (see Musiek & Lee, 1999). This potential can be used for the measurement of both central involvement as well as hearing sensitivity. The MLR is advantageous in that it provides information regarding the integrity of the CANS through the level of the primary auditory cortex. Similar to the ABR, a click stimulus or tone pip is used to evoke the MLR; however, there are some differences in recording parameters. The MLR is typically reserved for those individuals with normal periph-

eral hearing sensitivity who present with deficits that suggest involvement of the CANS beyond the generator sites for the ABR. It is recommended that a click stimulus be presented at a level of 70 dB nHL at a rate of approximately 10 clicks/second. The MLR also is obtained with slightly different filter settings (i.e., 20 or 30 to 1500 Hz). For the purposes of neurodiagnostic information, it is highly recommended that noninverting electrodes be placed at C_3, C_z, and C_4 in order to obtain information regarding the laterality of the response.

The authors' recommended procedures for waveform analysis with respect to the MLR includes evaluation of the Na and Pa waveforms (Figure 3–9). The Na waveform is the first major negative peak following wave V of the ABR, which is then followed by the first major positive

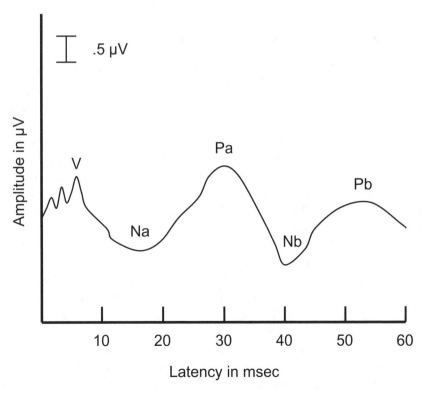

Figure 3–9. An example of a normal middle latency response.

peak labeled Pa. These waveforms typically occur in the first 70 msec following stimulation. In the opinion of the authors, the following criteria should be used for evaluating the MLR response: (1) the absence or presence of the response, (2) the absence or presence of an electrode effect, and (3) the absence or presence of an ear effect. An electrode effect is observed when there is a significant amplitude difference among the responses measured at the C_3 and C_4 electrodes sites for the Na-Pa complex. The ear effect is documented when there is significant difference in amplitude between the left and right ears at a particular electrode site for the Na-Pa complex. According to Musiek and colleagues (1999), amplitude differences in excess of 20 to 50% (depending on the criteria employed by the clinician), can be considered as abnormal for either ear or electrode effects. The 50% difference is the criterion adopted by the authors of this book for documenting abnormal results; however, further research is needed to corroborate this data. Of the two indices, it has been the authors' clinical experience that the electrode effect is the more sensitive of the two measures. Note that the above indices relate primarily to amplitude abnormalities of the response. This is different than the analysis of the ABR where one relies heavily on the latency measures for determination of abnormality. With respect to the MLR, abnormal amplitudes are the strongest indicator of pathology. However, latency may be used as an indicator of possible CANS involvement if the latency of the Pa peak exceeds 32 msec at any electrode site for a stimulus presented at 70 dB nHL to individuals with normal hearing sensitivity. Again, individuals using this procedure are encouraged to use their own norms as latency and amplitude measures can vary across averagers.

The late auditory evoked response potentials (LAER) like the MLR provide information regarding the neural integrity of the primary auditory cortex, as well as secondary association areas (see Hall, 2007; Musiek & Lee, 1999). The same electrode montage that is employed with the MLR is recommended for the LAERs; however, differences in recording parameters should be employed. The repetition rate of the LAER is reduced to around 1 click per second in order to maximize responses from the auditory cortical centers. Filters are also reduced significantly down to approximately 1 to 30 Hz for clinical cases. As this response occurs much later, a larger time window (>500 msec) is required to capture the response in its entirety. Unlike the previously mentioned potentials, the stimulus paradigm recommended for obtaining this response is different in that an oddball paradigm is employed (wherein two different frequencies are presented). In the classic oddball paradigm, a stimulus designated as the frequent tone is presented 80% of the time and a rare tone occurs 20% of the time. The patient is asked to keep track of the target (rare) stimuli. In some instances, the examiner may wish to record the late potentials without the P300. In this case, the use of the oddball paradigm just described is not necessary as the earlier potentials do not require that the patient attend to and recognize a difference between the stimuli being presented. So these potentials can be elicited with a single stimulus.

The primary waveforms examined for the late potentials are the N1, P2, and P3 (also referred to as the P300) waveforms with these waveforms occurring at latencies of approximately 100, 200, and 300 msec, respectively (Figure 3–10). The analysis of these waveforms is based on the latency of the response. However,

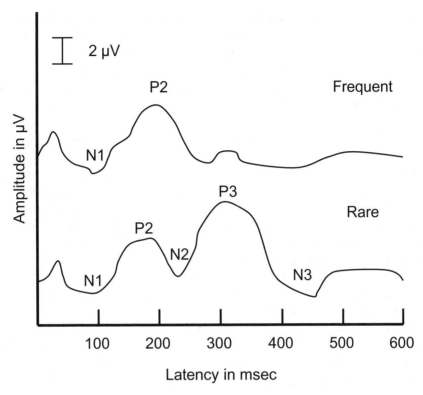

Figure 3–10. *An example of a normal late auditory evoked response, including the P3 (P300).*

amplitude measures can be applied when there is an obvious difference in amplitudes across the electrodes. Those applying the late potentials clinically need to establish their own norms. The following provides some general guidelines for interpretation of LAER measures. The most sensitive index for the LAER in the opinion of the present authors is an amplitude difference of 50% for the N1–P2 complex between electrodes, similar to what was discussed for the MLR. Additional indices related to latency and amplitude measurements are as follows: (1) the presence or absence of a response, (2) the absolute latencies of the various responses mentioned above, and (3) the amplitude measures for the N2–P3 and P3–N3 in addition to the N1–P2 response. Abnormality can be based on the following criteria: (1) absent waveforms, (2) nonreplicable waveforms, (3) N1 latency greater than 120 msec, (4) P2 latency greater than 228 msec, and (5) P3/P300 latency greater than 350 msec for young adults with good hearing sensitivity (Musiek et al., 1994; Musiek & Lee, 1999; Picton, 2011). Given the demyelination that occurs in the CANS after the fourth decade of life, it is recommended that approximately 10 msec be added to the P3 latency for each additional decade of life after the fourth decade (see Picton, 2011, for review). Again, these criteria are intended as only a general guide. More research is needed to corroborate these findings.

Electrophysiologic tests of cochlear and retrocochlear involvement provide clinicians with both powerful and useful diagnostic measures. The good sensitivity and specificity of these tests certainly supports their clinical use. Table 3–4 provides information regarding the sensitivity and specificity data used by the authors with respect to the use of auditory EPs for patients with confirmed lesions of the CANS (see Hall, 2007; Musiek, 1991; Musiek, Charette, Kelly, Lee, & Musiek, 1999; Musiek & Lee, 1999).

The MLR and LAERs are highly underutilized in the opinion of the authors. Although historically used primarily in the research arena, we believe that these procedures have an important and critical role in diagnostic audiology, as well as in the (re)habilitation of individuals diagnosed with neuroaudiologic disorders. The clinician, however, needs to have in depth knowledge and experience to apply these procedures accurately. If the reader desires a more thorough review of auditory evoked potentials, they are referred to Hall (2007), Musiek and Lee (1999), and Picton (2011).

Vestibular Assessment

Although the focus of this book is on auditory disorders, it is relevant to discuss tests of vestibular function and their role in diagnostic audiology. Given the

relationship between auditory and vestibular structure and function, there are many disorders which affect both systems. Often, those individuals with auditory disorders have comorbid vestibular involvement making it necessary for the audiologist to have knowledge of such assessment tools. The following section provides an overview of common vestibular assessment tools used clinically (for a more detailed review of vestibular assessment the reader is encouraged to refer to Jacobson & Shepard, 2008).

By far the most widely utilized measures of vestibular function are electronystagmography (ENG) and videonystagmography (VNG). The primary difference between these is the use of electrode (ENG) versus video (VNG) recordings. These measures assess the integrity of the vestibular system by evaluating both voluntary and involuntary eye movements. Evaluation of eye movements provides insight into the function or dysfunction of the vestibular system. This is because the ENG and VNG procedures are a direct measure of the vestibulo-ocular reflex and can provide information regarding differential diagnosis for four variables or domains: (1) normal versus abnormal vestibular function, (2) peripheral versus central system involvement, (3) right-

Table 3–4. Sensitivity and Specificity Data Associated with Auditory Evoked Potentials Based on the Authors' Literature Review of Reports of Lesions of the CANS

Test	Sensitivity	Specificity
ABR	High 80s–Low 90s	92%
MLR	50–73%	85%
N1–P2	70%	75%
P300	80%	68%

sided versus left-sided involvement, and (4) compensated versus uncompensated function. Within the ENG and VNG procedures, there are three primary subtests, which include oculomotor, positional, and caloric tests.

Oculomotor tests include a subgroup of tracking tests that assess saccadic, smooth pursuit, and optokinetic tracking (see Leigh & Zee, 2006). This subgroup of tests provides information regarding the contributions of the cerebellum and offers the most insight into possible central involvement. However, the examiner should use caution when administering these tests because age, fatigue, and a variety of medications can affect their results. The first of these eye movements,

which is routinely measured, are the saccades. Saccadic eye movements involve examining the velocity, accuracy, and latency with which the eyes can lock onto a target (Figure 3–11). The smooth pursuit response, unlike the saccades, is not a reflexive response, but rather a measure of the ability of the eyes to maintain gaze while tracking a response. This response, as seen in Figure 3–12, is obtained by having the patient fixate and track a target, which moves smoothly between the left and right visual fields resulting in a sinusoidal tracing. The smooth pursuit response is evaluated based on velocity, symmetry, and phase. Both slow and fast rates of stimulation are typically employed. The final oculomotor test used in the battery of

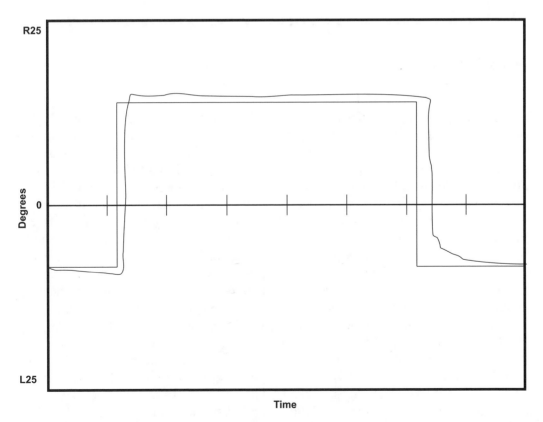

Figure 3–11. An example of a normal saccadic eye movement tracing.

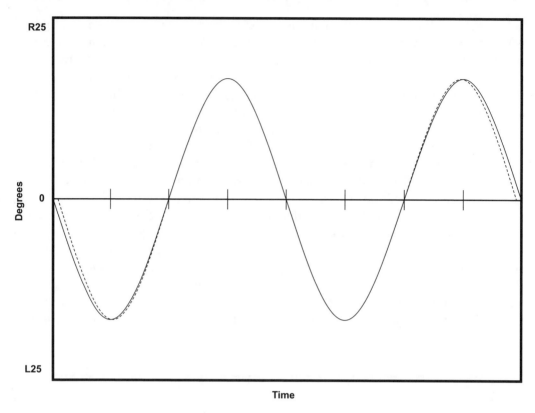

Figure 3–12. *An example of a normal smooth pursuit tracking tracing.*

measures is optokinetic tracking. This evaluates the reflexive abilities of the vestibular system with respect to moving stimuli in a full visual field (90%). The parameter for analysis is velocity gain of the eye movement in both the left and right directions for both slow and fast rates of stimulation. An example of a fast rate of optokinetic stimulation is seen in Figure 3–13. Abnormalities on any of the above oculomotor measures would suggest possible central nervous system involvement.

Positional and positioning tests constitute the second group of subtests within the ENG/VNG evaluation. Positional tests examine the response of the vestibular system when there are changes in head and body positions (see Brandt, 1990). This is different than the positioning tests,

which are intended to investigate the presence of benign paroxysmal positional vertigo (BPPV). Both of the measures, however, are intended to detect nystagmus when nystagmus should not be present. The positional tests typically are performed by having the patient lay in the supine, head left/right, and body left/right positions. Initially this is accomplished with vision denied. If nystagmus is detected with vision denied, then the vision-enabled condition is administered. When positional tests induce nystagmus in the vision-denied condition only, but the nystagmus is suppressed with vision, peripheral involvement is suspected. However, if nystagmus is observed for both conditions, or is direction changing, then possible central involvement should

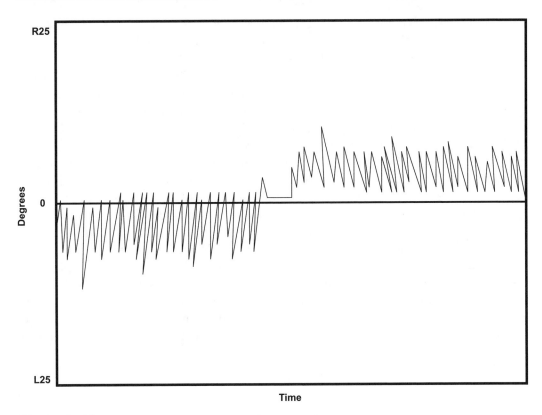

Figure 3–13. An example of a normal optokinetic tracing.

be further investigated. As indicated earlier, positioning tests are primarily used to investigate for possible BPPV (otolith debris in the posterior or horizontal semicircular canals). This information is obtained by performing several different maneuvers with the most widely used being the Dix Hallpike maneuver, in which the examiner looks for nystagmus when the posterior semicircular canal is oriented vertically. This is achieved by having the patient lie in a supine position with the neck extended and rotated toward the affected ear.

Caloric testing is perhaps the hallmark vestibular test (Barber & Stockwell, 1980; Stockwell, 1997). This is the only measure that can differentiate right-sided versus left-sided involvement as it is the only test that has the ability to evaluate only one vestibular system at a time. Its purpose is to determine the presence of a response, and if a response is detected, if there is an asymmetry between the responses of the two ears. Patients are seated in a supine position at a 30° angle. Each ear is stimulated independently in both a warm and cool condition using either water or air that is heated and/or cooled depending on the test condition. This procedure offers a direct measure of the function of the horizontal semicircular canals and is intended to induce nystagmus that is evaluated for the strength and symmetry of the response between the two ears. Two measures, ear weakness and directional preponderance, can be extracted from the responses. Caloric weakness is assessed by comparing the responses from the right ear (right warm and right cool) with those from the left ear (left warm and left cool) (Figure 3–14). Directional preponderance can also be derived from the caloric response by comparing the amplitude of the right-beating (right warm and left cool) to the left-beating (right cool and left warm) nystagmus. If no response is present or the response is severely reduced, then ice water stimulation is often attempted.

Vestibular evoked myogenic potentials (VEMPs) is a relative new comer to the world of diagnostic audiology. This test assesses vestibular system function through the use of evoked potentials (see Zapala & Brey, 2004). Specifically, it evaluates the saccular and afferent inferior vestibular nerve functions, and provides clinicians with information that is not readily available by means of the ENG or VNG. Therefore, it provides additional information with respect to differential diagnosis of site of lesion. There are many VEMP measurement techniques, which have been reported. Typically, however, this response is obtained with either a click or 500-Hz tone-burst stimulus. A rarefaction stimulus is presented usually at around 100 dB nHL and at a rate of around 5 stimuli per second. A noninverting electrode is commonly placed on the mid-sternocleidomastoid muscle and the patient must have sustained muscle contraction during recording in order to observe a waveform. Most clinicians will have the patient sustain this contraction by

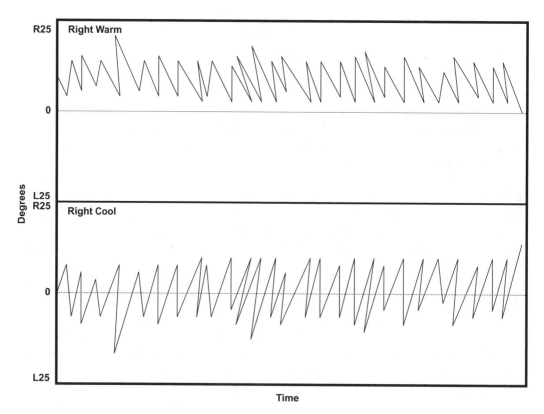

Figure 3–14. An example of normal bithermal caloric responses.

having the patient lie in the supine position while turning the head in the opposite direction of the test ear, and slightly lifting the head off of the table. The normal response characteristics is a large positive peak (P1 or P13) followed by a large negative peak (N1 or N23) (Figure 3–15).

Although there is variability among patients with respect to the amplitude of the response, the VEMP is typically very large and robust in nature and is usually on the order of 15 to 180 µV. The VEMP response is unique in that the patients serve as their own control with respect to determining the normality of the response. That is to say, that the right-sided and left-sided responses are compared to each other and an asymmetry ratio is calculated, where the asymmetry ratio equals $100(A_L-A_S)/(A_L+A_S)$. This measure appears to be sensitive to diseases that present with both vestibular and auditory involvement, including Ménière's disease, vestibular schwannoma, superior canal dehiscence syndrome, and multiple sclerosis (Akin & Murnane, 2008).

The battery of tests described above are standard protocol for ENG/VNG assessment of vestibular (dys)function. However, some variations are used in many clinics. Regardless, this is perhaps the strongest tool for the assessment of the vestibular system in that it provides general information regarding (ab)normality of the response, peripheral versus central involvement, and side of lesion information.

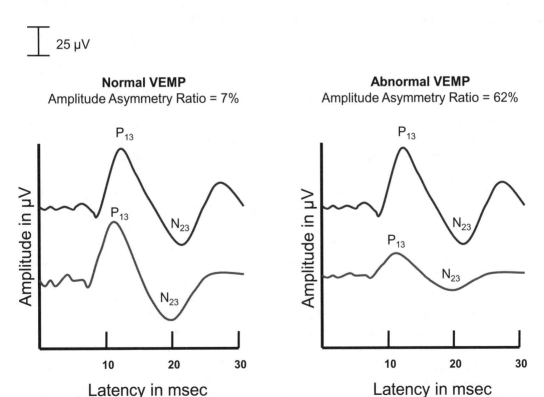

Figure 3–15. Examples of normal (left panel) and abnormal (right panel) vestibular evoked myogenic responses for the left and right sides.

BASICS OF COMPUTED TOMOGRAPHY AND MAGNETIC RESONANCE IMAGING

Imaging has developed into a valuable tool for diagnosing and characterizing congenital and pathologic conditions affecting the auditory system. Computed tomography (CT) and magnetic resonance (MR) imaging by far are the two most widely utilized procedures in the evaluation of the auditory system.

Computed Tomography

Computed tomography is an imaging procedure that utilizes X-rays and their absorption properties to generate two-dimensional images of the body. Using a loaf of bread as an example, a conventional X-ray would allow inspection of the bread as a whole, whereas a CT scan would provide evaluation of the individual slices that make up the loaf of bread. Unlike conventional X-rays, CT utilizes a "beam" or "fan" of X-rays that pass through the patient and then are detected by a series of "detectors" located on the other side of the patient. As the X-rays pass through the patient's body they are absorbed or attenuated to varying degrees based on the different compositions of the various body parts (e.g., bone, soft tissue, air, etc.). To create the CT image, the X-ray "beam" is rotated around the patient and the varying amounts of X-ray attenuation are recorded by the detectors. This process is then repeated multiple times as the patient passes through the CT scanner (typically by automated movement of the patient table), allowing for acquisi-

tion of several "slices" within the patient. Through complex mathematical analysis, the data collected by the detectors are used to assign varying shades of gray to different portions of the body and allows for generation of a series of images. This, of course, is a simplistic characterization with most modern scanners able to assign gray scale assignments to sample areas (voxels) as small as 0.4 mm in thickness.

Compared with conventional X-rays, CT provides very good contrast resolution and tissue discrimination, primarily by reducing the interference caused by overlapping structures. It is analogous to having five vehicles lined up "bumper-to-bumper," with the first vehicle being a bus and the next four being compact cars. Viewed from the front, the cars would be obscured by the mass of the bus, but if one were to walk in a circle (rotate) around the vehicles, the five separate vehicles would be readily apparent.

Computed tomography scans employ a black-white numerical scale measured in Hounsfield units (HU). The name for the CT values was chosen in honor of Sir Godfrey Hounsfield, the "father" of CT, who developed the first clinical scanner in 1972 (Wolbrast, 1993). Very dense structures such as bone have very high HUs (up to +1000), with less dense structures such as air having very low HUs (as low as −1000). In addition to the natural contrast provided by varying soft tissues and their respective differences in X-ray attenuation (densities), CT scans can often be "enhanced" by the addition of intravascular or oral contrast agents. Oral contrast is most commonly utilized for abdominal and pelvic applications, but intravascular contrast does have applications for imaging of the auditory system (Table 3–5). Currently, nonionic, iodinated contrast

Table 3–5. Indications for Intravascular Contrast Administration During Computed Tomography Imaging

Suspected Tumor	Paragangliomas (glomus tumors)
	Meningiomas
	Schwannomas
	Epidermoid and arachnoid cysts
Intracranial extension or involvement	Otitis media and mastoiditis
	Dural sinus thrombosis
Vascular abnormalities/anomalies	Vascular loops
	Anterior inferior cerebellar artery (AICA) syndrome
	Aberrant internal carotid artery
	Jugular bulb diverticulum, dehiscence

agents are the most frequently utilized intravascular agents for CT applications. These have the advantages of being readily available, relatively inexpensive (when compared with gadolinium, see MR imaging section), and have a reasonable safety profile with a low incidence of allergic reaction. Care, however, must be taken in using these agents, as iodinated agents can have a nephrotoxic effect, particularly in patients with compromised renal function.

Dedicated imaging of the temporal bone with CT should consist of a tailored sequence combining a small field of view, a high-resolution matrix (e.g., 512 × 512), and a thin section acquisition. Current CT scanners are capable of acquiring images slices in the range of 0.4- to 1.0-mm thickness, allowing for optimal multiplanar reconstructions (MPRs) in any imaging plane (Figure 3–16a). "True" coronal images (Figure 3–16b) of the temporal bone can be obtained by scanning the patient in a prone position with the

neck extended, or in the supine position with the neck extended (possibly requiring hanging the patient's head off the back of the table). However, obtaining "true" axial and coronal CT images not only requires patient cooperation for proper positioning, but also essentially doubles the radiation dose, as each scan must be performed separately. As such, most imaging centers opt for a single axial acquisition and MPRs in the coronal or sagittal planes. This not only limits the radiation exposure for the patient, but it also keeps imaging time to a minimum, with scan times generally lasting 60 seconds or less.

The axial images (Figure 3–17) should be obtained or reconstructed as MPRs along a plane 30° superior to the anthropologic baseline (i.e., the line intersecting the infro-orbital rim and the external auditory canal) and the coronal images should be obtained at a 90° perpendicular angle to the axial images (Chakeres & Augustyn, 2003). Both the axial and

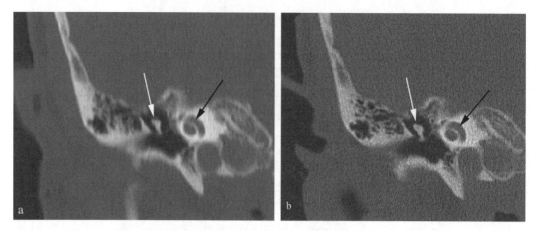

Figure 3–16. *A multiplanar reconstruction (MPR) computed tomography (CT) image of the temporal bone showing part of the middle ear ossicles* (white arrow) *and the cochlea* (black arrow) (**a**) *and a" true" coronal image of the same structures* (**b**).

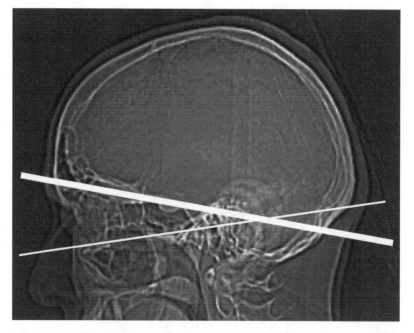

Figure 3–17. *CT scout image (axial cut) in the saggital plane showing the 30-degree plane* (heavy line) *on which MPRs should be constructed in reference to the anthropologic baseline (see text).*

coronal images should be reconstructed at 1- to 2-mm slice thickness. Supplemental intravenous contrast administration may be added to the protocol, particularly in evaluating for soft tissue masses/tumors, but this should probably be reserved for patients with a contraindication to MR imaging.

Magnetic Resonance Imaging

Magnetic resonance imaging provides true multiplanar imaging, with superb soft tissue delineation, all without the use of ionizing radiation. The procedure is based on the principle that hydrogen nuclei (protons) tend to align along a magnetic field. This principle is similar to how a dial on a compass aligns with the magnetic field of the earth. When a patient is placed within the MR scanner (magnet), the protons within the individual's body align along the magnetic field of the scanner. Various "pulses" can then be applied to the field, and the time for the protons to re-align within the magnetic field is called the *relaxation time*. The concentration of protons within various parts of the body (voxels), will determine the net relaxation times (e.g., T1, T2) for that particular voxel. Based on the relaxation times, various gray-scale assignments can be given to the voxels to generate an image.

Tesla (T) is the unit of measurement used to define the strength of the magnetic field within an MR scanner. Most clinical MR scanners have magnetic strengths ranging from 0.5 to 3.0 tesla. For reference, the earth's magnetic field is around 30 microtesla, and the large magnets utilized in "junk yards" to transport scrap metal and cars are only 0.3 tesla. Higher field strength magnets (e.g., 3T) provide increased signal-to-noise ratios (and thus reduced scan times) and superior resolution relative to midfield strength magnets (e.g., 1.5T). As they become more available commercially, the demand and utility of imaging the auditory system with high-field scanners (e.g., 3T and higher) assuredly will increase owing to the increased resolution ability of these more powerful magnetic fields.

Most MR protocols consist of a combination of *T1-weighted* and *T2-weighted* images in multiplanar acquisition. In routine MR imaging of the brain, T1-weighted images are considered best at defining anatomy and any distortion of normal structures owing to its superior soft tissue discrimination. T1-weighted images are also useful after the administration of intravenous contrast agents, as areas of abnormal enhancement become bright after contrast administration. Currently, the gadolinium-based contrast agents are most widely used clinically and traditionally have been thought to have an excellent safety profile with an extremely low incidence of anaphylactic allergic reaction. However, recently, an association between nephrogenic systemic fibrosis (NSF) and gadolinium contrast agents used for MR imaging has become a concern in patients with renal insufficiency. T2-weighted images are more sensitive to changes in water concentration, and thus are best for delineating areas of edema. In contrast to CT, with which coronal and sagittal imaging generally requires a MPR, MR imaging has the advantage of being able to acquire images in any plane (e.g., axial, coronal, sagittal, oblique). However, the added resolution and multiplanar capability comes at a time cost, with each sequences (e.g., T1, T2) requiring several minutes for acquisition. Thus, most MR examinations require around 30 to 60 minutes of scan time, depending on the complexity of the examination. As such, patient compliance and cooperation can be significant limitations of MR imaging, as the patient must remain motionless during the several minutes needed to acquire each sequence acquisition. For this reason, many patients will require some form of sedation to complete their examination. Patient claustrophobia issues, which may occur in some patients due to the small confined area within the scanner, often can be resolved with sedation or the use of "open" magnets that deviate from the traditional "tube" design, but the open magnets may be of decreased field strength (0.5 to 1.0 T) and thus have decreased resolution.

Dedicated imaging of the temporal bone and auditory system with MR imaging requires clinical input to ensure that the proper study is performed. For example, one might want to include an MR angiogram (arterial or venous) when evaluating for *pulsatile tinnitus*, as vascular anomalies may be best appreciated on these examinations. Magnetic resonance imaging of the auditory system is most frequently employed in cases of an acquired *sensorineural hearing loss*, spe-cifically when evaluating for tumors (e.g., schwannomas) associated with the vestibular and cochlear nerves. Dedicated imaging of the auditory system, referred to as an "internal auditory canal" protocol at most institutions, consists of T1 imaging (both without and after intravenous contrast administration) with thin-section acquisition in the axial and coronal planes. Additionally, imaging should include "fluid sensitive" T2 images utilizing a high-resolution matrix and a small field of view (Figure 3–18). The high-resolution T2 images can be acquired in multiple planes, providing exquisite detail of the vestibular and cochlear nerves, and are often used as a "screening" technique for vestibular schwannomas, obviating

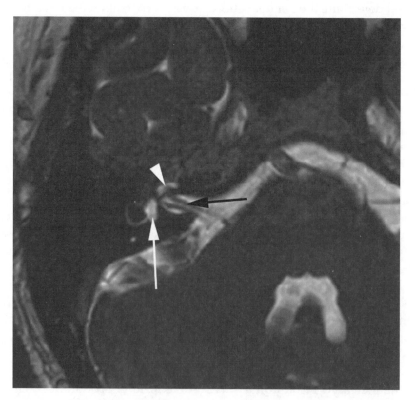

Figure 3–18. Magnetic resonance imaging (MRI) axial T2-weighted sequence image at the level of the internal auditory canal showing the cochlear nerve (black arrow) and fluid-filled cochlea (white arrowhead) and vestibule (white arrow).

the need for contrast. The vestibular and cochlear nerves can be seen surrounded by cerebral spinal fluid in the cerebellopontine angle and the internal auditory canal. Fluid signal within the labyrinthine structures can also be assessed on the T2 sequences, with the loss of the normal bright fluid signal intensity indicating a pathologic process. Similar approaches can be applied to the imaging of various brain structures as well. Generally, T1 imaging both without and following intravenous contrast is utilized in the evaluation of sensorineural hearing loss to avoid misinterpreting a congenital lesion (e.g., lipoma) as a neoplasm with only postcontrast or T2 imaging.

Normal Anatomy and Clinical Applications of CT and MR Imaging in the Evaluation of the Auditory System

Sound is produced when vibrational forces from the tympanic membrane are transmitted to the ossicular chain, and then into the vestibule via the oval window. With modern imaging techniques, the ossicles can generally be discriminated (Figure 3–19). The cochlea is a shell-like structure composed of two and one-half turns, which should be visible as the apical, middle, and basal turns. The vestibule represents the common chamber at the base of the semicircular canals. The round

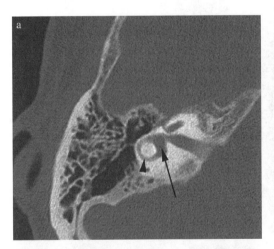

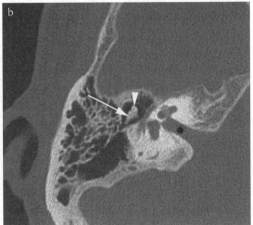

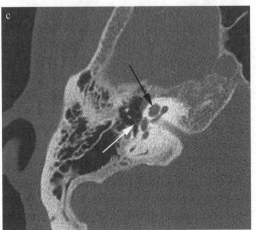

Figure 3–19. *Temporal bone axial CT image showing the vestibule* (black arrow), *horizontal semicircular canal* (black arrowhead), *and basal turn of the cochlea* (**a**). *A more inferior axial view demonstrating the internal auditory canal* (black asterisk), *head of the malleus* (white arrowhead), *short process of the incus* (white arrow), *and the second turn of the cochlea* (**b**). *At the level of the apical turn of the cochlea* (black arrow), *the stapes can be visualized* (white arrow) (**c**).

window is situated at the basal turn of the cochlea, with the oval window situated at the vestibule. The vibrational forces delivered to the cochlea are converted to energy "potentials" within the labyrinthine structures that synapse with the neural fibers that eventually make up the cochlear nerve. The cochlear nerve then courses through the internal auditory canal, through the cerebellopontine angle, to enter the brainstem (cochlear nuclei).

Computed tomography scans of the "temporal bone" provide excellent detail of the normal bony anatomy of the auditory system, including the internal auditory canal, the labyrinthine structures, the ossic-

ular chain, the middle ear cavity, and the external auditory canal. Pathology is manifested mainly as alterations in the bony morphology (e.g., destruction, erosion) of the temporal bone and its components.

Magnetic resonance imaging performed with an "internal auditory canal" protocol will provide excellent visualization of the facial and the vestibular and cochlear nerves (see Figure 3–18). Pathology is generally manifested as a soft tissue "lesion" of one of the nerves, with increased conspicuity of the lesion after administration of gadolinium-contrast agents (Figure 3–20). Additionally, lesions of the brainstem affecting the auditory

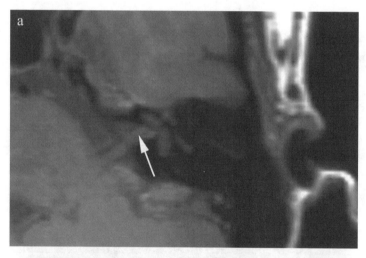

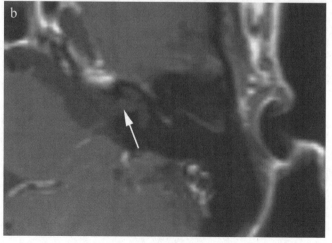

Figure 3–20. An axial T1 MRI *showing the seventh and eighth cranial nerves* (a) *and with gadolinium contrast enhancement* (b).

nuclei are best seen with MR imaging. Althougth the labyrinthine structures are visible with MR imaging, it currently does not afford the same detail as CT.

Computed tomography imaging has advantages over MR imaging in that it is readily available, with scanners located in nearly every hospital and most sizeable outpatient clinics. As previously stated, CT is fast; thus scans of diagnostic quality can generally be obtained in agitated or confused patients (e.g., trauma), as well as in infants/children without the need for sedation. The procedure provides excellent characterization of bony abnormalities, and thus is preferred for evaluation of fractures and ossicular disruption (Figure 3–21), bony destruction associated with soft tissue tumors (e.g., cholesteatoma), and bony abnormalities associated with congenital hearing loss (e.g., vestibular-cochlear dysplasia, Figure 3–22). Relative

to MR imaging, the cost of CT imaging is significantly less.

The disadvantages of CT imaging are most notable in its use of ionizing radiation, limited "true" multiplanar capability (although this is becoming less of an issue with high-quality MPRs), and poor evaluation of internal auditory canal pathology (notably vestibular schwannomas) secondary to artifact from adjacent bone. If intravenous contrast is indicated, the risk of an anaphylactoid reaction is higher with iodinated contrast agents relative to gadolinium, and, in cases of renal insufficiency, care must be taken to avoid potentially adverse effects and worsening renal function.

Advantages of MR imaging lie in its lack of ionizing radiation, superior soft tissue discrimination, true multiplanar capability, and safer contrast agent. The superior soft tissue discrimination afforded

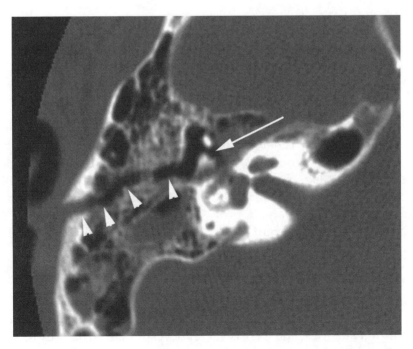

Figure 3–21. An axial temporal bone CT scan image showing the course of a fracture (white arrowheads) of the temporal bone and disarticulation of the ossicles (white arrow).

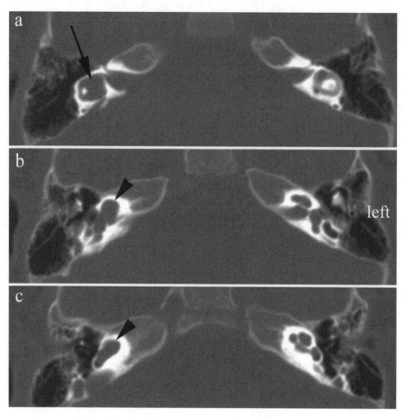

Figure 3–22. *An axial temporal bone CT scan image demonstrating right cochleovestibular dysplasia (arrows) compared with normal left inner ear structures from three different anatomic locations (**a**, **b**, and **c**). The vestibule is widely dilated with abnormal semicircular canals and the cochlea appears as a common cavity instead of the normal 2½ turns.*

by MR imaging makes it ideal for the evaluation of internal auditory canal pathology (e.g., schwannomas, Figure 3–23) and for soft tissue tumors (e.g., paragangliomas, Figure 3–24). The addition of an MR angiogram may help the evaluation of vascular anomalies (e.g., aberrant internal carotid artery, jugular diverticulum/dehiscence).

Disadvantages of MR imaging include longer scan times requiring patient compliance (and possibly sedation), more limited availability than CT, and increased cost. Once thought to be extremely safe, gadolinium-based contrast agents now have been associated with adverse effects (e.g., nephrogenic systemic fibrosis) in many patients with renal insufficiency. In addition to patients with renal insufficiency, other patients also may have a contraindication to MR imaging. Although not a complete listing of all of the contraindications for MR imaging, Table 3–6 lists some of the major contraindications.

In central auditory assessment, MR imaging is an important tool to corroborate test findings. Key individual auditory and vestibular structures of the central nervous system can be visualized readily with MR imaging (Figures 3–25 and 3–26).

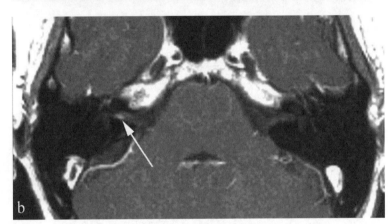

Figure 3–23. *Axial MRI images demonstrating a small intracanalicular vestibular schwannoma. This lesion appears as a dark-filling defect on T2-weighted images (white arrow) (a) and as a white enhancing lesion on contrasted T1 weighted images (white arrow) (b).*

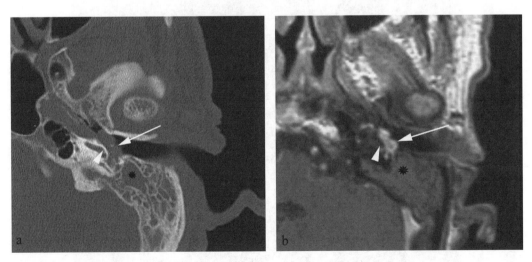

Figure 3–24. *Complementary axial CT (a) and contrasted T1-weighted MRI (b) images at the same level demonstrating an enhancing lesion (possible paraganglioma) filling the middle ear space (white arrow) adjacent to the tympanic segment of the facial nerve (white arrowhead). Opacification of the mastoid is also present (black asterisk) in both images; however, the MRI helps to differentiate between the enhancing lesion and fluid collection due to middle ear obstruction.*

Table 3–6. Absolute and Relative Contraindications to MR Imaging

Absolute	Cochlear implant
	Cardiac defibrillator
	Cardiac pacemaker, pacer dependent
	Metallic foreign body in critical location (e.g., eye)
	Certain cerebral aneurysm clips
Relative	Cardiac pacemaker, non-pacer-dependent
	Pregnancy
	Unstable patient
	Combative patient (consider general anesthesia if scan imperative)

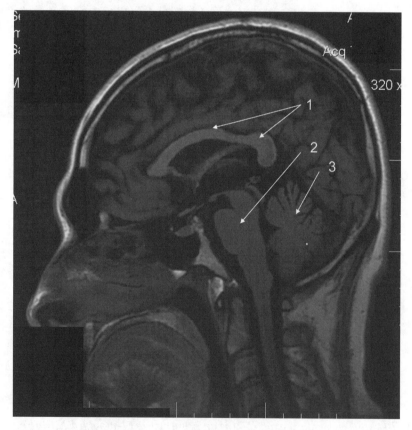

Figure 3–25. *A midline, sagittal view of an MRI of the brain showing some key structures such as the corpus callosum (1), the pons (2), and the cerebellum (3), as well as a clear depiction of the gyri and sulci at the brain's surface.*

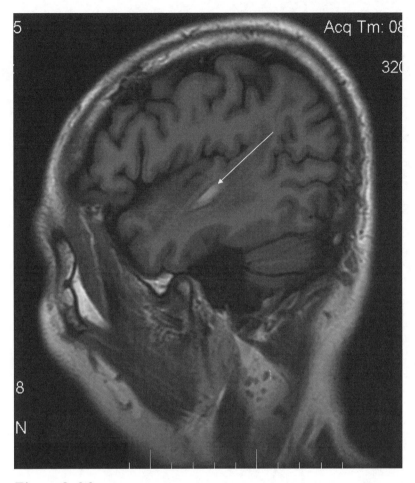

Figure 3–26. *MRI of a brain with a left temporal lobe lesion positioned near and including parts of Heschl's gyrus (see text).*

Figure 3–25 is an image of a normal brain showing several key structures. In Figure 3–26 the effects of a stroke can be noted in the inferior portion of Heschl's gyrus. This patient demonstrated abnormal findings on behavioral and electrophysiologic central auditory tests, which were corroborated by the imaging test results.

Computed tomography and MR imaging often play complementary roles in the evaluation of various auditory conditions, with each having relative advantages in characterizing a particular component of the disease process. Although not absolute, and certainly subject to change with continued advances in imaging techniques, Table 3–7 provides a template as to which imaging study should be performed in the initial evaluation of suspected auditory pathology.

Table 3–7. Disorders of the Auditory System and the Respective Roles of CT and MR Imaging in Their Diagnoses

Pathologic Process	CT	MRI
Congenital hearing loss	++	-
Progressive/acquired hearing loss	+	++
Vestibular-cochlear dysplasias	++	+
External auditory canal atresia	++	-
Otosclerosis	++	-
Superior semicircular canal dehiscence	++	-
Cholesteatoma (preoperative)	++	+
Recurrent cholesteatoma (postoperative)	+	++
Trauma	++	-
Schwannomas (e.g., vestibular, facial)	-	++
Meningiomas	+	++
Epidermoid and arachnoid cysts	+	++
Paragangliomas (glomus tumors)	++	++
Petrous apex cholesterol granulomas	+	++
Vascular abnormalities/anomalies	+	++

Note. ++ Modality of Choice, + Alternative Modality, – Limited Utility.

SUMMARY

The above tutorial is intended to provide the reader with a simple orientation with respect to the tools available to the clinician to aid in the diagnosis of disorders of the auditory system. Even the simplest measure, such as tympanometry, provides key information regarding auditory system function or dysfunction. One cannot stress enough how important these measures are in guiding audiologists and otolaryngologists in making the correct diagnosis in order to aid in appropriate audiologic and medical management and rehabilitation.

Acknowledgment. The authors gratefully acknowledge the contributions of Curtis A. Given, II, MD, Director of Neurointerventional Services, Central Baptist Hospital, Lexington, Kentucky to this chapter.

REFERENCES

Akin, F. W., & Murnane, O. D. (2008). Vestibular myogenic potentials. In G. P. Jacobson &

N. T. Shepard (Eds.), *Balance function assessment and management* (pp. 405–434). San Diego, CA: Plural.

American Academy of Audiology. (2010). *Diagnosis, treatment and management of children and adults with central auditory processing disorders.* Retrieved 6/15/11 from http://www.audiology.org/resources/documentlibrary/Documents/CAPD%20Guidelines%208-2010.pdf.

American Speech-Language-Hearing Association. (1997). *Guidelines for audiologic screenings*. Retrieved 6/15/11 from: http://www.asha.org/docs/html/GL1997-00199.html#sec1.3.5

Baran, J. A., & Musiek, F. E. (1999). Behavioral assessment of the central auditory system. In F. E. Musiek & W. F. Rintelmann (Eds.), *Contemporary perspectives in hearing assessment* (pp. 375–415). Boston, MA: Allyn & Bacon.

Barber, H. O., & Stockwell, C. W. (1980). *Manual of electronystagmography* (2nd ed.). St. Louis, MO: Mosby.

Brandt, T. (1990). Positional and positioning vertigo and nystagmus. *Journal of Neurological Sciences, 9*(1), 3–28.

Bush, M. L., Jones, R. O., & Shinn, J. B. (2008). Auditory brainstem response threshold differences in patients with vestibular schwannoma: A new diagnostic index. *Ear, Nose, and Throat Journal, 87*(8), 458–462.

Cameron, S., Brown, D., Keith, R., Martin, J., Watson, C., & Dillon, H. (2009). Development of the North American Listening in Spatialized Noise-Sentences test (NA LiSN-S): Sentence equivalence, normative data, and test-retest reliability studies. *Journal of the American Academy of Audiology, 20*(2), 128–146.

Cameron, S., & Dillon, H. (2007). Development of the Listening in Spatialized Noise-Sentences Test (LISN-S). *Ear and Hearing, 28*(2), 196–211.

Chakeres, D. W., & Augustyn, M. A. (2003). Temporal bone: Imaging. In P. M. Som & H. D. Curtin (Eds.), *Head and neck imaging* (4th ed., pp. 1093–1108). St. Louis, MO: Mosby.

Ferraro, J. A. (2000). Electrocochleography. In R. J. Roeser, M. Valente, & H. Hosford-Dunn (Eds.), *Audiology: Diagnosis* (pp. 425–451). New York, NY: Thieme.

Fifer, R. C., Jerger, J. F., Berlin, C. I., Tobey, E. A., & Campbell, J. C. (1983). Development of a dichotic sentence identification test for hearing-impaired adults. *Ear and Hearing, 4*(6), 300–305.

Hall, J. W., 3rd. (2007). *New handbook of auditory evoked responses.* Boston, MA: Allyn & Bacon.

Jacobson, G. P., & Shepard, N. T. (Eds.). (2008). *Balance function assessment and management.* San Diego. CA: Plural.

Jerger, J. (1970). Clinical experience with impedance audiometry. *Archives of Otolaryngology, 92*(4), 311–324.

Jerger, J., & Jerger, S. (1980). Measurement of hearing in adults. In M. M. Paparella & D. A. Shumrick (Eds.), *Otolaryngology* (2nd ed., pp. 1225–1262). Philadelphia, PA: W. B. Saunders.

Katz, J. (1962). The use of staggered spondaic words for assessing the integrity of the central auditory nervous system. *Journal of Auditory Research, 2,* 327–337.

Keith, R. W. (2000). *Random Gap Detection Test.* St. Louis, MO: Auditec.

Kemp, D. T. (1978). Stimulated acoustic emissions from within the human auditory system. *Journal of the Acoustical Society of America, 64*(5), 1386–1391.

Leigh, R. J., & Zee, D. S. (2006). *The neurology of eye movements* (4th ed.). New York, NY: Oxford University Press.

Lister, J. J., Roberts, R. A., & Lister, F. L. (2011). An adaptive test of temporal resolution: Age effects. *International Journal of Audiology, 50*(6), 367–374.

Lynn, G. E., Gilroy, J., Taylor, P. C., & Leiser, R. P. (1981). Binaural masking-level differences in neurological disorders. *Archives of Otolaryngology, 107*(6), 357–362.

Margolis, R. H., & Heller, J. W. (1987). Screening tympanometry: Criteria for medical referral. *Audiology, 26*(4), 197–208.

Margolis, R. H., & Hunter, L. L. (2000). Acoustic immittance measurements. In R. J. Roeser, M. Valente, & H. Hosford-Dunn (Eds.),

Audiology diagnosis (pp. 381–424). New York, NY: Thieme.

Margolis, R. H., Hunter, L. L., & Giebink, G. S. (1994). Tympanometric evaluation of middle ear function in children with otitis media. *Annals of Otology, Rhinology, and Laryngology, 163*(Suppl.), 34–38.

Musiek, F. E. (1983). Results of three dichotic speech tests on subjects with intracranial lesions. *Ear and Hearing, 4*(6), 318–323.

Musiek, F. E. (1991). Auditory evoked responses in site-of-lesion assessment. In W. F. Rintelmann (Ed.), *Hearing assessment* (2nd ed., pp. 383–428). Austin, TX: Pro-Ed.

Musiek, F. E., Baran, J. A., & Pinheiro, M. L. (1990). Duration pattern recognition in normal subjects and patients with cerebral and cochlear lesions. *Audiology, 29*(6), 304–313.

Musiek, F. E., Baran, J. A., & Pinheiro, M. L. (1994). *Neuroaudiology: Case studies.* San Diego, CA: Singular.

Musiek, F., Charette, L., Kelly, T., Lee, W. W., & Musiek, E. (1999). Hit and false-positive rates for the middle latency response in patients with central nervous system involvement. *Journal of the American Academy of Audiology, 10*(3), 124–132.

Musiek, F. E., & Chermak, G. D. (2007). *Handbook of central auditory processing disorder (Vol. 1). Auditory neuroscience and diagnosis.* San Diego, CA: Plural.

Musiek, F. E., Gollegly, K. M., Kibbe, K. S., & Verkest-Lenz, S. B. (1991). Proposed screening test for central auditory disorders: Follow-up on the dichotic digits test. *American Journal of Otology, 12*(2), 109–113.

Musiek, F. E., & Lee, W. W. (1999). Auditory middle and late potentials. In F. E. Musiek & W. F. Rintelmann (Eds.), *Contemporary perspectives in hearing assessment* (pp. 243–272). Boston, MA: Allyn & Bacon.

Musiek, F. E., & Pinheiro, M. L. (1985). Dichotic speech tests in the detection of central auditory dysfunction. In M. L. Pinheiro & F. E. Musiek (Eds.), *Assessment of central auditory dysfunction: Foundations and clinical correlates* (pp. 201–218). Baltimore, MD: Williams & Wilkins.

Musiek, F. E., & Pinheiro, M. L. (1987). Frequency patterns in cochlear, brainstem, and cerebral lesions. *Audiology, 26*(2), 79–88.

Musiek, F. E., Shinn, J. B., & Jirsa, R. (2007). The auditory brainstem response in auditory nerve and brainstem dysfunction. In R. F. Burkard, M. Don, & J. J. Eggermont (Eds.), *Auditory evoked potentials: Basic principles and application* (pp. 291–312). Baltimore, MD: Lippincott Williams & Wilkins.

Musiek, F. E., Shinn, J. B., Jirsa, R., Bamiou, D. E., Baran, J. A., & Zaidan, E. (2005). GIN (Gaps-In-Noise) test performance in subjects with confirmed central auditory nervous system involvement. *Ear and Hearing, 26*(6), 608–618.

Nozza, R. (2003). The assessment of hearing and middle ear function in children. In C. D. Bluestone et al. (Eds.). *Pediatric otolaryngology* (4th ed., Vol. 2, pp. 190–229). Philadelphia, PA: W. B. Saunders.

Picton, T. (2011). *Human auditory evoked potentials.* San Diego, CA: Plural.

Robinette, M. S., & Glattke, T. J. (Eds.). (2002). *Otoacoustic emissions: Clinical applications.* New York, NY: Thieme.

Schmidt, R. J., Sataloff, R. T., Newman, J., Spiegel, J. R., & Myers, D. L. (2001). The sensitivity of auditory brainstem response testing for the diagnosis of acoustic neuromas. *Archives of Otolaryngology-Head and Neck Surgery, 127*(1), 19–22.

Shinn, J. B., Chermak, G. D., & Musiek, F. E. (2009). GIN (Gaps-In-Noise) performance in the pediatric population. *Journal of the American Academy of Audiology, 20*(4), 229–238.

Stockwell, C. W. (1997). Vestibular testing: Past, present, future. *British Journal of Audiology, 31*(6), 387–398.

Willeford, J. (1977). Children's performance on the SSW test and Willeford battery: Interim clinical data. In R. W. Keith (Ed.), *Central auditory dysfunction* (pp. 43–72). New York, NY: Grune & Stratton.

Wilson, R. H., & Margolis, R. H. (1999). Acoustic reflex measurements. In F. E. Musiek & W. F. Rintelmann (Eds.), *Contemporary perspectives in hearing assessment* (pp. 131–166). Boston, MA: Allyn & Bacon.

Wilson, R. H., Preece, J. P., Salamon, D. L., Sperry, J. L., & Bornstein, S. P. (1994). Effects of time compression and time compression plus reverberation on the intelligibility of Northwestern University Auditory Test No. 6. *Journal of the American Academy of Audiology, 5*(4), 269–277.

Wolbrast, A. B. (1993). *Physics of radiology.* Norwalk, CT: Appleton & Lange.

Zapala, D. A., & Brey, R. H. (2004). Clinical experience with vestibular evoked myogenic potentials. *Journal of the American Academy of Audiology, 15*(3), 198–215.

Zappia, J. J., O'Connor, C. A., Wiet, R. J., & Dinces, E. A. (1997). Rethinking the use of auditory brainstem response in acoustic neuroma screening. *Laryngoscope, 107*(10), 1388–1392.

4

Outer and Middle Ear Disorders

INTRODUCTION

The outer (external) and middle ear comprise the receptive and transformer structures for the auditory system. The external ear includes the auricle or pinna and the external auditory canal. The external auditory canal is a skin-lined opening that ends at the eardrum or tympanic membrane. The subcutaneous support of the outer third of the external canal is cartilage, whereas the medial two-thirds of the canal, adjacent to the tympanic membrane, is bony. The tympanic membrane has three cellular layers: the lateral squamous cell layer, the middle fibrous layer, and the medial respiratory epithelial layer. The tympanic membrane is held in position by a bony trough of the medial external auditory canal, in which a fibrous ligament called the annulus resides. The superior portion of the membrane lacks a fibrous layer and is referred to as the pars flaccida; the rest of the membrane is referred to as the pars tensa.

The middle ear is an aerated space that begins laterally with the tympanic membrane and ends medially with the bony encasement of the cochlea and the vestibule. The middle ear space is divided into separate regions based on their relationships to the tympanic membrane annulus. The protympanum is the anterior-most space of the middle ear and it contains the opening of the Eustachian tube, which connects the middle ear to the nasopharynx. The mesotympanum is on the same plane as the tympanic membrane and it contains the handle of the malleus, the long process of the incus, the stapes, the oval and round windows, and the tympanic segment of the facial nerve. The hypotympanum is inferior to the annulus and is the typical location of the bony covering of the jugular bulb; however, this bulb may lack a bony covering creating a risk of jugular bulb injury during middle ear surgery. The epitympanum is above the tympanic membrane and is closely related to the pars flaccida portion of the tympanic membrane. This space contains the head of the malleus and the short process of the incus and is confluent with the air cells of the mastoid portion of the temporal bone by an opening called the antrum. The external and middle ears are surrounded by vital neural and vascular structures that can become involved in the disease processes that affect the ear. (For more information on the anatomy and physiology of the outer and middle ears, see Musiek and Baran, 2007, and Chapter 2, Structure and Function of the Auditory and Vestibular Systems.)

A wide variety of diseases, both congenital and acquired, can affect this portion of the auditory system resulting in significant hearing dysfunction. As a whole, diseases of the external and middle ears are quite prevalent and account for a large portion of health care resources. This chapter examines a selection of the diseases and conditions that affect the external and/or middle ears.

AURAL ATRESIA

Introduction

Aural atresia is a condition in which the external auditory canal (EAC) fails to develop properly, resulting in an abnormally closed or absent canal (see also Chapter 9, Hereditary and Congenital Hearing Loss). Any interruption of the embryologic development of the EAC can result in atresia with varying degrees of severity. This condition is usually congenital in nature; however, acquired atresia can also occur and is most commonly related to chronic infections of the external auditory canal.

Symptoms

Atresia of the external auditory canal is typically discovered during a newborn screening examination. The condition is characterized by the absence of an external auditory canal or the presence of a blind pouch in the canal, and may involve one or both ears. Microtia, which is the malformation or absence of the pinna, is frequently present with aural atresia; however, the pinna is normal in many patients with this condition. The middle ear also may be involved in individuals with aural atresia. In these cases, the tympanic membrane typically is absent and the ossicles may be significantly malformed or completely absent. In addition, the inner ear may be malformed; however, this condition is less common than external and/or middle ear malformations due to the separate and distinct embryologic development of the inner ear. When the EAC is shallow or blunted, the atresia may not be identified at birth and diagnosis is often delayed until entrance into school. In these cases, a routine hearing screening test administered in school may identify hearing loss and ultimately lead to the medical diagnosis of aural atresia.

The absence of an external canal results in a conductive hearing loss, and in the event that the condition is bilateral and left untreated, the patient is likely to experience significant speech and language delays. The external canal, if not completely absent, may be as small as a pinpoint in size and this narrowing or stenosis of the ear canal may lead to the collection of epithelial skin cells in the external auditory canal, known as an external canal cholesteatoma, which can result in inflammation, pain, and/or discharge. Other systemic congenital anomalies may be present, but special attention should be paid to craniofacial anomalies, such as cleft palate, which may be an important consideration during perioperative airway management (see Schuknecht, 1989).

Incidence and Prevalence

Congenital aural atresia generally occurs in 1 out of 10,000 to 20,000 live births. Typically, males are affected more than females and unilateral atresia is approximately three times more common than bilateral atresia (De la Cruz & Chandraseckhar, 1994). Also, the right ear tends to be involved more frequently than the left ear and the atretic portion of the external canal is more frequently bony rather than membranous (Jahrsdoerfer, 1978).

Etiology and Pathology

This condition is primarily a congenital disease that may occur in conjunction with a number of syndromes (e.g., Pierre Robin, CHARGE, VATER, Goldenhar, and Treacher Collins). Anomalies of the ear tend to occur in conjunction with other craniofacial malformations due to their common embryologic origins. Five branchial arches and their associated structures form the major structures of the head and neck. The ossicles begin to develop in the 4th gestational week and this process continues to the 16th gestational week, when the ossicles reach adult size. During the 8th gestational week, the first brachial groove forms a plug of cells that migrates medially to oppose the developing middle ear cleft. The plug of cells begins to hollow out to form an epithelial lined external auditory canal during the 6th month of gestation. Any interruption during this external and middle ear development typically results in ossicular malformation or atresia of the canal (see Lambert, 1998).

Site of Lesion

The severity and location of aural atresia can be classified in a number of ways. A commonly used classification system was described by Schuknecht (1989). Type A, or meatal atresia, involves the lateral cartilaginous portion of the canal, which is extremely narrowed in the atretic ear preventing sloughing skin cells and cerumen to exit the external canal. These sloughing skin cells can form a cyst, which then can erode soft tissue and bony structures. Type B, or partial atresia, involves a narrowing of the cartilaginous and bony portions of the canal. In this condition, the narrowed ear canal typically allows visualization of the tympanic membrane, but malformations of the ossicles are common. Type C, or total atresia, involves complete atresia of the cartilaginous and bony portions of the canal; however, the mastoid and middle ear are aerated. The bone adjacent to the middle ear is referred to as the atretic plate. The tympanic membrane is typically absent and the ossicles are fused and frequently adherent to the atretic plate. Type D, or hypopneumatic atresia, is similar to type C; however, the mastoid is poorly pneumatized and the facial nerve has an aberrant course within the temporal bone.

Audiology

The audiologic evaluation of an individual with atresia can be difficult, but it is a critical component of the diagnostic workup, especially in the case of pediatric patients.

Audiologic evaluation is accomplished through two different approaches that are dependent on the presence of either unilateral or bilateral atretic involvement. Either way, when evaluating an infant or a young child, the recommended approach is through the use of the auditory brainstem response (ABR). Most individuals with atresia present with a significant conductive hearing loss on the involved side. If a patient presents with involvement of only one ear, auditory sensitivity should be determined initially for the normal or nonatretic ear. This may be accomplished using a traditional click stimulus ABR in combination with frequency-specific ABR tone-bursts in order to establish the level of hearing sensitivity across a range of frequencies. Once this has been established, it is recommended that bone conduction testing be performed on the atretic side with masking delivered to the uninvolved ear.

In cases of bilateral atresia, bone conduction ABR is critical in determining serviceable hearing; however, it is nearly impossible to determine with any degree of certainty, which is the better hearing ear due to presence of the bilateral conductive loss and related masking dilemmas.

Medical Examination

Atresia of the external auditory canal is typically found during a routine neonatal screening examination shortly after birth, as it may be heralded by microtia. The examination of aural atresia begins with inspection and palpation of the head and neck. The patient may have dysmorphic features or craniofacial anomalies that may require further workup and intervention prior to addressing the aural atresia (e.g., Pierre Robin sequence with cleft palate). Otologic examination involves inspection

and palpation of the auricle with careful photographic documentation of any degree of microtia. One must also examine facial nerve function as the facial nerve may have a highly variable course in atretic ears. Examination of the external auditory canal may be limited, but an attempt to evaluate the canal must be made. The use of a microscope to inspect the canal may uncover a stenotic or narrowed meatus and allow for cleaning of cerumen and squamous debris. Computed tomography (CT) scanning is vital in determining the location and severity of the compromise, as well as to aid in preoperative planning. The gold standard imaging procedure is a high-resolution CT scan of the temporal bone with 1- to 2-mm slices.

Audiologic Management

Audiologic management in cases of atresia varies depending on a variety of factors (i.e., unilateral versus bilateral atresia, hearing sensitivity of the nonatretic ear, the extent of the atresia, the age of the patient, etc.). If serviceable hearing is documented through pure-tone testing, a bone conduction hearing aid is often a viable option in many cases (Declau, Cremers, & Van de Heyning, 1999). Keeping in mind, however, that if the nonatretic ear demonstrates any degree of hearing loss, this should be managed with traditional amplification. For preschool and school-age children, utilization of an FM system should be considered in order to provide them with the best possible signal-to-noise ratio.

Medical Management

The type of treatment utilized for aural atresia is based on the severity of disease. Documentation of audiologic function must occur early in the evaluation of these patients, whether by bone conduction audiometry or evoked auditory responses. Careful examination of the CT scan must be performed. Lack of sensorineural function and/or the presence of a malformed inner ear are contraindications for surgical intervention. Jahrsdoerfer and colleagues developed a 10-point grading scale of temporal bone anatomy that is used commonly today in determining candidacy for surgical intervention (Jahrsdoerfer, Yeakley, Aguilar, Cole, & Gray, 1992). The grading scale is based on giving a point for the normal radiographic appearance of specific temporal bone structures, such as the ossicles, the mastoid, and the course of the facial nerve. The only exception is the stapes, which if normal is given 2 points. A score of 5 or less disqualifies a patient from surgical intervention.

Surgical correction of the atretic ear canal is difficult and requires a combination of skill and experience. Typically, microtia is surgically addressed by a reconstructive surgeon prior to the creation of a new external auditory canal. Microtia repair usually occurs when the child reaches 6 or 7 years of age and aural atresia repair is performed 1 to 2 years later. Patients with incomplete atresia or stenotic ear canals require careful cleaning of the canal and close follow-up to prevent cholesteatoma formation. If the canal cannot be cleaned adequately, then surgical correction becomes necessary.

Repair of the atretic canal involves a postauricular incision and the drilling of a new external auditory canal within the temporal bone while carefully avoiding the mastoid air cells, the middle cranial fossa dura mater, and the facial nerve. Once the middle ear is reached, careful inspection of the ossicles is performed.

A tympanic membrane graft is fashioned from temporalis fascia and draped over the ossicles. A skin graft is then carefully placed into position to provide the lining for the newly created canal. Patients are followed closely as outpatients and debridement of the canal is performed frequently in the clinic using a microscope.

Patients who are poor reconstructive surgical candidates based on their scores on the Jahrsdoerfer grading scale may be candidates for surgical implantation of a bone-anchored hearing aid. However, patients must have a significant audiologic reserve to be candidates for the placement of this type of device. The process involves the placement of a metal implant in the temporal bone to which a hearing aid can be attached. Similar to a bone-conduction hearing aid, an anchored aid directly conducts sound through the temporal bone to the cochlea. A body processor is worn to increase the gain of a bone-anchored aid.

EUSTACHIAN TUBE DYSFUNCTION

Introduction

Eustachian tube anatomy and function is vital as it connects the middle ear space with the nasopharynx and dysfunction of this connection can lead to significant otologic disease (Bluestone, 1998). The middle ear opening to the Eustachian tube is located in the anterior medial aspect of the middle ear. The proximal one-third of the tube passes through the petrous portion of the temporal bone. The distal two-thirds is primarily cartilaginous and terminates in the superior lateral aspect of the nasopharynx. Redundant cartilage of this tube protrudes into the nasopharynx and is referred to as the *torus tubarius*. Two muscles, the tensor veli palatini and the levator veli palatini, which have attachments to the palate, are responsible for active dilation of the distal portion of the Eustachian tube. Bluestone describes the three physiologic functions of the Eustachian tube as: (1) ventilation of the middle ear, (2) protection from the nasopharynx, and (3) clearance of secretions of the middle ear.

The Eustachian tube is a dynamic structure that is closed at rest but opens passively in response to changes in atmospheric pressure and actively in response to activities such as sneezing, swallowing, or yawning. The tube also can be opened forcibly by autoinsufflation. If the tube fails to open or becomes blocked, the air within the middle ear is absorbed, creating a vacuum or a negative pressure condition. This negative pressure leads to retraction of the tympanic membrane and may lead ultimately to further disease of the middle ear (e.g., otitis media). In some individuals, the tube may be abnormally patent (i.e., open), which is referred to as a patulous Eustachian tube.

Symptoms

The symptoms of Eustachian tube dysfunction depend on the type of dysfunction present. Occlusion of the tube that results in negative middle ear pressure typically results in a sensation of pain and pressure in the ear as the tympanic membrane retracts. Patients also indicate difficulty in "popping" their ears by autoinsufflation and they may also experience tinnitus and disequilibrium. Chronic occlusion of the tube may lead to the development of serous fluid collection within the middle ear, a condition referred to as otitis media with effusion. This effusion leads to a conductive hearing loss and the fluid may become infected leading to acute otitis media. Persistent effusion with associated conductive hearing loss may affect speech and language development in children (Dhooge, 2003).

Patients with patulous Eustachian tubes experience autophony, which is the perception of one's own breath and speech as being excessively loud. This perception of increased loudness of one's breath and speech is due to the existence of a persistently patent or open tube.

Incidence and Prevalence

According to Bluestone (2004), Eustachian tube dysfunction affects 70 to 90% of children by the age of 2 years. He also reported that Eustachian tube dysfunction is more common in children less than 5 years of age, and in males, Native Americans, and patients with lower socioeconomic status.

Etiology and Pathology

Middle ear disease is extremely prevalent in children and can be attributed primarily to a developing Eustachian tube. The fundamental difference between pediatric and adult Eustachian tube anatomy accounts for the increase in dysfunction of this tube in children as compared to adults. The Eustachian tube is shorter in children than in adults and it reaches adult size by 7 years of age (Sadler-Kimes, Siegel, & Todhunter, 1989). In addition, the tube slopes approximately 10° from the horizontal plane of the skull base in infants and young children compared with a 45° slope that is noted in adults (Proctor, 1967). These differences can have a detrimental effect on middle ear ventilation, protection, and clearance.

Obstruction of the tube may be due to intrinsic inflammation within the nasal cavity, middle ear, or the tube itself. Tobacco use, gastroesophageal reflux, nasal polyps, allergic rhinitis, chronic sinusitis, and upper respiratory infections are common causes of this inflammation. Functional obstruction can also occur in children with cleft palate defects because the peritubal muscles are unable to effectively open the distal portion of the Eustachian tube. Extrinsic obstruction of the Eustachian tube may result from the presence of a mass within the nasopharynx, such as a nasopharyngeal carcinoma or adenoid hypertrophy.

Patulous Eustachian tube has been associated with extensive weight loss and pregnancy, which may deplete peritubal soft tissue mass or change tissue characteristics, respectively, allowing the tube to abnormally remain open. In addition, neurologic insult, such as a stroke, and degenerative neurologic disorders, such as multiple sclerosis, may lead to muscle atrophy allowing for abnormal tube patency.

Site of Lesion

The site of pathology leading to Eustachian tube dysfunction may lie on multiple levels. The primary pathology may reside within the nasal cavity as described above with either inflammation or a mass effect obstruction. In addition, the tube can be obstructed due to inflammation within the tube itself, or it functionally may not open due to peritubal muscle dysfunction.

Audiology

Traditional audiologic evaluation typically includes tympanometry to assess middle ear function (see Chapter 3, Audiologic, Vestibular, and Radiologic Procedures). Tympanometry was first reported in the assessment of Eustachian tube dysfunction in the late 1960s (Holmquist, 1969) and has been an integral part of the evaluation since that time (Leo, Piacentini, Incorvaia, & Consonni, 2007). A number of tests can be performed with tympanometric procedures to measure Eustachian tube function. These generally require doing a baseline tympanogram, then creating positive and/or negative pressure in the ear canal and asking the patient to swallow several times. Following this procedure, the tympanogram is retraced. If the peak pressure changes, the Eustachian tube is functioning. If there is no change in the peak pressure, the findings suggest that the Eustachian tube is not functioning.

During tympanometric testing, individuals with patulous Eustachian tubes often show oscillations that correspond to the patient's breathing patterns (inhalations and exhalations), with these oscillations becoming more notable with hard breathing (see Fowler & Shanks, 2002, for more discussion).

When using regular tympanometry, patients who present with Eustachian tube dysfunction (exclusive of patulous tubes) often present with either negative pressure and/or reduced compliance. In addition, a traditional audiologic evaluation including pure-tone threshold testing, speech recognition thresholds, and word recognition testing is recommended to determine if the Eustachian tube dysfunction has impaired the patient's hearing sensitivity. If hearing loss is present, it will be either conductive or mixed in nature (dependent on whether or not a preexisting sensorineural loss is present).

Medical Examination

A thorough examination of the head and neck is vital to diagnosing the etiology of Eustachian tube dysfunction. Otoscopy with pneumatic insufflation is key to determining the appearance of the tympanic membrane, the presence of an effusion, and the compliance of the tympanic membrane. Rhinoscopy assists in identifying nasal masses or inflammatory conditions. A thorough evaluation of the nasopharynx is mandatory and can be accomplished by indirect nasopharyngoscopy or by direct inspection with a flexible nasopharyngoscope. A Valsalva test involves forced expiration with a closed mouth and an occluded nose while the tympanic membrane is inspected. A tympanic membrane bulging laterally as the middle ear space is filled with air indicates a patent Eustachian tube. A Politzer test involves inspection of the tympanic membrane while air is injected into the nasopharynx as the patient swallows. The tympanic membrane should respond in a manner similar to the Valsalva test.

Radiographic evaluation with plain film lateral view x-ray of nasopharyngeal soft tissue may reveal adenoid hypertrophy or other nasopharyngeal masses. Computed tomography and magnetic resonance imaging (MRI) can clearly delineate skull base anatomy and pathology and is routinely utilized in evaluation of masses of the nasopharynx.

Audiologic Management

In most instances, Eustachian tube dysfunction is managed otologically. Audiologic support for this is primarily diagnostic.

Medical Management

Management of Eustachian tube dysfunction depends on the etiology. Inflammatory conditions such as allergies or upper respiratory infections are typically treated medically with oral steroids, intranasal steroid sprays, antihistamines, decongestants, and/or allergy immunotherapy. Obstruction, whether intrinsic or extrinsic, that has been refractory to medical management typically is treated with myringotomy with placement of a pressure equalization (PE) tube to bypass the Eustachian tube and to equalize the pressure between the middle ear and the external environment (Bluestone, 2004). There also are handheld devices that deliver a stream of air to the nasal cavity while the patient swallows that can be used to help equalize pressure. While swallowing, air is diverted into the Eustachian tube, which then can ventilate the middle ear (Silman & Arick, 1999). The use of these devices is not common at this time. Initial clinical experiences appear to be favorable but further evaluation and assessment is needed before these devices are routinely recommended for treatment of Eustachian tube dysfunction.

Case 4–1: Eustachian Tube Dysfunction

History

This 52-year-old male reported 6 weeks of chronic aural fullness and pressure with no noticeable hearing loss. He also reported occasional tinnitus, which he described as a "cracking" sound. No other significant audiologic or otologic symptoms were reported.

Audiology

Routine pure-tone testing revealed hearing thresholds within normal limits for both ears and excellent word recognition performance was noted bilaterally (Figure 4–1).

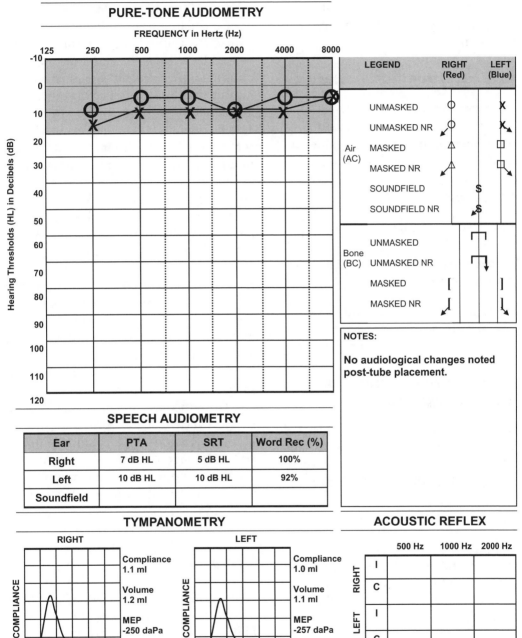

DISORDER: Eustachian Tube Dysfunction

PURE-TONE AUDIOMETRY

SPEECH AUDIOMETRY

Ear	PTA	SRT	Word Rec (%)
Right	7 dB HL	5 dB HL	100%
Left	10 dB HL	10 dB HL	92%
Soundfield			

TYMPANOMETRY

RIGHT
Compliance 1.1 ml
Volume 1.2 ml
MEP -250 daPa

LEFT
Compliance 1.0 ml
Volume 1.1 ml
MEP -257 daPa

ACOUSTIC REFLEX

NOTES:

No audiological changes noted post-tube placement.

Figure 4–1. Pure-tone, speech audiometry, and tympanometry results for a 52-year-old male with Eustachian tube dysfunction (Case 4–1).

Tympanometry indicated normal volume and compliance bilaterally with excessive negative pressure (Type C tympanograms) in both ears.

Medical Examination Result

The patient presented with normal appearing mastoids, pinnae, ear canals, and tympanic membranes without evidence of fluid, perforation, or retraction.

Impression

Suspected Eustachian tube dysfunction.

Audiologic Recommendations and Management

It was recommended that the patient follow up with an otolargynologist, with subsequent audiologic follow-up as necessary.

Medical Recommendations and Management

Following medical and audiologic evaluation it was recommended that the patient undergo a bilateral PE tube placement under local anesthesia in the office.

Additional Comments

The patient received significant benefit from the bilateral PE tube placement, with relief of his pressure and aural fullness symptoms noted post-tube placement bilaterally.

OTITIS MEDIA

Introduction

Otitis media refers to inflammation of the middle ear and involves a broad range of disease processes. This inflammation, which is typically preceded by some form of Eustachian tube dysfunction, is accompanied by a fluid collection (or effusion) behind the tympanic membrane. In acute otitis media, a purulent effusion develops rapidly due to bacterial colonization and is characterized by systemic symptoms. This purulent effusion may resolve into a serous effusion (a collection of fluid in the middle ear space) before complete resolution occurs. The presence of a serous effusion for more than 30 days, regardless of etiology, is referred to as chronic otitis media with effusion. The condition where either three or more bouts of acute otitis media occur within 6 months or four or more episodes of acute otitis media occur in 1 year is referred to as recurrent acute otitis media. Chronic suppurative otitis media refers to persistent inflammation and disease of the middle ear and is discussed further in the cholesteatoma section.

Otitis media is ubiquitous and may be due to a variety of etiologies. Otitis media accounts for one of the most common pediatric diagnoses made by primary care providers and results in a significant consumption of health care funds annually (Bluestone, 2004).

Symptoms

Acute otitis media typically is accompanied by fever, otalgia, pressure, and irritability. These symptoms may be decreased or absent in older patients. Although acute otitis media usually is responsive to antimicrobial therapy, complications that can occur include meningitis, labyrinthitis, petrositis, brain abscess, facial paralysis, and coalescent mastoiditis. Any evidence of mental status change in the case of acute otitis media or of a failure of symptoms to improve after appropriate medical treatment should raise the suspicion of one of these complications.

The presence of an effusion also causes a conductive hearing loss. In some cases, chronic otitis media with effusion may be completely asymptomatic with the exception of a conductive hearing loss.

Incidence and Prevalence

Acute otitis media is extremely prevalent and one study reports an incidence of over 90% in both Caucasian and African American children in the first 2 years of life. Up to age 3, children generally experience at least one episode of acute otitis media per year (Bluestone & Klein, 2007). This disease is more common in young children and occurs much less frequently in children over the age of 6 years (O'Neill, Roberts, & Bradley Stevenson, 2006). The rates of acute otitis media are higher in children with repeated exposure to large numbers of other children, such as in daycare settings (Paradise et al., 1997).

Otitis media with effusion typically presents in children less than 6 years of age and may be secondary to upper respiratory infections or acute otitis media (Rovers, Schilder, Zielhuis, & Rosenfeld, 2004). The rate of middle ear effusion is reported to be higher in pediatric patients in an ICU setting than in other settings (Derkay, Bluestone, Thompson, & Kardatske, 1989), and the incidence of chronic otitis media with effusion is reported to range from 15 to 20% (Zielhuis, Rach, van den Bosch, & van den Broek, 1990).

Etiology and Pathology

An upper respiratory viral infection commonly occurs in conjunction with acute otitis media and results in a breakdown of the protection that the nasal mucosa provides against bacterial infection (Henderson et al., 1982). The primary cause of otitis media is Eustachian tube dysfunction. When bacteria are allowed to colonize the middle ear space, otitis media occurs. The most common bacterial pathogens are *Strepococcus pneumoniae*, *Haemophilus influenzae*, and *Moraxella catarrhalis* (Bluestone, Stephenson, & Martin, 1992). Conditions that impair immune system function, such as diabetes or HIV, can increase the risk of infection. Anatomic abnormalities of the Eustachian tube secondary to craniofacial conditions such as cleft palate also increase risk of acute otitis media. Tobacco smoke exposure, adenoid hypertrophy, lower socioeconomic status, and group daycare attendance are additional risk factors. Finally, chronic infectious or inflammatory granulomatous diseases such as tuberculosis or Wegener's granulomatosis, induce exudation of fluid from the middle ear mucosa, which can lead to the development of otitis media.

Site of Lesion

Otitis media, by definition, is located primarily in the middle ear; however, as previously described, its etiology depends on Eustachian tube dysfunction as bacteria typically migrate or reflux into the middle ear from the nasopharynx. Due to the confluent relationship between the middle ear and the mastoid, an effusion that fills the middle ear typically extends into the mastoid as well. In the situation of acute otitis media, increasing middle ear pressure due to accumulating purulent effusion can lead to perforation of the tympanic membrane and drainage of pus into the external auditory canal (Bluestone & Klein, 2003).

Audiology

The audiologic examination for the patient with otitis media typically includes tympanometry and routine audiologic evaluation appropriate to the patient's age (Aithal, Aithal, & Pulotu, 1995). Tympanometry, although first introduced by Metz in the mid 1940s (Metz, 1946), truly began its clinical integration in the early 1970s. Tympanometry allows for evaluation of the middle ear status with most patients with otitis media presenting with negative pressure and/or reduced compliance. As the disease progresses, tympanograms change from a negative pressure peak early on to a flat tympanometric configuration with significant fluid accumulation in the middle ear at advanced stages of the disease. The audiologic evaluation often reveals a conductive or mixed hearing loss (depending if a preexisting sensorineural loss is present). The configuration of the loss is usually flat with a slight low-frequency tilt (i.e., poorer hearing thresholds in the low frequencies when compared to the high frequencies). This ascending contour is often noted at the beginning of the disease process as the tympanic membrane and the ossicular chain increase in stiffness with decreasing middle ear pressure. As the fluid in the middle ear accumulates over time, a mass effect may result and the configuration becomes flat as the high frequencies also are compromised. The degree of hearing loss is usually in the mild range (20 to 40 dB HL), but it can fluctuate considerably (Jerger & Jerger, 1981).

Medical Examination

Pneumatic otoscopy is key to the diagnosis of otitis media. In acute otitis media, the tympanic membrane appears red and bulging; however, the purulent middle ear effusion behind the eardrum may not be easily visualized due to thickening of the tympanic membrane. Chronic otitis media with effusion is characterized by clear honey-colored fluid in the middle ear. A thorough examination of the upper aerodigestive tract is indicated to identify associated diseases and/or the etiologic causes for otitis media. In addition, the palate must be examined if an adenoidectomy is being considered. Performing an adenoidectomy on a patient with a cleft palate or a submucous cleft can lead to velopharyngeal insufficiency and nasal reflux.

A unilateral effusion in adults, due to the low incidence of otitis media, without a clear precipitating event is a concerning finding. A thorough evaluation of the nasopharynx in these cases must be performed to rule out a neoplasm. Appendixes 4A through 4D provide examples of a normal tympanic membrane, as well as eardrums with a variety of otologic conditions.

Audiologic Management

Audiologic management is reserved for cases in which hearing loss is present and traditional medical management is unsuccessful. Hearing loss typically ranges from mild to moderate depending on the state of the disease. In such cases, either traditional or bone conduction/anchored hearing aids are highly successful. However, long-term complications can evolve and patients should be made aware of this possibility (Hobson et al., 2010). Most patients with purely conductive hearing losses present with excellent word recognition abilities (90–100%); therefore, amplification will provide the additional gain needed for everyday functioning for patients for whom medical intervention is unsuccessful or contraindicated. It should be kept in mind that long-standing conductive hearing loss is a form of auditory deprivation, which in some cases can affect higher order auditory processes. If central auditory dysfunction secondary to auditory deprivation is suspected, then a central auditory processing assessment should be completed and appropriate management procedures implemented (see Chapter 7, Disorders Affecting the Central Auditory Nervous System).

Medical Management

Acute otitis media can resolve spontaneously; however, the use of oral antibiotics helps to shorten the duration of symptoms and prevent complications of otitis media. Compared with simple observation, treatment of acute otitis media with antibiotics results in a 25% decrease in pain in children less than 2 years of age (Rovers et al., 2006). Treatment of acute otitis media with antibiotics, such as amoxicillin, cephalosporins, and macrolides, are directed at the most common organisms found in the middle ear. However, there is some concern regarding the frequent usage of antimicrobial drugs and the bacterial resistance that can result (Goossens, Ferech, Vander Stichele, & Elseviers, 2005).

Recurrent acute otitis media is typically treated with myringotomy and PE tube placement. Currently, tympanostomy (PE) tube placement is recommended in the event of three or more separate episodes of acute otitis media in 6 months or 4 or more episodes in 12 months (Bluestone & Klein, 2003). The placement of the PE tube allows for adequate aeration of the middle ear space preventing the accumulation of an effusion. Tympanostomy tubes also alleviate many of the symptoms of acute otitis media when it occurs. A great variety of tubes are available commercially that differ in size, duration of effectiveness, and composition. Tubes that remain in place longer have a higher risk of leaving a tympanic membrane perforation.

Chronic otitis media with effusion is unlikely to respond to antibiotics (Rosenfeld & Post, 1992); however, this fluid may resolve spontaneously. Observation of nonacute effusion for 3 months is recommended, unless the patient is at risk for speech and language delay. In children at risk, tympanostomy tube placement is recommended.

Adenoidectomy is also a key component of the treatment of otitis media. This procedure has been shown to decrease the morbidity of otitis media (Gates, Avery, Prihoda, & Cooper, 1987). This surgical procedure is performed in cases of persistent or recurrent otitis media following an initial trial with tympanostomy tubes.

Case 4–2: Otitis Media

History

This 3-year-old female was seen for an audiologic evaluation following a failed preschool hearing screening test. The patient's parents reported that their daughter had a history of occasional otitis media and a speech and language delay with no other significant audiologic or neurologic symptoms reported.

Audiology

Pure-tone testing was completed using conditioned play audiometric procedures. Test results documented a mild conductive hearing loss in both ears (Figure 4–2A). Tympanometry revealed little or no compliance bilaterally (Type B tympanograms) and word recognition was excellent for both ears.

DISORDER: Otitis Media Pre-Op

PURE-TONE AUDIOMETRY

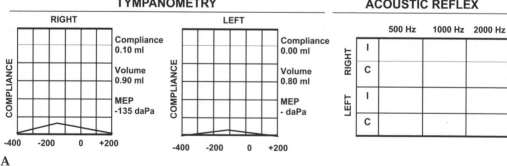

Ear	PTA	SRT	Word Rec (%)
Right	27 dB HL	25 dB HL	100%
Left	38 dB HL	30 dB HL	92%
Soundfield			

SPEECH AUDIOMETRY

TYMPANOMETRY

RIGHT — Compliance 0.10 ml, Volume 0.90 ml, MEP -135 daPa

LEFT — Compliance 0.00 ml, Volume 0.80 ml, MEP - daPa

ACOUSTIC REFLEX

A

Figure 4–2. Pure-tone air and bone conduction thresholds and tympanometry results for a 3-year-old with bilateral otits media (Case 4–2). Results are shown for both preoperative testing (**A**) and postoperative testing (**B**). continues

DISORDER: Otitis Media Post-Op

PURE-TONE AUDIOMETRY

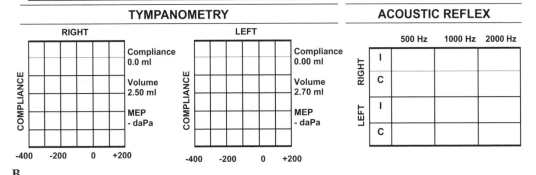

FREQUENCY in Hertz (Hz)

LEGEND		RIGHT (Red)	LEFT (Blue)
Air (AC)	UNMASKED	◯	X
	UNMASKED NR		
	MASKED	△	□
	MASKED NR		
	SOUNDFIELD	S	
	SOUNDFIELD NR		
Bone (BC)	UNMASKED		
	UNMASKED NR		
	MASKED	[	]
	MASKED NR		

NOTES:

SPEECH AUDIOMETRY

Ear	PTA	SRT	Word Rec (%)
Right	5 dB HL	5 dB HL	100%
Left	8 dB HL	5 dB HL	100%
Soundfield			

TYMPANOMETRY

RIGHT

Compliance 0.0 ml
Volume 2.50 ml
MEP - daPa

LEFT

Compliance 0.00 ml
Volume 2.70 ml
MEP - daPa

ACOUSTIC REFLEX

		500 Hz	1000 Hz	2000 Hz
RIGHT	I			
	C			
LEFT	I			
	C			

B

Figure 4–2. continued

119

Medical Examination Result

The patient presented with normal appearing mastoids, pinnae, and ear canals; however, evaluation of the tympanic membranes with a microscope revealed excessive purulent fluid bilaterally.

Impression

Recurrent otitis media with effusion.

Audiologic Recommendations and Management

Reevaluation following medical intervention.

Medical Recommendations and Management

It was recommended that the patient undergo bilateral PE tube placement.

Additional Comments

A postoperative audiogram revealed normal peripheral hearing bilaterally (Figure 4–2B).

Case 4–3: Otitis Media

History

An 83-year-old male with a history of presbycusis was evaluated due to a decrease in his hearing sensitivity and the report of a right-sided aural fullness following an upper respiratory infection lasting 6 months.

Audiology

Test results indicated a mild sloping to severe sensorineural hearing loss in the left ear (Figure 4–3A) and a moderate to severe mixed hearing loss in the right ear. Tympanometry revealed normal pressure, volume, and compliance for the left ear (Type A tympanogram) and reduced compliance and negative pressure with normal volume for the right ear (Type B tympanogram). Word recognition was fair bilaterally.

Medical Examination Result

The patient presented with a normally appearing mastoid, pinna, and ear canal for the left side; however, evaluation of the right tympanic membrane microscopically revealed dullness with excessive fluid.

Impression

Otitis media with effusion in the right ear.

Audiologic Recommendations and Management

Reevaluation following medical intervention.

Medical Recommendations and Management

It was recommended that the patient undergo unilateral PE tube placement in the right ear under local anesthesia in the office.

Additional Comments

One month following PE tube placement, the patient's postoperative audiogram revealed a symmetric sensorineural hearing loss with recovery of the conductive component in the right ear. The tympanogram was flat with large volume (Figure 4–3B).

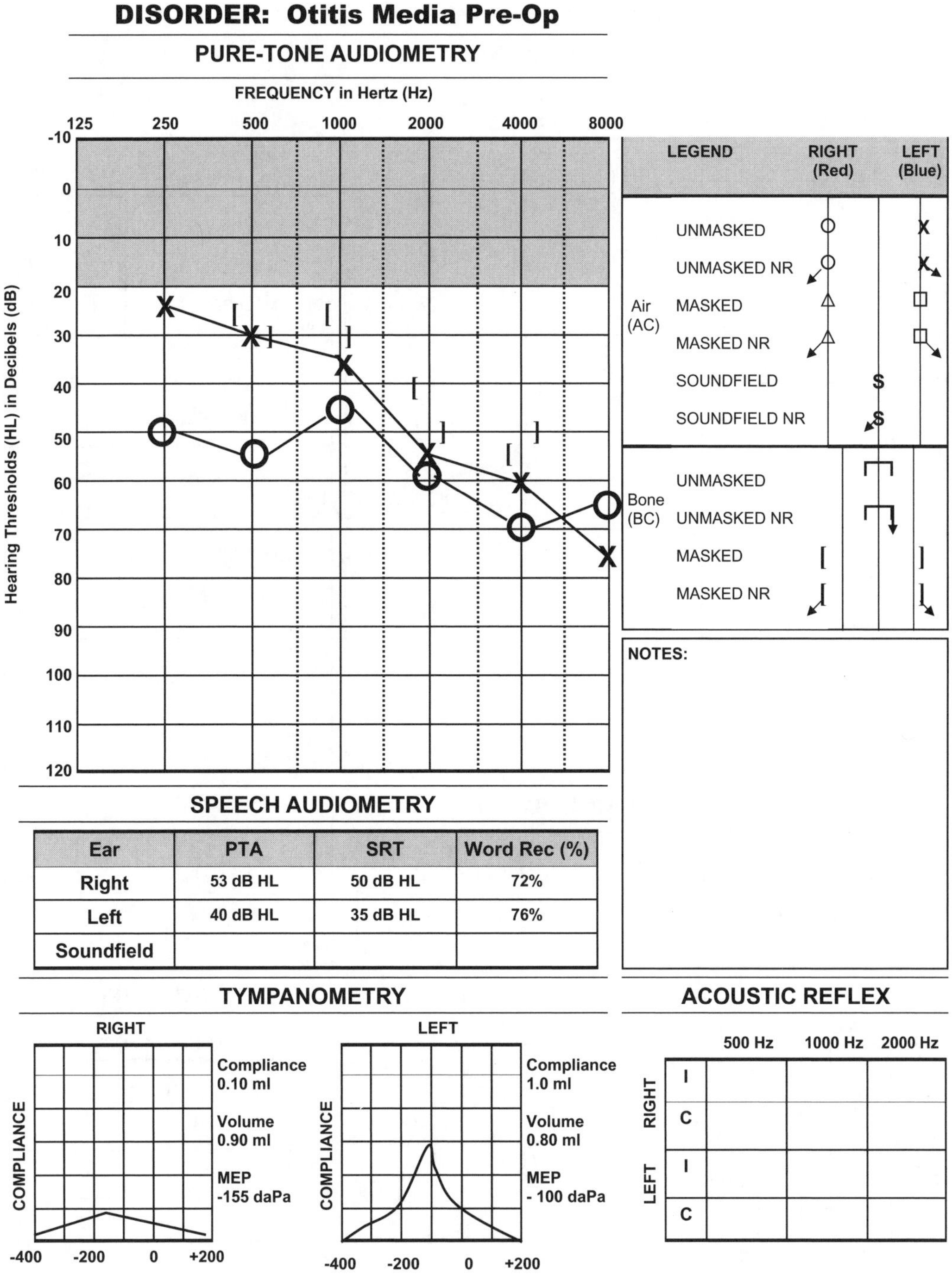

DISORDER: Otitis Media Pre-Op
PURE-TONE AUDIOMETRY
FREQUENCY in Hertz (Hz)
125 250 500 1000 2000 4000 8000
-10 0 10 20 30 40 50 60 70 80 90 100 110 120
Hearing Thresholds (HL) in Decibels (dB)
LEGEND
RIGHT (Red)
LEFT (Blue)
Air (AC)
UNMASKED
UNMASKED NR
MASKED
MASKED NR
SOUNDFIELD
SOUNDFIELD NR
Bone (BC)
UNMASKED
UNMASKED NR
MASKED
MASKED NR
NOTES:
SPEECH AUDIOMETRY
Ear | PTA | SRT | Word Rec (%)
Right | 53 dB HL | 50 dB HL | 72%
Left | 40 dB HL | 35 dB HL | 76%
Soundfield
TYMPANOMETRY
RIGHT
COMPLIANCE
Compliance 0.10 ml
Volume 0.90 ml
MEP -155 daPa
-400 -200 0 +200
LEFT
COMPLIANCE
Compliance 1.0 ml
Volume 0.80 ml
MEP - 100 daPa
-400 -200 0 +200
ACOUSTIC REFLEX
500 Hz 1000 Hz 2000 Hz
RIGHT I C
LEFT I C

A

Figure 4–3. *Pure-tone air and bone conduction thresholds, speech audiometry, and tympanometry results for an 83-year-old male with otitis media in the right ear (Case 4–3). Results are shown for both preoperative testing (**A**) and postoperative testing (**B**).* continues

DISORDER: Otitis Media Post-Op

PURE-TONE AUDIOMETRY

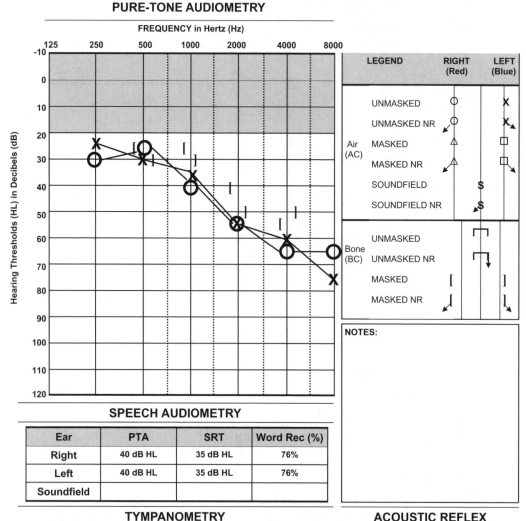

SPEECH AUDIOMETRY

Ear	PTA	SRT	Word Rec (%)
Right	40 dB HL	35 dB HL	76%
Left	40 dB HL	35 dB HL	76%
Soundfield			

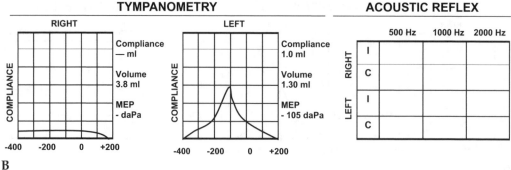

B

Figure 4–3. continued

CHOLESTEATOMA

Introduction

Chronic otitis media is a distinct entity from other forms of otitis media. This disease may manifest itself in the following conditions: persistent perforation of the tympanic membrane, erosion of the ossicles, middle ear granulation tissue, and cholesteatoma. The term, cholesteatoma, is used to describe a collection of keratin-producing squamous epithelial cells within the middle ear. The term, however, is a misnomer in that a cholesteatoma is not a neoplasm. Johannes Müller first described this condition in the 19th century as "a pearly tumor" (Müller, 1838) and presumably this label led to the coining of the term, cholesteatoma, which continues to be the term used for this middle ear pathology. A cholesteatoma contains viable and nonviable squamous epithelial cells with a blend of osteolytic enzymes, cholesterol crystals, and keratin debris.

The middle ear is lined primarily by respiratory cuboidal epithelium, whereas the external auditory canal is lined by squamous epithelial cells, and the tympanic membrane serves as a barrier between the two regions. Cholesteatomas can be either acquired or congenital. An acquired cholesteatoma refers to the collection of squamous epithelial cells that collect either adjacent to, or through, a compromised tympanic membrane to affect middle ear structure and function. There are two types: primary acquired cholesteatoma, which involves a squamous collection within a retracted tympanic membrane pocket, and secondary acquired cholesteatoma, which is characterized by squamous cell migration through a tympanic membrane perforation into the middle ear. A congenital cholesteatoma refers to the presence of squamous cells within the middle ear with no history of tympanic membrane perforation, otitis media, or Eustachian tube dysfunction (Canalis & Lambert, 2000).

Symptoms

Primary cholesteatomas are frequently clinically silent until they reach a size large enough to impinge on the ossicles, causing a conductive hearing loss. A secondary cholesteatoma with bacterial colonization leads to persistent foul-smelling otorrhea due to the presence of chronic inflammation and infection. As a retraction pocket with cholesteatomatous debris deepens in the middle ear space and extends into the mastoid, pain may be experienced and the ossicles may be eroded causing conductive hearing loss. Erosion of bone adjacent to the middle ear can lead to significant complications. An expanding cholesteatoma may damage the facial nerve along its course within the temporal bone leading to facial paralysis. In addition, a fistula of the labyrinth, specifically in the horizontal semicircular canal, may occur with resulting vertigo or dizziness. Finally, erosion of tegmen bone or an intravascular spread of colonized bacteria may lead to meningitis, brain abscess, or subdural empyema. These conditions may be heralded by neurologic symptoms, such as mental status changes, headache, and fever (Penido Nde et al., 2005).

Incidence and Prevalence

Otitis media is a ubiquitous disease; however, chronic otitis media with cholesteatoma is significantly less common.

Congenital cholesteatomas occur at an incidence rate of 0.12 per 100,000 (Tos, 2000). The annual incidence of acquired cholesteatomas in Caucasians has been found to be about 3 per 100,000 in children and 9.2 per 100,000 for people of all ages with a male predominance (Olszewska et al., 2004). Regarding the type of cholesteatoma, the mean age of children with congenital cholesteatomas is 5.6 years, and those with acquired cholesteatomas is 9 years (Nelson et al., 2002).

Etiology and Pathology

A congenital cholesteatoma is felt to be a remnant of embryonic epithelial cell nests trapped in the middle ear during development. Chronic otitis media with secondary cholesteatoma is a result of long-term Eustachian tube dysfunction. Recurrent infections of the middle ear space can irreversibly change the middle ear mucosa (Tos & Bak-Pedersen, 1972). This can change the nature of mucosa from a cuboidal respiratory epithelium to a squamous epithelium, which can deposit keratin debris in the middle ear, according to a metaplasia theory of cholesteatoma development (Sadé, Babiacki, & Pinkus, 1983).

Another mechanism of cholesteatoma formation is invagination of squamous epithelium within a retracted tympanic membrane. Chronic inflammation in the middle ear can lead to weakening of the fibrous layer of the tympanic membrane (Abramson & Huang, 1977). This weakened membrane can be easily retracted by negative middle ear pressure. The region of the tympanic membrane that lacks a fibrous layer, referred to as the pars flaccida, which is the superior portion of the membrane, is the most frequently retracted area. Squamous epithelium of the external layer of a healthy tympanic membrane typically migrates outward in a lateral-to-medial direction and sloughs in the external auditory canal, but when a membrane retraction develops this sloughing epithelium, keratin debris, and a host of bacteria are trapped in this pocket. This matrix of debris leads to further inflammation and may cause the formation of granulation tissue.

The bacteria in a cholesteatoma are diverse and recalcitrant to medical management. The primary organism of chronic otitis media is *Pseudomonas aeruginosa*. Pathogens such as *Staphylococcus aureus*, *Escherichia coli, Streptococcus epidermidis*, as well as a mix of anaerobes, also may be found within a cholesteatoma. Moisture within the pocket and the external ear create an ideal environment for bacterial growth. This pocket has a tendency to expand and tunnel into the middle ear and erode the bone that it comes into contact with by several different mechanisms, including mechanical pressure destruction, biochemical degradation from bacterial toxins or granulation tissue, and cellular absorption of bone by osteoclasts (Canalis & Lambert, 2000). The ossicles are frequently eroded by an expanding cholesteatoma. Other sites of bony erosion include the bone covering the horizontal portion of the facial nerve and the tegmen tympani and/or the tegmen mastoideum, which separate the middle ear and mastoid, respectively, from dura (Amar, Wishahi, & Zakhary, 1996).

Chronic marginal perforations of the tympanic membrane can result in squamous cell migration into the middle ear and the development of a secondary acquired cholesteatoma. In addition, traumatic perforation of the tympanic membrane, such as a blast injury or temporal bone fracture, may deposit keratin-forming squamous cells within the middle ear that may result in a secondary acquired cholesteatoma (Canalis & Lambert, 2000).

Site of Lesion

Cholesteatomas tend to develop in predictable locations in the middle ear and temporal bone. Embryonic cell nests may pathologically remain in the middle ear during development leading to a congenital cholesteatoma. Within the middle ear, this usually occurs in the anterior mesotympanum or the protympanum. A congenital cholesteatoma also may occur within the petrous apex of the temporal bone and usually is referred to as an epidermoid cyst.

The most common location of a primary acquired cholesteatoma is the posterior epitympanic space, also known as Prussak's space (Palva, Ramsay, & Böhling, 1996). A cholesteatoma in this region extends posteriorly into the mastoid by way of the antrum. In this confined space, the head of the malleus and the short process of the incus can easily be eroded by the disease process. The anterior aspect of the epitympanic space can also be involved by a cholesteatoma, which typically invades the mesotympanum anterior to the handle of the malleus. The posterior aspect of the pars tensa may also become retracted and result in a primary acquired cholesteatoma that extends into the posterior mesotympanum. In the same region, perforation of the tympanic membrane may be the site of development of a secondary acquired cholesteatoma. Cholesteatomas can also extend into the petrous portion of the temporal bone. Appendix 4E presents an example of tympanic membrane with a cholesteatoma.

Audiology

The audiologic examination for a patient with a cholesteatoma should involve routine tympanometry to evaluate middle ear function and comprehensive audiometry to determine hearing sensitivity. There is significant variability with respect to tympanometric results in patients with cholesteatoma, with this variability dependent on the degree of ossicular chain involvement. For cases with very little ossicular chain involvement, normal pressure, volume, and compliance may be observed. However, once the ossicular chain becomes involved, compliance is significantly reduced. Patients with no underlying sensorineural involvement generally present with a purely conductive hearing loss on the affected side. In rare cases, patients will present with normal peripheral hearing sensitivity (see Jerger & Jerger, 1981).

Medical Examination

A vital aspect of successful diagnosis and treatment of cholesteatoma involves obtaining a detailed otologic history. Documentation must be made of the history of otitis media as well as tympanostomy tube placement, which may indicate a long history of Eustachian tube dysfunction. The duration and character of otorrhea is also an important aspect of the otologic history. Due to the chronic nature and high recurrence rate of cholesteatomas, these patients may have had multiple operations. Previous surgical reports can provide vital clues to the initial presentation of the disease as well as to the extent of bone erosion caused by the disease processes. Inquiries should be made regarding a history of hearing loss, otalgia, tinnitus, and vertigo.

A thorough head and neck examination should accompany a careful otologic examination. Otomicroscopy is used to thoroughly clean the external canal of drainage and debris. In early stages of chronic otitis media, the epitympanic area of the tympanic membrane may have a shallow retraction pocket. Determination of the depth of the pocket and the presence of keratin debris should be made. As this pocket expands, the depth of the pocket cannot be visualized and successful removal of all of the debris is uncertain. The debris within the pocket may be of differing consistencies and color; however, classically, a cholesteatoma looks like white cake icing. Granulation tissue may be present in this region. If it is present, it is beefy red in color and has a propensity to bleed when manipulated. This granulation tissue may also appear polypoid and this polyp may extend into the external auditory canal. Bone erosion typically occurs along the scutum or posterior bony wall and ossicular erosion may be identified when any debris has been removed. Pneumatic otoscopy with a fistula test can also reveal bony erosion of the horizontal semicircular canal. A tuning fork exam may indicate a significant conductive hearing loss.

The utilization of imaging in the case of chronic otitis media varies greatly among otologists. Radiographic imaging of the temporal bone can be helpful in delineating anatomy and may provide some information regarding the extent of disease. High-resolution thin slice CT of the temporal bone without contrast is frequently utilized if there are atypical symptoms, complications of otitis media, or suspicion of bony erosion of the tegmen, facial nerve, or the labyrinth. Computed tomography scans can also be particularly useful in preoperative planning for revision surgical procedures.

Audiologic Management

Similar to other middle ear disorders, patients with cholesteatomas will require amplification if traditional medical management is unsuccessful.

Medical Management

Chronic otitis media requires close clinical follow-up. Subtle changes on examination or in history may herald progression of the disease. With the use of otomicroscopy, retraction pockets can be evaluated and cleaned regularly. Some retractions may remain stable for years without progression or development of an invasive cholesteatoma, and monitoring may be the best treatment option for those that are poor surgical candidates. Generally, observation of a chronically diseased ear is not recommended for children. Avoidance of water exposure to the external auditory canal can be helpful in decreasing moisture within a retraction pocket and thus decrease bacterial overgrowth. Ototopical drops composed of antibiotics with or without steroids are commonly used to treat persistent drainage and inflammation associated with chronic otitis media with cholesteatoma. Placement of a PE tube can aerate the middle ear and may prevent progression of tympanic membrane retraction. Although medical treatment can alleviate the symptoms of cholesteatomas, it does not address the etiology of the problem. Irreversible damage to the middle ear, which is the case in chronic otitis media with cholesteatoma, requires surgical intervention. The purpose of surgical treatment of cholesteatoma is to create a safe dry ear. A secondary goal of surgical intervention is the restoration of hearing. Tympanoplasty is a surgical procedure in which disease is removed from the middle ear and a weakened or perforated tympanic membrane is repaired. Auricular perichondrium, with or without cartilage, and temporalis fascia are commonly used to repair and reinforce the tympanic membrane. Mastoidectomy, which may be performed along with tympanoplasty, involves the removal of chronic disease within the mastoid air cells. A complete mastoidectomy, or canal wall up (CWU) mastoidectomy, involves careful removal of the cholesteatoma and diseased mucosa within the air cells of the mastoid by drilling the cholesteatoma and any diseased mucosa away. The posterior canal wall is left intact in this procedure and candidates for this procedure have an aerated mastoid and reasonable Eustachian tube function. It is imperative to remove all of the cholesteatoma during the procedure because even a microscopic remnant of squamous debris within the mastoid or middle ear can lead to a recurrence. It is impossible to evaluate the mastoid cavity in the clinic following a CWU mastoidectomy, thus a re-look procedure is recommended in 6 to12 months to inspect for recurrent disease. During a re-look procedure, the status of the ossicles can be examined and ossiculoplasty can be performed to restore ossicular continuity and function, if needed. A CWU mastoidectomy can only be performed in a reliable patient as failure to follow up can result in devastating progression of recurrent disease. The advantage of a CWU mastoidectomy is that the anatomy of the external auditory ear and tympanic membrane is restored; thus, water exposure of the external auditory canal following the surgical procedure is safe. The ear that has undergone a CWU mastoidectomy also can be amplified with a hearing aid more easily than one that has undergone alternative treatments. Historically, mastoidectomy included removal of the posterior wall of the external auditory canal to create a wide-open cavity that could easily be cleaned and evaluated for recurrence in a clinic setting. This procedure is now called a modified radical mastoidectomy or canal wall down (CWD) mastoidectomy. The indications for this procedure are the presence of recurrent disease, a labyrinthine fistula, extensive destruction of the posterior canal wall by cholesteatoma, cholesteatoma in an only hearing ear, recurrent disease following CWU mastoidectomy, a sclerotic mastoid, or a patient who is unreliable or unlikely to follow through with a re-look procedure. The disadvantage of a CWD mastoidectomy is that the ear must remain dry or significant infection can occur within the cavity. Also, the mastoid bowl must be examined regularly in clinic to remove debris as this cavity cannot be self-cleaning by nature. This procedure typically provides a safe ear in which recurrence can be caught easily and removed without significant risk or discomfort to the patient (Bennett, Warren, & Haynes, 2006).

Case 4–4: Cholesteatoma

History

This 70-year-old male with a long-standing history of mastoiditis and meningitis was seen for re-evaluation due to the presence of chronic discharge from both ears for the past 2 years. The patient's medical conditions had resulted in diminished hearing and he previously had been fitted with binaural amplification, which he continues to use.

Audiology

A comprehensive audiologic examination revealed a severe to profound mixed hearing loss in the left ear and a profound mixed hearing loss in the right ear (Figure 4–4). Word recognition was good for the left ear, but could not be evaluated for the right ear. Tympanometry indicated reduced compliance bilaterally (Type B tympanograms) with a large volume noted for the left ear.

Medical Examination Result

The patient presented with an anterior tympanic membrane perforation on the left side. The right tympanic membrane presented no visible landmarks due to thickening. A CT examination was ordered, which revealed a significant cholesteatoma in the right ear. The cholesteatoma had eroded a significant amount of bone and had exposed the dura on the right side. The left ear continued to present with chronic infection.

Impression

Unilateral cholesteatoma.

Audiologic Recommendations and Management

It was recommended that the patient continue with the use of binaural amplification following medical management.

Medical Recommendations and Management

Following medical and audiologic evaluation, it was recommended that the patient undergo a right radical mastoidectomy.

Additional Comments

The patient chose to undergo the recommended surgical procedure (i.e., right radical mastoidectomy). Results of that surgery revealed an extensive cholesteatoma, which had eroded much of the cochlea and the horizontal semicircular canal in the right ear. This was likely the source of the patient's prior history of meningitis. The patient has done well since the surgery; however, no improvement in hearing was observed postoperatively.

Case 4–5: Cholesteatoma

History

This 9-year-old male presented with a long-standing history of intermittent drainage and recurrent infection in the left ear. No other significant audiologic or otologic symptoms were reported.

Audiology

A comprehensive audiologic examination revealed normal peripheral hearing sensitivity for the right ear and a severe

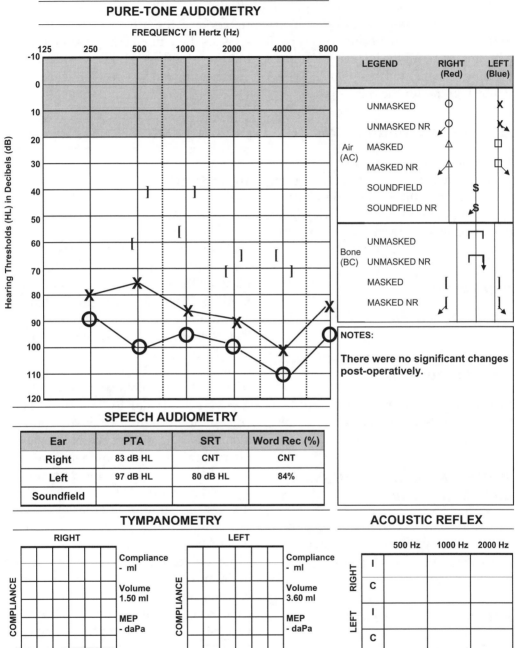

DISORDER: Cholesteatoma Pre- & Post-Op

PURE-TONE AUDIOMETRY

SPEECH AUDIOMETRY

Ear	PTA	SRT	Word Rec (%)
Right	83 dB HL	CNT	CNT
Left	97 dB HL	80 dB HL	84%
Soundfield			

NOTES:

There were no significant changes post-operatively.

TYMPANOMETRY

ACOUSTIC REFLEX

Figure 4–4. *Pure-tone air and bone conduction results, speech audiometry, and tympanometry for a 70-year-old male with a right-sided cholesteatoma (Case 4–4).*

rising to mild conductive hearing loss for the left ear (Figure 4–5). Word recognition was excellent bilaterally. Tympanometry indicated reduced compliance (Type B tympanogram) for the left ear and normal pressure, volume, and compliance (Type A tympanogram) for the right ear.

Medical Examination Result

The patient presented with an obvious pars flaccida cholesteatoma extending into the attic in the left ear and a normal appearing mastoid, pinna, ear canal, and tympanic membrane without fluid, perforation, or retraction in the right ear.

Impression

Left-sided cholesteatoma.

Audiologic Recommendations and Management

Reevaluation and possible amplification for the left ear following medical management.

Medical Recommendations and Management

It was recommended that the patient undergo left mastoidectomy and tympanoplasty with possible ossicular chain reconstruction.

Additional Comments

The patient's parents chose to have their son undergo the recommended surgery. Results of that surgery revealed an extensive cholesteatoma, which required revision 5 months postoperatively. Audiologic test results following surgery revealed

significant improvement in hearing sensitivity, as well as improved middle ear function in the affected ear (see Figure 4–5). As the patient still presented with a mild hearing loss on the left side, a mild gain hearing aid was recommended.

GLOMUS TUMORS

Introduction

Glomus tumors are benign slow-growing highly vascularized neoplasms that may occur in various regions of the body. They are the second most common benign neoplasm of the temporal bone, after the vestibular schwannoma. The understanding and resulting treatment of glomus tumors has evolved dramatically in the past century. In 1941, while examining a series of human temporal bones, Stacy Guild identified a discrete collection of capillary-size vessels similar to the carotid body adjacent to the jugular bulb and coursing along the tympanic branch of the glossopharyngeal nerve (Jacobson's nerve) and the auricular branch of the vagus nerve (Arnold's nerve). He referred to these masses as "glomus jugularie" (Guild, 1941). Rosenwasser recognized Guild's description and gave confirmation of a distinct disease process as he reported on the removal of a glomus jugulare tumor in 1945 (Rossenwasser, 1945). Initially, it was thought that glomus tumors were vascular in origin; however, they actually arise from a collection of neuroendocrine paraganglial cells originating from neural crest cells and are surrounded by a dense collection of capillaries and venules. These tumors have also been referred to as paragangliomas.

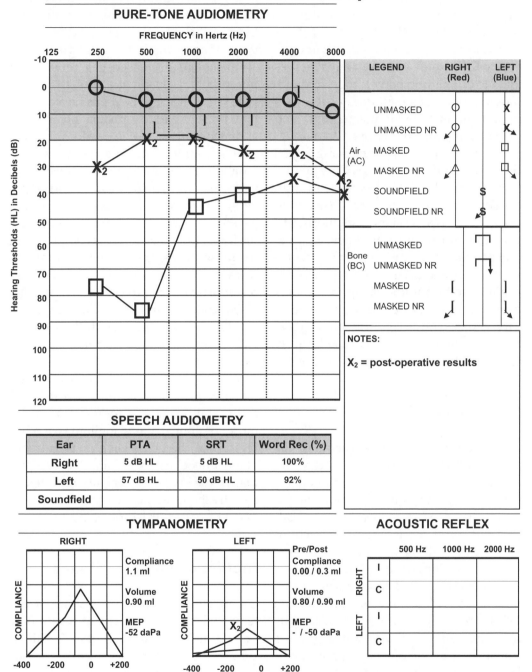

DISORDER: Cholesteatoma Pre- & Post-Op

PURE-TONE AUDIOMETRY

SPEECH AUDIOMETRY

Ear	PTA	SRT	Word Rec (%)
Right	5 dB HL	5 dB HL	100%
Left	57 dB HL	50 dB HL	92%
Soundfield			

NOTES:

X₂ = post-operative results

TYMPANOMETRY

RIGHT
Compliance 1.1 ml
Volume 0.90 ml
MEP -52 daPa

LEFT
Pre/Post Compliance 0.00 / 0.3 ml
Volume 0.80 / 0.90 ml
MEP - / -50 daPa

ACOUSTIC REFLEX

Figure 4–5. Pure-tone air and bone conduction results, speech audiometry, and tympanometry for a 9-year-old with a left-sided cholesteatoma (Case 4–5). Results are shown for both preoperative and postoperative testing. Postoperative pure-tone thresholds are indicated by X₂ for the left ear. Right ear test results remained unchanged.

Paragangliomas may be present throughout the body, but temporal bone tumors are classified based on their location. Cervical paragangliomas occur adjacent to the carotid artery or cranial nerves and include carotid body tumors and glomus vagale. Paragangliomas of the temporal bone include glomus jugulare and glomus tympanicum tumors. Glomus jugulare tumors develop from paranglial tissue within the adventitia of the jugular bulb (Gulya, 1993) and may extend from the skull base into and through the temporal bone to cause significant morbidity. Glomus tympanicum tumors develop from paraganglion adjacent to either Jacobson's nerve or Arnold's nerve and typically are confined to the middle ear space but may extend into the mastoid or external auditory canal. The ascending pharyngeal artery provides the primary blood supply to glomus tumors of the temporal bone.

Symptoms

The symptoms of glomus tumors of the temporal bone are variable and develop gradually due to a slow growth pattern. As a glomus tympanicum tumor fills the middle ear, conductive hearing loss, otalgia, and aural fullness may be encountered. The hallmark symptom of this highly vascular lesion is pulsatile tinnitus, which is reported to be present in 76% of patients (Woods, Strasnick, & Jackson, 1993). Any patient with pulsatile tinnitus must be fully evaluated for a glomus tumor. Destruction of the tympanic membrane and bleeding can occur but are uncommon. Expansion of the tumor within the mastoid can compromise the facial nerve leading to paralysis, and erosion of the labyrinth can occur resulting in vertigo and sensorineural hearing loss. A glomus jugulare tumor may also affect other cranial nerves, most commonly the contents of the jugular foramen. Glossopharyngeal nerve injury typically presents as an absent or decreased gag reflex with potential for dysphagia due to loss of pharyngeal sensation. Vagus nerve injury may present with dysphagia, hoarseness, and recurrent aspiration due loss of laryngeal sensation and unilateral vocal fold paralysis. The accessory nerve, which innervates the sternocleidomastoid and trapezius, can present as neck and shoulder weakness when it is compromised. Finally, the hypoglossal nerve can be compromised resulting in ipsilateral tongue paralysis. Intracranial extension of the tumor can result in mental status changes, headache, visual changes, and strokelike symptoms.

Glomus tumors, due to their neuroendocrine origin, may secrete vasoactive catecholamines, which when present in significant amounts may cause hypertension, palpitations, diaphoresis, and arrhythmias. These symptoms are much more common in paragangliomas of other regions of the body, such as an adrenal gland pheochromocytoma. Paragangliomas of the head and neck are reported to be actively hormone secreting in less than 4% of the cases (Erickson et al., 2001).

Incidence and Prevalence

Glomus tumors are rare lesions of the temporal bone and occur at a rate of 1 per 1.3 million people (Moffat & Hardy, 1989). Paragangliomas typically are isolated lesions, but other tumors, such as contralateral lesions, carotid body tumors, or glomus vagale tumors, can occur in up to 10% of patients (Spector, Ciralsky, & Ogura, 1975). Neoplasms of neural crest cell origin may also be found in

7% of these patients (Spector, Maisel, & Ogura, 1974). Glomus tumors are more common in Caucasians and in women (O'Leary, Shelton, Giddings, Kwartler, & Brackmann, 1991). They also have a predilection to be transmitted in an autosomal dominant pattern with variable penetrance within families and these patients are at a higher risk of multiple tumors (Horn & Hankinson, 1994).

Etiology and Pathology

Glomus tumors are composed of two cells types. Chief cells, which are the neuroendocrine cells, are filled with vasoactive compounds that can be secreted as described above. Sustentacular cells are similar to Schwann cells and support the chief cells. This cluster of cells is surrounded by a dense network of capillaries and venules. This tumor is typically benign, slow growing, and travels along the path of least resistance. Traveling through haversian canals of the bone and within mastoid air space, these tumors gradually erode the temporal bone. They can place vital neural and vascular structures at risk with their diffuse yet insidious growth; thus, appropriate management of these tumors has involved multidisciplinary innovation and collaboration.

Metastasis of glomus tumors occurs in approximately 1 to 4% of the patients (Borsanyi, 1962; Brown, 1985) and this condition appears to be more prevalent in those with familial inheritance of the disease.

Site of Lesion

Glomus tympanicum tumors are found in the middle ear space and originate from paraganglia traveling along Jacobson's or Arnold's nerve on the promontory, which is the bone overlying the basal turn of the cochlea (Appendix 4F). Glasscock and Jackson developed a classification system for these tumors based on their location within the middle ear space and surrounding areas (Table 4–1) (Jackson, Glasscock, & Harris, 1982).

Glomus jugular tumors develop from the adventitia of the jugular bulb just below the hypotympanum. Two separate location classification systems have been developed. Fisch first described in 1979 a classification system that does not distinguish between jugulare and tympanicum tumors, but simply describes tumor extension (Table 4–2) (Oldring & Fisch, 1979). Glasscock and Jackson later offered their jugular classification system (Table 4–3) (Jackson et al., 1982). Both systems are used widely.

Table 4–1. Glasscock-Jackson Glomus Tympanicum Classification (1982)

Type I	Mass limited to the promontory
Type II	Mass fills the middle ear space
Type III	Mass fills the middle ear and extends into mastoid
Type IV	Mass fills middle ear, mastoid, and extends into the external auditory canal

Table 4–2. Fisch Glomus Classification (1982)

Class A	Mass limited to the middle ear
Class B	Mass limited to the middle ear and mastoid without destruction of bone in the infralabyrinthine compartment
Class C1	Mass extends into infralabyrinthine compartment with destruction of the jugular foramen and jugular bulb
Class C2	Mass extends into infralabyrinthine compartment with involvement of vertical portion of the carotid canal
Class C3	Mass extends into infralabyrinthine compartment with involvement of the horizontal portion of the carotid canal
Class D1	Mass with up to 2 cm of intracranial extension
Class D2	Mass with greater than 2 cm of intracranial extension
Class D3	Mass with inoperable intracranial extension

Table 4–3. Glasscock-Jackson Glomus Jugulare Classification (1982)

Type I	Mass involving the jugular bulb, middle ear, and mastoid
Type II	Mass extends under the internal auditory canal
Type III	Mass extends into the petrous apex
Type IV	Mass extends into the clivus or infratemporal fossa

Audiology

On audiologic examination, patients may present with virtually any pattern of hearing loss (conductive, mixed, or sensorineural); however, in rare cases, the patient may present with normal peripheral hearing sensitivity. In a retrospective investigation, conductive hearing loss accounted for nearly 76% of the hearing losses observed (Fayad, Keles, & Brackmann, 2010). Additionally, tympanometry may yield a variety of test results, but has demonstrated utility in the evaluation of these vascular lesions (Leveque, Bialostozky, Blanchard, & Suter, 1979). One unique sign that may be observed during tympanometry is a pulsating beat, which can be seen throughout the immittance recordings. This pulsation is typically synchronous with the patient's heart beat (Jerger & Jerger, 1981).

Medical Examination

The examination of a patient with a glomus tumor must be careful and thorough. Vital sign documentation may uncover hypertension or tachycardia present from a secreting tumor. Otoscopic examination may reveal a bluish or reddish mass behind the tympanic membrane. Upon insufflation of the membrane one may see a blush of the mass, which is known as Brown sign (Karas & Kwartler, 1993). A glomus tumor may erode through the membrane and present as a mass within the external auditory canal. Biopsy of a polyp or mass within the external auditory canal is not advised in the outpatient clinic due to the risk of brisk bleeding. A thorough cranial nerve exam during the head and neck exam is vital to document deficits due to tumor extension.

If a secreting tumor is suspected, laboratory tests should include a 24-hour urine test. This test can detect vasoactive tumor products, such as vanillylmandelic acid and epinephrine derivatives.

Imaging studies are vital to correct diagnosis and management of patients with glomus tumors. Computed tomography scans of the temporal bone and skull base with contrast can provide evidence of bone erosion by the tumor and additionally help to document the extent of the compromise. Magnetic resonance imaging (MRI) with contrast provides definition of the tumor itself and delineates the presence and degree of intracranial extension. The typical appearance of the tumor is a "salt and pepper" pattern, which is due to flow voids within vessels of the tumor. Angiography is also helpful in the diagnosis and may be combined with treatment by embolization.

Audiologic Management

Audiologic management is dependent on surgical outcome and degree of involvement. Patients who present with favorable outcomes following surgery resulting in essentially no hearing loss will only need to be monitored audiologically. However, patients who continue to present with peripheral involvement or who have complications following surgery may benefit from traditional amplification.

Medical Management

Typically, glomus tympanicum tumors are treated surgically. The removal of tumors in Glassock-Jackson classes I and II may be removed through a tympanoplasty approach. A laser is sometimes utilized to assist with hemostasis. Surgical intervention for classes III and IV tumors may involve a mastoidectomy. Complete excision is important in these cases as small remnants of tumor can create a sizable recurrence.

Glomus jugulare tumor treatment has become controversial. Treatment options, other than observation, include radiation therapy, surgery, or a combination of both. Because these are slow growing tumors many patients may opt for observation for a period of time. However, radiation treatment of glomus jugulare tumors is recommended as the primary treatment in some institutions (Saringer, Khayal, Ertl, Schoeggl, & Kitz, 2001; Sheehan, Kondziolka, Flickinger, & Lunsford, 2005). Patients with advanced disease or advanced age may benefit from primary radiation. One study found a difference of 10% in treatment failures between radiation and surgery favoring radiation (Carrasco & Rosenman, 1993). Surgery for glomus jugulare tumor is extensive in nature and not without complication. The approach is based on the extension of the tumor and is quite variable. Some basic elements present in surgical management of Glasscock-Jackson types I and II tumors involve identification and ligation of the internal jugular vein in the neck. Similarly, the sigmoid sinus is identified and occluded. A mastoidectomy to access the tumor is performed, which may involve mobilization of the facial nerve. Tumor margins are identified and the tumor is removed carefully. Types III and IV tumors require access to the deep portion of the temporal bone, skull base, and potentially to the intracranial space. A defect within the surgical site can be reconstructed using multiple techniques. A significant complication of this surgery includes damage to cranial nerves. Dysfunction of previously functioning cranial nerves occurs postoperatively in 25 to 50% of patients (Pensak & Jackler, 1997). Many surgeons opt to not surgically remove tumors when the patient develops dysfunction of these lower cranial nerves as surgery places them at significant risk. Vagus nerve damage leading to chronic aspiration and even to feeding tube dependence can be devastating to patients of any age. During preoperative angiography, embolization of feeding arterial vessels can be performed and can assist with decreasing the amount of bleeding during surgical resection.

Combination of surgery and radiation may be a beneficial option. Incomplete removal of tumor is typically treated with postoperative radiation. Patel and colleagues reported on complication rates in patients with combination therapy and found that the incidence of facial and lower cranial nerve injury was similar to those rates from traditional infratemporal fossa resections (Patel, Sekhar, Cass, & Hirsch, 1994).

Case 4–6: Glomus Tumor

History

This 44-year-old female presented with a persistent left-sided pulsatile tinnitus.

She indicated that the tinnitus was initially faint, mild, and intermittent, but that over the past 2 years it had become very noticeable and constant. No other significant audiologic or otologic history was reported.

Audiology

Audiologic test results demonstrated normal peripheral hearing sensitivity and excellent word recognition bilaterally (Figure 4–6). Tympanometry revealed normal volume and compliance for the right ear, with borderline normal middle ear pressure (−105 daPa). For the right ear, the tympanogram was of unusual shape, showing high compliance with normal middle ear pressure and volume measures.

Medical Examination Result

The patient presented with a normal appearing mastoid, pinna, external auditory canal, and tympanic membrane on the right side. The left ear canal presented with erythematous changes of the posterior canal wall with a bulging erythematous pulsatile mass posteriorly-inferiorly and within the posterior portion of the tympanic membrane. Results from the CT evaluation demonstrated a very large vascular lesion (2.4 cm) with expansion into and erosion of the skull base.

Impression

Large left-sided glomus jugulare tumor.

Audiologic Recommendations and Management

Reevaluation following medical intervention.

DISORDER: Glomus Tumor Pre- & Post-Op

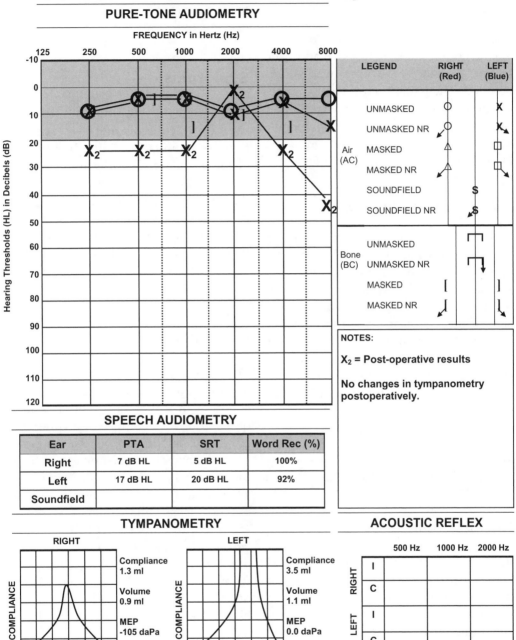

PURE-TONE AUDIOMETRY

SPEECH AUDIOMETRY

Ear	PTA	SRT	Word Rec (%)
Right	7 dB HL	5 dB HL	100%
Left	17 dB HL	20 dB HL	92%
Soundfield			

NOTES:

X₂ = Post-operative results

No changes in tympanometry postoperatively.

TYMPANOMETRY

RIGHT — Compliance 1.3 ml, Volume 0.9 ml, MEP -105 daPa

LEFT — Compliance 3.5 ml, Volume 1.1 ml, MEP 0.0 daPa

ACOUSTIC REFLEX

Figure 4–6. Pure-tone air and bone conduction results, speech audiometry, and tympanometry for a 44–year-old female with a glomus tumor on the left side (Case 4–6). Postoperative findings are indicated by X₂ for the left ear and right ear test results remained the same.

Medical Recommendations and Management

A CT scan was recommended to evaluate the middle ear structures. In addition, surgical excision of the tumor was recommended. The patient underwent the recommended surgery where a combined jugular vein, jugular bulb, sigmoid sinus, and infratemporal fossa resection of the large glomus tumor was performed.

Additional Comments

After surgery, there was a decrease in pure-tone hearing (X_2) (see Figure 4–6). However, speech recognition remained excellent bilaterally. Although the patient did well following surgery, she has had significant recurrence of the tumor and has undergone multiple surgeries for continued removal of the lesion. Interestingly, she has had little loss of hearing in light of the extensive tumor involvement (see Figure 4–6).

OTOSCLEROSIS

Introduction

In 1704 Valsalva first identified a fixed stapes during a cadaveric dissection (Canalis, 1990). Subsequently, Toynbee studied many cases of stapes fixation and found the fixation to exist around the margins of the oval window (Toynbee, 1841). Politzer (1894) is known for the first histologic evaluation of otosclerosis by demonstrating abnormal bone of the otic capsule. Otosclerosis is a metabolic bone-remodeling disease of the temporal bone. It primarily affects the otic capsule and the ossicles. A change in the character and composition of the bone results in hearing loss.

Symptoms

The hallmark symptom of otosclerosis is conductive hearing loss. Typically, the loss is unilateral initially, but often becomes bilateral with time. Tinnitus may also be present; however, vertigo or dizziness is uncommon. If the disease is progressive, sensorineural hearing loss or deafness may develop. A family history is usually positive for this disease process and a history of chronic otitis media is typically absent.

Incidence and Prevalence

This disease is the most common cause of adult conductive hearing loss. It is more common in Caucasian patients and an otosclerotic focus of disease is present in 10% of this population, but approximately 1% of the overall population is affected by the disease (Levin, Fabian, & Stahle, 1988). Women are more commonly affected by the disease than men (Cawthorne, 1955) and the disease typically presents between the 2nd and 4th decades of life, but it may present at any age. Pregnancy seems to accelerate the presentation of the disease; thus, this may be a reason for the higher prevalence in women. The disease has an autosomal dominant transmission pattern with incomplete penetrance.

Etiology and Pathology

In the endocondral bone of the otic capsule affected areas become highly vascularized and the bone is resorbed. Immature bone is laid down in this area and eventually becomes mineralized. This happens in discrete areas throughout the otic capsule leaving a mosaic pattern. When this occurs around the oval window, the stapes footplate becomes fixed and fails to conduct sound into the cochlear efficiently. If the cochlea becomes involved, a sensorineural component to the hearing can also occur, resulting in a mixed hearing loss (Doherty & Linthicum, 2004).

Site of Lesion

The most common site of otosclerotic bone is an area just anterior to the stapes footplate, referred to as the fissula ante fenestrum. This is the site that can fix the footplate in position causing a conductive hearing loss. Another focus of otosclerosis can be the round window, which can be completely obliterated by the disease. Recent research indicates that cochlear otosclerosis involves damage to the spiral ligament, thus leading to progressive sensorineural hearing loss (Doherty & Linthicum, 2004).

Audiology

Careful audiologic evaluation is a key component to the diagnosis and management of otosclerosis. Comprehensive audiometry should include air and bone conduction, as well as speech threshold and word recognition testing. The hallmark audiologic finding in patients with otosclerosis is a conductive hearing loss. The amount of conductive involvement often correlates with the degree of stapes fixation. One cannot discuss audiologic patterns of otosclerosis without mention-

ing the Carhart notch. First described by Carhart in 1950, the Carhart notch has been routinely observed in otosclerotic patients. This notch results in a reduction of bone conduction thresholds, particularly at 2000 Hz; however, it may be observed at alternative frequencies. This notch in the bone conduction thresholds is attributed to abnormal mechanical effects on the middle ear system secondary to stapes fixation. Often, the pure-tone air-conduction audiogram shows an ascending configuration. This is likely related to the increased stiffness of the middle ear system and is termed the "stiffness tilt" (Hannley, 1993).

Speech recognition typically is excellent in patients who present with purely conductive involvement; however, patients who have comorbid sensorineural involvement may show diminished word recognition abilities correlated to the degree of pathology. Tympanometry results in these patients will often be normal or demonstrate reduced compliance (Jacobson & Mahoney, 1977; Sutherland &Campbell, 1990). However, in many of the cases with normal compliance, the width of the tympanogram shape is reduced (Ivy, 1975). Immittance audiometry typically will yield elevated or absent acoustic reflexes (Probst, 2007). However, a general exception to this rule is for patients early in the clinical course of the disease. These individuals can present with reflexes at normal or near normal levels. However, an unusual negative deflection often is observed in their tracings at both the onset and the offset of the eliciting stimulus (Rane, Yut, & Berger, 1978).

Audiologic findings are particularly important in cases where surgical intervention is being considered. Successful surgery will often result in partial or complete closure of the presurgical air-bone gap.

Medical Examination

Examination of the otosclerotic ear reveals a normal tympanic membrane with normal mobility. In active forms of the disease, which are characterized by hypervascularity and bone resorption, the promontory may have a reddish hue that can be visualized on otoscopic exam. This is known as Schwartze's sign (House, 1997). Tuning fork exam, which should include 256, 512, and 1024 Hz, gives an estimation of the degree of conductive hearing loss. Some have recommended the use of CT imaging in conductive hearing loss evaluation; however, this is not commonly used unless conflicting information or physical findings are found.

Audiologic Management

Audiologic management depends on three factors: (1) medical management, (2) presurgical peripheral involvement, and (3) postsurgical outcome measures. Some patients may not be surgical candidates for a variety reasons, and for those patients, traditional amplification may be an appropriate intervention strategy to assist with hearing difficulties. In some instances, patients undergoing surgery may present with pre-existing, comorbid sensorineural involvement. In these instances, patients will routinely require amplification following medical intervention even if the air-bone gap is closed. Appropriate counseling is critical in these circumstances.

Medical Management

Historically, surgical management of this disease has been a source of controversy. Kessel first treated otosclerosis with sta-pes mobilization in 1878 (Kessel, 1878); however, stapes operations fell out of favor during the late 19th century in the majority of the medical community. The early 20th century saw many advances in techniques for treating this disease process. Lempert introduced a one-stage fenestration of the horizontal semicircular canal that became widely popular (Lempert, 1938). Shea permanently changed the treatment of otosclerosis by describing an operation involving removal of the stapes and placement of a wire prosthesis from the incus to the oval window grafted with a vein graft (Shea, 1958).

The primary indication for surgical intervention of otosclerosis is the presence of a conductive hearing loss of more than 25 dB HL and the presence of a negative 512-Hz Rinne test without evidence of otitis media (McKenna & de Venecia, 2007). Contraindications include surgery in an only hearing ear, active Ménière's disease, otitis media, or otitis externa, and tympanic membrane perforations. Surgical intervention involves exploration of the middle ear, typically approached through the ear canal, to confirm the presence of a fixed footplate. Once this is confirmed the fixed footplate can be addressed by two main techniques. A stapedectomy involves the removal of a portion or the entire stapes footplate, grafting the open oval window, and placement of a prosthesis from the long process of the incus to the graft. A stapedotomy involves removal of the stapes superstructure, creating a hole in the fixed footplate with a drill or a laser, and placing a prosthesis from the incus to the stapedotomy site. This procedure can be done under general anesthesia or under local anesthesia with intravenous sedation. Immediate postoperative complications for these procedures include facial nerve damage, disarticulation of the incus, failure to correct the hearing loss, chorda tympani injury, cerebral spinal fluid (CSF) leak, vertigo, and granuloma formation. The complication of most concern is sensorineural hearing loss, which can be complete, and is the result of trauma to the vestibule during the procedure. Profound sensorineural hearing loss occurs in less than 1% of patients undergoing surgery for otosclerosis (House, 1997). Conductive hearing loss can occur in a delayed fashion due to the prosthesis moving from the correct position. However, if done correctly, stapes surgery is highly restorative and rewarding.

Case 4–7: Otosclerosis

History

This 42-year-old female reported a history of progressive hearing loss bilaterally, with the hearing sensitivity in the right ear perceived to be poorer than in the left ear. The patient also reported unilateral tinnitus in the right ear with no other audiologic or otologic history reported.

Audiology

The patient presented with a moderate, rising to mild mixed hearing loss bilaterally with the right ear demonstrating poorer thresholds than the left ear (Figure 4–7A). Tympanometry revealed normal pressure, volume, and compliance for both ears (Type A tympanograms) and word recognition was excellent bilaterally.

Medical Examination Result

The patient presented with normal appearing mastoids, pinnae, ear canals, and tympanic membranes without fluid, perforation, or retraction. Given the patient's history, the audiometric findings (i.e., an air-bone gap greater than 20 dB), and the fact that the patient had a reversal of the tuning fork examination, otosclerosis was highly suspected.

Impression

Bilateral otosclerosis.

Audiologic Recommendations and Management

It was recommend that the patient followup with an otolargynologist. Depending on the outcome, possible bilateral amplification should be considered.

Medical Recommendations and Management

The patient was given the options of either using hearing aids or undergoing surgery to close the air-bone gap in the right ear and she elected to have the surgery. A stapedectomy for correction of the conductive hearing loss in the right ear was performed.

Additional Comments

The patient chose to undergo the recommended surgical procedure. The surgery included a right stapedectomy. Postoperative test results demonstrated a complete closure of the preoperative air-bone gap in the right ear (Figure 4–7B). The left ear continues to present with a mixed hearing loss due to otosclerosis and is being considered for stapedectomy in the future.

DISORDER: Otosclerosis Pre-Op

PURE-TONE AUDIOMETRY

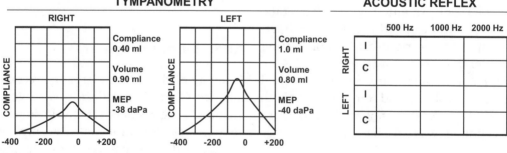

SPEECH AUDIOMETRY

Ear	PTA	SRT	Word Rec (%)
Right	57 dB HL	50 dB HL	100%
Left	42 dB HL	40 dB HL	100%
Soundfield			

TYMPANOMETRY

RIGHT
Compliance 0.40 ml
Volume 0.90 ml
MEP -38 daPa

LEFT
Compliance 1.0 ml
Volume 0.80 ml
MEP -40 daPa

ACOUSTIC REFLEX

	500 Hz	1000 Hz	2000 Hz
RIGHT I			
RIGHT C			
LEFT I			
LEFT C			

A

Figure 4–7. Pure-tone air and bone conduction results, speech audiometry, and tympanometry for a 42-year-old female with otosclerosis (Case 4–7). Results are shown for both preoperative testing (**A**) and postoperative testing (**B**). Note: otosclerosis was confirmed for the right ear and diagnosed as probable in the left ear. continues

DISORDER: Otosclerosis Post-Op

PURE-TONE AUDIOMETRY

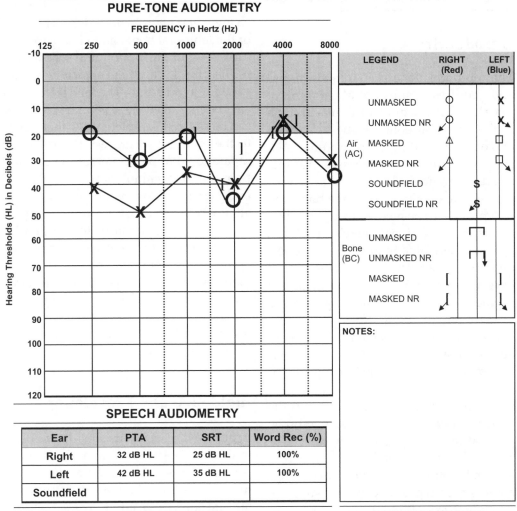

SPEECH AUDIOMETRY

Ear	PTA	SRT	Word Rec (%)
Right	32 dB HL	25 dB HL	100%
Left	42 dB HL	35 dB HL	100%
Soundfield			

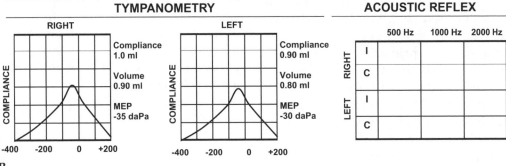

B

Figure 4–7. continued

143

TEMPORAL BONE TRAUMA

Introduction

The temporal bone is extremely dense and requires a substantial amount of force to cause fracture or trauma. Trauma of the temporal bone can be of various etiologies, including blunt trauma, penetrating trauma, compressive trauma, and barotrauma. Blunt trauma may or may not involve fracture of the bone and is typically associated with automobile accidents, recreational vehicle accidents, falls, and assaults. Strangely, one report describes a man struck in the lateral head by a species of flying fish, which resulted in fracture and sudden hearing loss and vertigo (Goldenberg, Karam, Danino, Flax-Goldenberg, & Joachims, 1998). Penetrating injuries carry a poor prognosis and may be due to gunshot injuries or stabbings. Compressive injuries involve a sudden increase of pressure within the ear canal resulting in tympanic membrane perforation. Etiologies include blast injuries and being slapped or struck across the ear. Barotrauma involves the development of negative middle ear pressure due to descent from high altitudes or ascension during diving. Middle ear damage and a perilymph fistula may occur. This chapter deals primarily with temporal bone fractures due to their higher incidence than the other forms of temporal bone trauma. Temporal bone trauma is rarely an isolated injury and typically is a part of multisystem trauma, which can create diagnostic and therapeutic difficulties.

Symptoms

Patients who suffer temporal bone trauma often are afflicted with a variety of other injuries, specifically intracranial injuries. This may result in severe mental status changes and neurologic deficits. Fractures of the temporal bone may violate the otic capsule resulting in profound sensorineural hearing loss, which typically is irreversible, and vertigo. The facial nerve can also be impinged by a bone fragment or can be severed completely. Further injury to the middle ear can result in ossicular separation, tympanic membrane perforation, and the accumulation of blood in the middle ear, known as hemotympanum, all of which can cause a conductive hearing loss. Vascular injury to the jugular venous system or the carotid artery can occur as well. Bloody otorrhea is a common symptom of temporal bone trauma. Any compromise of the dura and tegmen can result in a CSF leak, which may manifest as otorrhea or rhinorrhea (Brodie & Thompson, 1997).

Incidence and Prevalence

Automobile accidents result in head trauma in 75% of cases, and are the most common cause of a temporal bone fracture. High-risk behaviors are also a significant source of trauma. These fractures are more common in men with a peak incidence in the 3rd and 4th decades of life. Other common causes of temporal bone fractures include assaults, falls, motorcycles accidents, bicycle accidents, and gunshot wounds (Brodie & Thompson, 1997).

Etiology and Pathology

A temporal bone fracture is the result of significant force to the lateral aspect of the skull. A force of more than 1800 pounds per square inch is involved in fracturing the skull. Fracture patterns were described by Ulrich in 1926 as longitudinal or transverse based on the direction of the fracture in relationship to the long axis of the petrous portion of the temporal bone (Ulrich, 1926). Longitudinal fractures are more prevalent and account for 70 to 80% of temporal bone trauma. Facial nerve paralysis occurs in approximately 20% of longitudinal fractures (Ghorayeb &Yeakley, 1992; McGuirt & Stool, 1992; Nicol & Johnstone, 1994; Shapiro, 1979; Williams, Ghorayeb, &Yeakley, 1992). When blunt force is applied to the lateral portion of the skull a longitudinal fracture occurs. Transverse fractures are less common, but facial nerve injury occurs approximately 50% of the time. Force applied to the frontal bone can transmit force to the medial aspect of the temporal bone resulting in a transverse fracture. Penetrating trauma typically results in comminution of bone and classic fracture patterns are not as helpful in defining the fracture patterns in these patients as distinct fracture lines may not be observed.

Site of Lesion

The longitudinal and transverse fracture classification is helpful, but another classification has been developed to describe the status of the otic capsule (Dahiya et al., 1999). This system is more helpful in predicting outcomes following the injury. An otic capsule sparing fracture is similar to the longitudinal fracture line and the cochlea and vestibule remain intact. An otic capsule violating fracture has a fracture line extending into the cochlea or vestibule and is associated with a significantly higher incidence of sensorineural hearing loss and/or vertigo. Fractures of the temporal bone may involve several locations that lead to symptoms. Injury of

the facial nerve typically occurs near the geniculate ganglion and the nerve is tethered in position at that point; however, injury can occur at any location along the path of the facial nerve. The ossicles also may be affected and even disarticulated. The incudostapedial joint is the most common site of dislocation during temporal bone fractures and this site of compromise is more commonly associated with a longitudinal fracture (Appendix 4G). In addition, the jugular bulb and carotid artery can be involved by fractures, which usually are caused by penetrating trauma.

Audiology

Initial evaluation in patient with temporal bone trauma occurs once the patient is stable and should include otoscopy, comprehensive audiometry, and tympanometry. Initial otoscopic evaluation of the temporal bone patient is crucial in determining if the external auditory meatus is clear. Often, these patients will present with fluid or blood matter in the external auditory meatus, which must first be cleaned prior to proceeding with the audiologic evaluation. The comprehensive evaluation should include both air and bone conduction threshold tests to determine the type of hearing impairment, if a hearing loss is present. Patients with temporal bone fractures may present with a variety of hearing profiles, including conductive, sensorineural, and mixed. Speech audiometry should be agreement with pure-tone findings. Tympanometry is often warranted and results will vary from normal to reduced compliance (fluid or blood in the tympanum) to hypermobility (ossicular disarticulation) depending on the extent of the involvement. (For additional information on ossicular disarticulation, see the discussion provided below under the heading, Other Disorders Affecting the Outer and Middle Ears.)

On occasion, electroneuronography (ENoG) is needed in cases of facial nerve involvement. In such circumstances, it is important to wait at least 72 hours before performing the ENoG to allow Wallerian degeneration (neural degeneration that results when the axon separates from the cell body) to occur. In addition, the ENoG should be completed within 21 days of the trauma as intervention after this time is not likely to be successful. Through direct electrical stimulation, the audiologist is able to determine the integrity of the facial nerve function.

Medical Examination

Initial evaluation of a trauma patient requires application of the ABCs of cardiopulmonary resuscitation. Once stabilized, a secondary survey and thorough exam can be performed. Inspection of the scalp and skull for lacerations is important. One may visualize bruising around the mastoid process, referred to as Battle's sign, or bruising around the eyes, known as raccoon sign (Herbella, Mudo, Delmonti, Braga, & Del Grande, 2001). These bruising patterns are indicative of a skull base fracture. Inspection of the ear may be difficult as the canal may be occluded with blood and debris. If the tympanic membrane is visualized, one should inspect for a bluish bulge of the membrane that results from blood filling the middle ear space, a condition known as hemotympanum. Cerebral spinal fluid may be found leaking from the ear; however, if the tympanic membrane is intact CSF may tract down the Eustachian tube causing rhinorrhea. A thorough cranial nerve examination as a part of the head and neck exam is impor-

tant. Facial nerve function and the onset of facial weakness should be documented. Radiographic imaging is typically performed via a high-resolution CT scan of the temporal bone with thin slices. This scan typically provides the information necessary to guide clinical decisions and predict outcomes. The fracture pattern can be identified and surrounding anatomy can be delineated from this CT scan.

Audiologic Management

If there are residual effects of the temporal bone trauma, including conductive, mixed, or sensorineural hearing loss that have not been or cannot be medically treated, then appropriate audiologic rehabilitative actions should be undertaken. This could include amplification via air or bone conduction hearing aids and appropriate audiologic follow-up for monitoring of the hearing loss and audiologic rehabilitation, if indicated.

Medical Management

The role of medical and surgical intervention is to manage complications caused by temporal bone fractures. Not all fractures require intervention. Fractures isolated to the mastoid air cells or the squamous portion of the temporal bone generally are observed clinically. When examining a traumatized external auditory canal, any debris in the canal should be carefully removed. Infections can occur in this setting; thus, antibiotic ear drops are frequently used. A perforated tympanic membrane may heal within a few weeks to months. If the perforation lasts longer, then a tympanoplasty should be performed along with evaluation of the middle ear to ensure that no squamous debris has been implanted within the middle ear space.

Conductive hearing loss in the setting of temporal bone fracture must be followed closely with serial examinations. Hemotympanum may cause a conductive hearing loss, but it generally resolves within a few months and does not require intervention. Ossicular dislocation or disarticulation may occur and may be hidden by the hemotympanum; however, a traumatically separated joint may rejoin with time. If a conductive hearing loss remains 6 months following the incident, then a middle ear exploration with inspection of the ossicles should be performed. When the facial nerve is injured, it is critical that the degree of weakness and the onset of paralysis be determined. Weakness of the nerve carries an excellent prognosis, but prognosis in cases with complete paralysis depends on the onset of the symptom. Delayed onset paralysis has a better prognosis (>90% regain function) than paralysis that occurs at the time of the insult. An ENoG should be performed after 48 hours after the injury and more than 90% degeneration within 6 days is associated with a poorer outcome. Treatment options for facial paralysis include high dose steroids, which are felt to decrease edema around the nerve, or with surgical decompression, which involves removal of bone surrounding the nerve to relieve pressure on the nerve. There is no statistically significant difference in surgical and conservative treatments; however, the key is to operate on those with suspected transected nerves (Brodie & Thompson, 1997). When paralysis is immediate and ENoG reveals more than 90% degeneration, the suspicion for a transected nerve is high. A decompression of the facial nerve can be performed via a translabyrinthine approach in those with profound sensorineural hearing loss or via a combined transmastoid and supralabyrinthine approach in those with otic capsule sparing fractures. The time of decompression is variable, but typically it occurs within 1 week (Brodie &Thompson, 1997).

A CSF leak can be a persistent and serious problem. Most leaks are likely to close in 7 to 10 days and conservative treatment is recommended, which involves elevation of the head of the bed and lumbar drain. If the leak continues, it is imperative to locate the site of the leak. A CT cisternogram provides contrast of the CSF from the surrounding anatomy and helps to locate the leak. Intrathecal fluorescein or a radioactive carrier can be used if CT is unsuccessful. More than 90% of leaks close spontaneously (Brodie & Thompson, 1997). It is important to note that there is a much greater risk of meningitis in leaks lasting longer than 7 days. However, prophylactic antibiotics have significantly lowered the rate of meningitis in these cases. Surgical repair of fistulas that persist must be preceded by determination of hearing status, presence of brain herniation, status of the ear canal, and location of the fistula. In the event of an otic capsule disrupting fracture, a radical mastoidectomy is performed with obliteration of the middle ear space. An otic capsule sparing fracture can be managed by a complete mastoidectomy and closing the tegmen leak. If the mastoid tegmen is the source of the leak, fascia can be placed over leak and fat or muscle is packed in the mastoid.

Tegmen tympani CSF leak is addressed via a middle cranial fossa craniotomy and rotation of a temporalis flap to cover the defect. If brain herniation is present, it is repaired by a combined mastoidectomy and craniotomy. If the external auditory canal is damaged with a CSF leak, then a radical mastoidectomy is performed to prevent cholesteatoma formation.

Patients with otic capsule disrupting fractures typically have sensorineural hearing loss that is irreversible. When these fractures are bilateral and patients have bilateral severe to profound sensorineural hearing loss, cochlear implants may be beneficial (Morgan, Cocker, & Jenkins, 1994).

Vertigo following temporal bone fracture is common and should be evaluated by electronystagmography (ENG). Patients may have a concussive membranous labyrinth injury that presents with positional vertigo with otherwise normal ENG findings. This type of injury is typically self-limiting. A massive vestibular labyrinth injury can be managed by vestibular suppressants and antiemetics and traumatic cupulolithiasis can be managed by an Epley maneuver. Finally, a perilymph fistula accompanied by vertigo and fluctuating SNHL is managed by a middle ear exploration with closure of the fistula.

Case 4–8: Ossicular Disarticulation or Dislocation

History

This 28-year-old male reported a unilateral hearing loss and tinnitus in the left ear following a motor vehicle accident. No other significant audiologic or otologic history was reported.

Audiology

The patient presented with essentially normal peripheral hearing sensitivity in the right ear, whereas the pure-tone audiogram for the left ear indicated borderline normal hearing through 500 Hz, sloping to a mild to moderate mixed hearing loss for the remaining frequencies (Figure 4–8). Tympanometry revealed normal pressure, volume, and compliance for the right ear (Type A tympanogram), and normal pressure and volume with hypercompliance for the left ear (Type A_d tympanogram). Word recognition was excellent bilaterally.

Medical Examination Result

Medical examination revealed normal appearing mastoids, pinnae, ear canals, and tympanic membranes without fluid, perforation, or retraction.

Impression

Suspected ossicular disarticulation.

Audiologic Recommendations and Management

It was recommend that the patient follow-up with an otolargynologist. Depending on the outcome, possible amplification for the left ear should be considered.

Medical Recommendations and Management

Following medical evaluation it was recommended that the patient undergo left middle ear exploration and possible ossicular reconstruction following a CT scan.

Additional Comments

Inspection of the CT scan revealed an incudomalleolar disarticulation and the patient chose to undergo surgery for

DISORDER: Ossicular Disarticulation

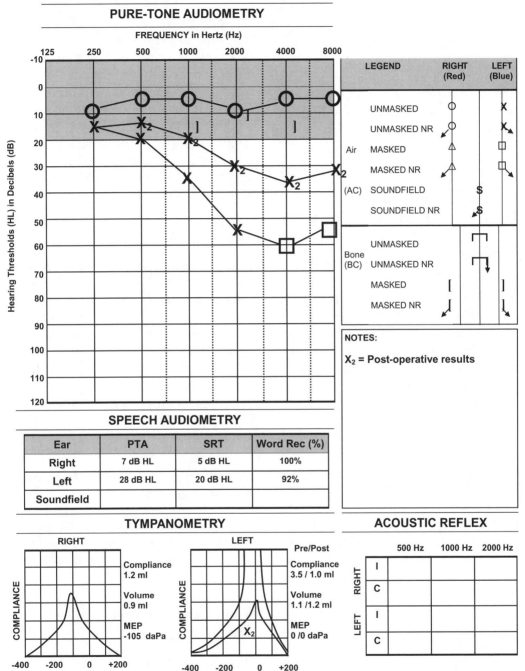

Figure 4–8. Pure-tone air and bone conduction results, speech audiometry, and tympanometry for a 28-year-old male who had sustained a head trauma resulting in disarticulation of the left ossicular chain (Case 4–8). Postoperative findings are indicated by X_2 for the left ear and right ear test results remained the same.

repair of the disarticulation. The surgery included a left tympanotomy with incus repositioning. Although the results of postoperative testing demonstrated a significant improvement in hearing sensitivity and middle ear compliance for the left ear following surgery, a mild conductive hearing loss remained for the high frequencies (see Figure 4–8) and the patient was fit with monaural amplification.

Case 4–9: Ossicular Disarticulation or Dislocation

History

A 14-year-old male was seen for a hearing evaluation and ENoG following an all terrain vehicle (ATV) accident. The patient suffered traumatic subarachnoid hemorrhage and bilateral temporal bone fractures resulting in facial nerve paralysis (grade VI), and a bilateral conductive hearing loss.

Audiology

An otoscopic check was unremarkable bilaterally. Tympanometry revealed normal pressure, volume, and compliance for the left ear and reduced compliance in the right ear (Figure 4–9A). Responses to pure-tone audiometry indicated a flat moderate conductive hearing loss in both ears and word recognition scores were excellent bilaterally. Reliability was considered to be good. In addition, an ENoG was performed to determine the degree of facial nerve involvement. Response to the ENoG demonstrated absent responses for both the left and right sides (Figure 4–9B). These findings indicated significant facial nerve involvement with total dysfunction bilaterally.

Medical Examination Result

The patient was evaluated after discussion with his parents and exploratory surgery was performed to determine the etiology of the conductive hearing loss. The right ear was chosen for exploration due to the patient's report of poorer hearing on that side in spite of relatively symmetrical hearing. Perioperative evaluation revealed disarticulation at the mallealincudal joint and a right-sided ossiculoplasty was performed.

Impression

Conductive hearing loss secondary to ossicular disarticulation and bilateral facial paralysis. It is of interest to note that tympanomentry was normal in one ear and reduced compliance was noted in the other. Usually, with disarticulations, hypercompliance is observed. Perhaps, the ossicular chain in this patient may have been subluxed, which could explain the unexpected tympanometric findings in this case.

Audiologic Recommendations and Management

It was recommended that the patient follow up with an otolargynologist, with subsequent audiologic follow-up as necessary.

Medical Recommendations and Management

This patient demonstrated very little complication as a result of the facial nerve paralysis. It was recommended that he continue to monitor hearing and facial nerve function.

DISORDER: Ossicular Disarticulation

PURE-TONE AUDIOMETRY

FREQUENCY in Hertz (Hz)

LEGEND		RIGHT (Red)	LEFT (Blue)
Air (AC)	UNMASKED	○	X
	UNMASKED NR	○	X
	MASKED	△	□
	MASKED NR	△	□
	SOUNDFIELD	$	
	SOUNDFIELD NR	$	
Bone (BC)	UNMASKED		⌐
	UNMASKED NR		
	MASKED	[	]
	MASKED NR		

NOTES:

SPEECH AUDIOMETRY

Ear	PTA	SRT	Word Rec (%)
Right	33 dB HL	40 dB HL	100%
Left	30 dB HL	30 dB HL	100%
Soundfield			

TYMPANOMETRY

RIGHT

Compliance .30 ml

Volume 1.1 ml

MEP - 85 daPa

LEFT

Compliance .70 ml

Volume 1.2 ml

MEP -15 daPa

ACOUSTIC REFLEX

		500 Hz	1000 Hz	2000 Hz
RIGHT	I			
	C			
LEFT	I			
	C			

A

Figure 4–9. Pure-tone air and bone conduction results, speech audiometry, and tympanometry (*A*) and ENoG results (*B*) for a 14–year-old male who had sustained a head injury (Case 4–9). continues

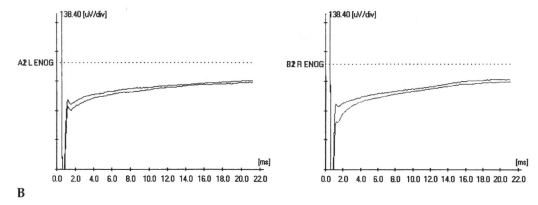

B

Figure 4–9. continued

Additional Information

There has been no significant improvement in the either the patient's hearing or facial nerve function. He continues to be monitored routinely and has obtained binaural amplification with significant benefit noted.

OTHER DISORDERS AFFECTING THE OUTER AND MIDDLE EARS

External Otitis

This is an infection of the ear canal and/or the pinna that is often noticed in the summer and is commonly caused by swimming in water with high counts of bacteria. It is typically caused by a bacterial invasion into the external ear canal. The most common bacteria is *pseudomonas*. External otitis can also be related to fungal infections, but these are relatively rare. In viewing the ear canal, mucopurulent matter is usually observed along with redness and swelling of the tissue involved. The patient will complain of severe discomfort, especially when the pinna is moved. Audiologically, there is seldom much of an effect on hearing unless swelling closes the ear canal. Following testing of patients with this disorder, sterilized cleaning or disposal of earphones (inserts) is in order. Treatment of the patient includes cleaning of the affected area and topical application of antibacterial agents. These antibacterial agents are sometimes combined with corticosteroids, which may provide better treatment than antibacterial applications alone (Castillo & Roland, 2007).

Exostoses and Osteomas

Exostoses are bony growths occurring in the medial (bony) portion of the ear canal (see Appendix 4H). These multiple bony growths seem to be related to cold water exposure and are often seen in swimmers. This is often a bilateral condition. Exostoses become bothersome only when they trap debris in the ear canal or they become so large that they impinge on the eardrum or block the ear canal. The presence of exostoses in the ear canal may make it difficult to visualize the tympanic membrane. If large enough to close off the ear canal, these growths can cause conductive hearing loss. The ear canal, especially if cerumen is present, can be blocked by pushing cerumen against the exostoses when ear inserts are used. So care must be exercised when using ear insert receivers with patients with exotoses. Management of these patients usually involves surgical removal of the exostoses (Parisier, Kimmelman, & Hanson, 1997).

Osteomas are also bony growths and are often confused with exostoses. These, however, are usually singular in number and are located more laterally in the canal. They are a true neoplasm that is a mix of bone and fibrous tissue and they tend to occur more often in children than in adults. Audiologically the same concerns exist for osteomas as those mentioned for exostoses. Osteomas occasionally can be removed in the otolaryngologist's office, but often a brief general anesthetic is required (Parisier et al., 1997).

Tympanic Membrane Perforation

Castillo and Roland (2007) provide a nice review of tympanic membrane perforations from which we draw information. These generally are related to trauma (blasts, penetrating injuries, head trauma, etc.) or infections, such as otitis media. Most tympanic membrane perforations will heal spontaneously unless they are large or are related to ongoing or recurring infections. They can occur in either the pars flaccida or pars tensa. However, if they occur in the pars flaccida, concern about cholesteatomas would be in order.

Long-standing perforations also herald concern over possible cholesteatomas. Small perforations generally do not yield hearing loss; however, large tympanic membrane perforations can result in up to 50 dB of hearing loss, although in most cases the hearing loss is much less severe. Increased volume measures during tympanometric testing are indications of tympanic membrane perforations unless the patient has a PE tube in place. Careful otoscopic exams should always be completed to determine if a tympanic membrane perforation is present. Care must also be taken during audiologic and vestibular (caloric) exams whenever a perforation is noted so that the tympanic membrane perforation is not further disturbed or contaminated. Treatment for tympanic membrane perforations that do not spontaneously heal is otologic surgical repair (see Appendix 4I for an example of a tympanic membrane perforation).

Tympanosclerosis

Tympanosclerosis is a condition in which white calcified plaques of connective tissue occur at and around the circumference of the tympanic membrane and/or the head of the malleus (Castillo & Roland, 2007) (See Appendix 4J for an example of tympanosclerosis). When these plaques are only on the tympanic membrane, the condition is called myringosclerosis, which is more common than tympanosclerosis. Both conditions are often associated with chronic otitis media and inflammatory processes of the middle ear. Myringosclerosis seldom yields a measurable hearing loss; however, tympanosclerosis can result in a measurable hearing loss especially if it involves the ossicular chain. In cases with measurable hearing loss, the hearing loss will be a conductive hearing loss and the tympanograms will typically reveal slightly reduced compliance (Castillo & Roland, 2007).

Ossicular Chain Dislocation

Ossicular chain dislocation or ossicular chain disarticulation can be a result of various types of trauma, congenital abnormalities, necrosis (secondary to chronic infections), and surgical interventions (Baylor College of Medicine, 2001; Castillo & Roland, 2007). The hearing loss noted in cases of ossicular chain dislocation typically is a conductive hearing loss; however, in some cases of head injury, the associated trauma may cause a subluxation of the ossicular chain with penetration into the cochlea, which results in a mixed hearing loss (Castillo & Roland, 2007). Audiology plays a key role in the diagnosis of ossicular chain dislocation in that near to maximum conductive loss is often observed in patients with ossicular chain dislocation and their tympanograms show hypercompliance, but no crossed acoustic reflexes even if hearing sensitivity is good in the acoustically stimulated ear. If the ossicular chain is subluxed or fibrous tissue has formed to keep the chain somewhat intact, the hearing may be relatively good with tympanograms showing reduced compliance and in some cases present acoustic reflexes, although often elevated (Jerger & Jerger, 1981). Treatment of ossicular chain dislocation is otologic surgery to repair the dislocation or disarticulation of the ossicular chain and to resolve the conductive hearing loss that has resulted from the disarticulated ossicular chain.

This surgical procedure involved is called ossiculoplasty (i.e., repair of the ossicular chain) and closure of the air-bone gap to 10 dB occurs slightly less than 75% of the time (Castillo & Roland, 2007).

SUMMARY

This chapter provided a brief overview of select conditions that affect the auditory system. Diseases of the external and middle ears are diverse in etiology and have profound effects on auditory function. Appropriate management of these diseases requires a combination of thorough history and physical examination, careful audiologic testing, and appropriate diagnostic imaging. A clear understanding of these conditions and appropriate management procedures can lead to improved auditory function and quality of life for patients.

Acknowledgment. The authors gratefully acknowledge the contributions of Matthew Bush, MD, Assistant Professor, Department of Otolaryngology, University of Kentucky, to this chapter.

REFERENCES

Abramson, M., & Huang, C. C. (1977). Localization of collagenase in human middle ear cholesteatoma. *Laryngoscope, 87*(5, Pt. 1), 771–791.

Aithal, V., Aithal, S., & Pulotu, L. (1995). Otitis media with effusion in children: An audiological case series study. *Papua and New Guinea Medical Journal, 38*(2), 79–94.

Amar, M. S., Wishahi, H. F., & Zakhary, M. M. (1996). Clinical and biochemical studies of bone destruction in cholesteatoma, *Journal of Laryngology and Otology, 110*(6), 534–539.

Baylor College of Medicine. (2001). *Bobby Alford's otolaryngology.* Retrieved 6/15/11 from http://www.bcm.edu/oto.

Bennett, M., Warren, F., & Haynes, D. (2006). Indications and technique in mastoidectomy. *Otolaryngologic Clinics of North America, 39*(6), 1095–1113.

Bluestone, C. (1998). Anatomy and physiology of the Eustachian tube. In C. Cummings, J. M. Fredrickson, L. A. Harker, C. J. Krause, M. A. Richardson, & D. E. Schuller (Eds.), *Otolaryngology: Head and neck surgery* (Vol. 3, pp. 3003–3025). St. Louis, MO: Mosby.

Bluestone, C. D. (2004). Studies in otitis media: Children's Hospital of Pittsburgh—University of Pittsburgh progress report—2004. *Laryngoscope, 114*(11 Pt. 3, Suppl. 105), 1–26.

Bluestone, C. D., & Klein, J. O. (2003). Otitis media and Eustachian tube dysfunction. In C. D. Bluestone, S. E. Stool, C. M. Alper, E. M. Arjmand, C. I. Casselbrant, J. E. Dohar, & R. F. Yellon (Eds.), *Pediatric otolaryngology* (4th ed., Vol. 1, pp. 474–686). New York, NY: W. B. Saunders.

Bluestone, C. D., & Klein, J. O. (2007). *Otitis media in infants and children.* Philadelphia, PA: W. B. Saunders.

Bluestone, C. D., Stephenson, J. S., & Martin, L. M. (1992). Ten-year review of otitis media pathogens. *Pediatric Infectious Disease Journal, 11*(8 Suppl.), S7–S11.

Borsanyi, S. J. (1962). Glomus jugulare tumors. *Laryngoscope, 72*, 1336–1345.

Brodie, H. A., & Thompson, T. C. (1997). Management of complications from 820 temporal bone fractures. *American Journal of Otology, 18*(2), 188–197.

Brown, J. S. (1985). Glomus jugulare tumors revisited: A ten-year statistical follow-up of 231 cases. *Laryngoscope, 95*(3), 284–288.

Canalis, R. F. (1990). Valsalva's contribution to otology. *American Journal of Otolaryngology, 11*(6), 420–427.

Canalis, R., & Lambert, P. (2000). *Chronic otitis media and cholesteatoma.* Philadelphia, PA: Lippincott Williams & Wilkins.

Carhart, R. (1950). Clinical application of bone conduction audiometry. *Archives of Otolaryngology, 51*(6), 798–808.

Carrasco, V., & Rosenman, J. (1993). Radiation therapy of glomus jugulare tumors. *Laryngoscope, 103*(11 Pt. 2, Suppl. 60), 23–27.

Castillo, M., & Roland, P. (2007). Disorders of the auditory system. In R. Roeser, M. Valente, & H. Hosford-Dunn (Eds.), *Audiology: Diagnosis* (2nd ed., pp. 82–87). New York, NY: Thieme.

Cawthorne, T. (1955). Otosclerosis. *Journal of Laryngology and Otology, 69*(7), 437–456.

Dahiya, R., Keller, J. D., Litofsky, N. S., Bankey, P. E., Bonassar, L. J., & Megerian, C. A. (1999). Temporal bone fractures: Otic capsule sparing versus otic capsule violating clinical and radiographic considerations. *Journal of Trauma, 47*(6), 1079–1083.

De la Cruz, A., & Chandraseckhar, S. S. (1994). Congenital malformation of the temporal bone. In D. E. Brackmann, S. Shelton, & M. A. Arriaga (Eds.), *Otologic surgery* (1st ed., pp. 69–84). Philadelphia, PA: W. B. Saunders.

Declau, F., Cremers, C., & Van de Heyning, P. (1999). Diagnosis and management strategies in congenital atresia of the external auditory canal. Study Group on Otological Malformations and Hearing Impairment. *British Journal of Audiology, 33*(5), 313–327.

Derkay, C. S., Bluestone, C. D., Thompson, A. E., & Kardatske, D. (1989). Otitis media in the pediatric intensive care unit: A prospective study. *Otolaryngology-Head and Neck Surgery, 100*(4), 292–299.

Dhooge, I. J. (2003). Risk factors for the development of otitis media. *Current Allergy and Asthma Reports, 3*(4), 321–325.

Doherty, J. K., & Linthicum, F. H., Jr. (2004). Spiral ligament and stria vascularis changes in cochlear otosclerosis: Effect on hearing level. *Otology and Neurotology, 25*(4), 457–464.

Erickson, D., Kudva, Y. C., Ebersold, M. J., Thompson, G. B., Grant, C. S., van Heerden, J. A., & Young, W. F., Jr. (2001). Benign paragangliomas: Clinical presentation and treatment outcomes in 236 patients. *Journal* of *Clinical Endocrinology and Metabolism,* 86(11), 5210–5216.

Fayad, J. N., Keles, B., & Brackmann, D. E. (2010). Jugular foramen tumors: Clinical characteristics and treatment outcomes. *Otology & Neurotology, 31*(2), 299–305.

Fowler, C. G., & Shanks, J. E. (2002). Tympanometry. In J. Katz (Ed.), *Handbook of clinical audiology* (5th ed., pp. 175–204), Philadelphia, PA: Lippincott Williams & Wilkins.

Gates, G. A., Avery, C. A., Prihoda, T. J., & Cooper, J. C., Jr. (1987). Effectiveness of adenoidectomy and tympanostomy tubes in the treatment of chronic otitis media with effusion. *New England Journal of Medicine, 317*(23), 1444–1451.

Ghorayeb, B. Y., & Yeakley, J. W. (1992). Temporal bone fractures: Longitudinal or oblique? The case for oblique temporal bone fractures. *Laryngoscope, 102*(2), 129–134.

Goldenberg, D., Karam, M., Danino, J., Flax-Goldenberg, R., & Joachims, H. (1998). Temporal bone fracture following blunt trauma caused by a flying fish. *Journal of Laryngology and Otology, 112*(10), 959–961.

Goossens, H., Ferech, M., Vander Stichele, R., & Elseviers, M. (2005). Outpatient antibiotic use in Europe and association with resistance: A cross-national database study. *Lancet, 365*(9459), 579–587.

Guild, S. R. (1941). A hitherto unrecognized structure, the glomus jugularis, in man. *Anatomical Record, 79*(Suppl. 1), 28.

Gulya, A. J. (1993). The glomus tumor and its biology. *Laryngoscope, 103*(11 Pt. 2, Suppl. 60), 7–15.

Hannley, M. T. (1993). Audiologic characteristics of the patient with otosclerosis. *Otolaryngologic Clinics of North America, 26*(3), 373–387.

Henderson, F. W., Collier, A. M., Sanyal, M. A., Watkins, J. M., Fairclough, D. L., Clyde, W. A., Jr., & Denny, F. W. (1982). A longitudinal study of respiratory viruses and bacteria in the etiology of acute otitis media with effusion. *New England Journal of Medicine, 306*(23), 1377–1383.

Herbella, F. A., Mudo, M., Delmonti, C., Braga, F. M., & Del Grande, J. C. (2001). "Raccoon eyes" (periorbital haematoma) as a sign of skull base fracture. *Injury, 32*(10), 745–757.

Hobson, J. C., Roper, A. J., Andrew, R., Rothera, M. P., Hill, P., & Green, K. M. (2010). Complications of bone-anchored hearing aid implantation. *Journal of Laryngology and Otology, 124*(2), 132–136.

Holmquist, J. (1969). Eustachian tube function assessed with tympanometry. A new testing procedure in ears with intact tympanic membrane. *Acta Otolaryngologica, 68*(6), 501–508.

Horn, K. L., & Hankinson, H. (1994). Tumors of the jugular foramen in neurotology. In R. K. Jackler & D. E. Brackmann (Eds.), *Neurotology* (pp. 1059–1068). St. Louis, MO: Mosby.

House, J. (1997) *Otosclerosis.* In G. B. Hughes & M. L. Pensak (Eds.), *Clinical otology* (2nd ed., pp. 241–249). New York, NY: Thieme.

Ivy, R. G. (1975). Tympanometric curves and otosclerosis. *Journal of Speech and Hearing Research, 18*(3), 554–558.

Jackson, C. G., Glasscock, M. E., Jr., & Harris, P. E. (1982). Glomus tumors. Diagnosis, classification, and management of large lesions. *Archives of Otolaryngology, 108*(7), 401–410.

Jacobson, J. T., & Mahoney, T. M. (1977). Admittance tympanometry in otosclerotic ears. *Journal of the American Audiology Society, 3*(2), 91–98.

Jahrsdoerfer, R. A. (1978). Congenital atresia of the ear. *Laryngoscope, 88*(9 Pt. 3, Suppl. 13), 1–48.

Jahrsdoerfer, R. A., Yeakley, J. W., Aguilar, E. A., Cole, R. R., & Gray, L. C. (1992). Grading system for the selection of patients with congenital aural atresia. *American Journal of Otology, 13*(1), 6–12.

Jerger, S., & Jerger, J. (1981). *Auditory disorders*: *A manual for clinical evaluation.* Boston, MA: Little Brown.

Karas, D. E., & Kwartler, J. A. (1993). Glomus tumors: A fifty-year historical perspectives, *American Journal of Otology, 14*(5), 495–500.

Kelemen, G. (1959). Aural embryopathies. *Annals of Otology, Rhinology, and Laryngology, 68*, 798–802.

Kessel, J. (1878). Uber das Mobilisieren des Steigbugels durch Ausschneiden des Trommelfelles, Hammers und Ambosses bei Undurchgangigkeit der tube. *Archiv fur Ohrenheilkunde, 13,* 69–72.

Lambert, P. R. (1998). Congenital aural atresia. In B. J. Bailey (Ed.), *Head and neck surgery-Otolaryngology* (2nd ed., pp. 1997–2009). Philadelphia, PA: Lippincott-Raven.

Lempert, J. (1938). Improvement of hearing in cases of otosclerosis: A new, one stage surgical technique. *Archives of Otolaryngology-Head and Neck Surgery, 28(1),* 42–67.

Leo, G., Piacentini, E., Incorvaia, C., & Consonni, D. (2007). Sinusitis and Eustachian tube dysfunction in children. *Pediatric Allergy and Immunology, 18*(Suppl. 18), 35–39.

Leveque, H., Bialostozky, F., Blanchard, C. L., & Suter, C. M. (1979). Tympanometry in the evaluation of vascular lesions of the middle ear and tinnitus of vascular origin. *Laryngoscope, 89*(8), 1197–1218.

Levin, G., Fabian, P., & Stahle, J. (1988). Incidence of otosclerosis. *American Journal of Otology, 9*(4), 299–301.

McGuirt, W. F., Jr., & Stool, S. E. (1992). Temporal bone fractures in children: A review with emphasis on long-term sequelae. *Clinical Pediatrics, 31*(1), 12–18.

McKenna, M., & de Venecia, R. (2007). Otosclerosis. In G. Hughes & M. Pensak (Eds.), *Clinical otology* (Vol. 3, pp. 258–271). New York, NY: Thieme.

Metz, O. (1946). The acoustic impedance measured on normal and pathological ears. *Acta Otolaryngologica, 33*(63 Suppl.), 29–48.

Moffat, D., & Hardy, D. (1989) Surgical management of large glomus jugulare tumours: Infra-and trans-temporal approach. *Journal of Laryngology and Otology, 103*(12), 1167–1180.

Morgan, W. E., Coker, N. J., & Jenkins, H. A. (1994). Histopathology of temporal bone fractures: Implications for cochlear implantation. *Laryngoscope, 104*(4), 426–432.

Müller, J. (1838). *Ueber den feineren Bau und die formen der krankhaften Geschwulste.* Berlin, Germany: G. Reimer.

Musiek, F. E., & Baran, J. A. (2007). *The auditory system: Anatomy, physiology, and clinical correlates.* Boston, MA: Allyn & Bacon.

Nelson, M., Roger, G., Koltai, P. J., Garabedian, E. N., Triglia, J. M., Roman, S., . . . Hammel, J. P. (2002). Congenital cholesteatoma: Classification, management, and outcome. *Archives of Otolaryngology-Head and Neck Surgery, 128*(7), 810–814.

Nicol, J. W., & Johnstone, A. J. (1994). Temporal bone fractures in children: A review of 34 cases. *Journal of Accident and Emergency Medicine, 11*(4), 218–222.

O'Leary, M. J., Shelton, C., Giddings, N. A., Kwartler, J., & Brackmann, D. E. (1991). Glomus tympanicum tumors: A clinical perspective. *Laryngoscope, 101*(10), 1038–1043.

Oldring, D., & Fisch, U. (1979). Glomus tumors of the temporal region: Surgical therapy. *American Journal of Otology, 1*(1), 7–18.

Olszewska, E., Wagner, M., Bernal-Sprekelsen, M., Ebmeyer, J., Dazert, S., Hildmann, H., & Sudhoff, H. (2004). Etiopathogenesis of cholesteatoma. *European Archives of Oto-rhino-laryngology, 261*(1), 6–24.

O'Neill, P., Roberts, T., & Bradley Stevenson, C. (2006). Otitis media in children (acute). *Clinical Evidence, 15,* 500–510.

Palva, T., Ramsay, H., & Böhling, T. (1996). Prussak's space revisited. *American Journal of Otology, 17*(4), 512–520.

Paradise, J. L., Rockette, H. E., Colborn, D. K., Bernard, B. S., Smith, C. G., Kurs-Lasky, M., & Janosky, J. E. (1997). Otitis media in 2253 Pittsburgh-area infants: Prevalence and risk factors during the first two years of life. *Pediatrics, 99*(3), 318–333.

Parisier, S., Kimmelman, C., Hanson, M. (1997). Diseases of the external auditory canal. In G. Hughes & M. Pensak (Eds.), *Clinical otology* (2nd ed., pp. 196–201), New York, NY: Thieme.

Patel, S. J., Sekhar, L. N., Cass, S. P., & Hirsch, B. E. (1994). Combined approaches for resection of extensive glomus jugulare tumors. A review of 12 cases. *Journal of Neurosurgery, 80*(6), 1026–1038.

Penido Nde, O., Borin, A., Iha, L. C., Suguri, V. M., Onishi, E., Fukuda, Y., & Cruz, O. L. (2005). Intracranial complications of otitis media: 15 years of experience in 33 patients. *Otolaryngology-Head and Neck Surgery, 132*(1), 37–42.

Pensak, M. L., & Jackler, R. K. (1997). Removal of jugular foramen tumors: The fallopian bridge technique. *Otolaryngology-Head and Neck Surgery, 117*(6), 586–591.

Politzer, A. (1894). Veber primare Erkankung der Knochernen Labyrinth Kapsel. *Ohrenheilkunde, 25,* 309–312.

Probst, R. (2007). Audiological evaluation of patients with otosclerosis. *Advances in Otorhino-laryngology, 65,* 119–126.

Proctor, B. (1967). Embryology and anatomy of the Eustachian tube. *Archives of Otolaryngology, 86*(5), 503–514.

Rane, R. L., Yut, J. P., & Berger, K. W. (1978). Negative needle deflection of the acoustic reflex in otosclerotics. *Journal of the American Audiology Society, 3*(6), 241–244.

Rosenfeld, R. M., & Post, J. (1992). Metaanalysis of antibiotics for the treatment of otitis media with effusion. *Otolaryngology-Head and Neck Surgery, 106*(4), 378–386.

Rosenwasser, H. (1945). Carotid body tumor of the middle ear and mastoid. *Archives of Otolaryngology, 41,* 64–67.

Rovers, M., Glasziou, P., Appelman, C., Burke, P., McCormick, D., Damoiseaux, R., . . . Hoes A. W. (2006). Antibiotics for acute otitis media: A meta-analysis with individual patient data. *Lancet, 368*(9545), 1429–1435.

Rovers, M. M., Schilder, A. G., Zielhuis, G. A., & Rosenfeld, R. M. (2004). Otitis media. *Lancet, 363*(9407), 465–473.

Sadé, J., Babiacki, A., & Pinkus, G. (1983). The metaplastic and congenital origin of cholesteatoma. *Acta Otolaryngologica, 96*(1–2), 119–129.

Sadler-Kimes, D., Siegel, M. I., & Todhunter, J. S. (1989). Age-related morphologic differences in the components of the Eustachian tube/middle ear system. *Annals of Otology, Rhinology, and Laryngology, 98*(11), 854–858.

Saringer, W., Khayal, H., Ertl, A., Schoeggl, A., & Kitz, K. (2001). Efficiency of gamma knife radiosurgery in the treatment of glomus jugulare tumors. *Minimally Invasive Neurosurgery, 44*(3), 141–146.

Schuknecht, H. F. (1989). Congenital aural atresia. *Laryngoscope, 99*(9), 908–917.

Shapiro, R. S. (1979). Temporal bone fractures in children. *Otolaryngology and Head and Neck Surgery, 87*(3), 323–329.

Shea, J. J., Jr. (1958). Fenestration of the oval window. *Annals of Otology, Rhinology, and Laryngology, 67*(4), 932–951.

Sheehan, J., Kondziolka, D., Flickinger, J., & Lunsford, L. D. (2005). Gamma knife surgery for glomus jugulare tumors: An intermediate report on efficacy and safety. *Journal of Neurosurgery, 102*(Suppl.), 241–246.

Silman, S., & Arick, D, (1999). Efficacy of a modified politzer apparatus in management of eustachian tube dysfunction in adults. *Journal American Academy of Audiology, 10*(9), 496–501.

Spector, G. J., Ciralsky, R. H., & Ogura, J. H. (1975) Glomus tumours in the head and neck: III. Analysis of clinical manifestations. *Annals of Otology, Rhinology, and Laryngology, 84*(1 Pt. 1), 73–79.

Spector, G. J., Maisel, R. H., & Ogura, J. H. (1974). Glomus jugulare tumors: II. A clinicopathologic analysis of the effects of radiotherapy. *Annals of Otology, Rhinology, and Laryngology, 83*(1), 26–32.

Sutherland, J. E., & Campbell, K. (1990). Immittance audiometry. *Primary Care, 17*(2), 233–247.

Tos, M. (2000). A new pathogenesis of mesotympanic (congenital) cholesteatoma. *Laryngoscope, 110*(11), 1890–1897.

Tos, M., & Bak-Pedersen, K. (1972). The pathogenesis of chronic secretory otitis media. *Archives of Otolaryngology, 95*(6), 511–521.

Touma, J. B., & Touma, B. J. (2006). *Atlas of otoscopy.* San Diego, CA: Plural Publishing.

Toynbee, J. (1841). Pathological and surgical observations on the diseases of the ear. *Medico-Chirurgical Transactions, 24,* 190–211.

Ulrich, K. (1926). Verletzungen des Gehororgans bei schadelbasisfrakturen (eine histologische und klinissche Studie). *Acta Otolaryngologica, 6*(Suppl.), 1–150.

Williams, W. T., Ghorayeb, B. Y., & Yeakley, J. W. (1992). Pediatric temporal bone fractures. *Laryngoscope, 102*(6), 600–603.

Woods, C. I., Strasnick, B., & Jackson, C. G. (1993). Surgery for glomus tumors: The Otology Group experience, *Laryngoscope, 103*(Suppl. 60), 65–70.

Zielhuis, G., Rach, G. H., van den Bosch, A., & van den Broek, P. (1990). The prevalence of otitis media with effusion: A critical review of the literature. *Clinical Otolaryngology and Allied Sciences, 15*(3), 283–288.

Appendix 4A

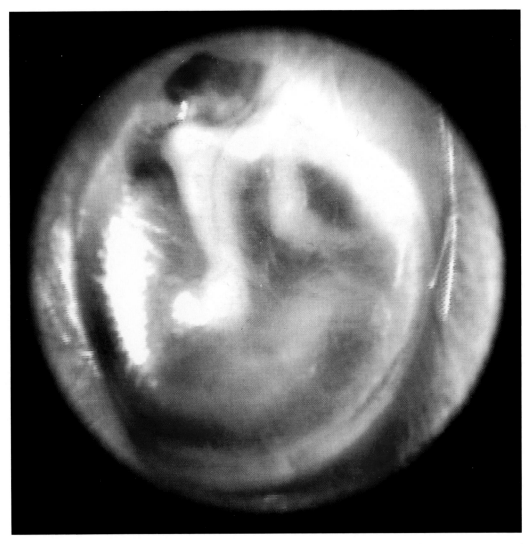

An example of a normal tympanic membrane. Reproduced with permission from Touma, J., and Touma, B., (2006), Atlas of otoscopy, *p. 3. Copyright © 2006 Plural Publishing, Inc.*

Appendix 4B

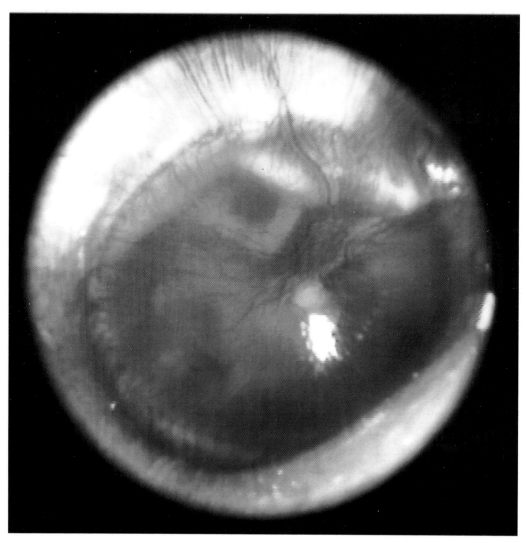

An example of an eardrum revealing serous otitis media. Reproduced with permission from Touma, J., and Touma, B., (2006), Atlas of otoscopy, *p. 11. Copyright © 2006 Plural Publishing, Inc.*

Appendix 4C

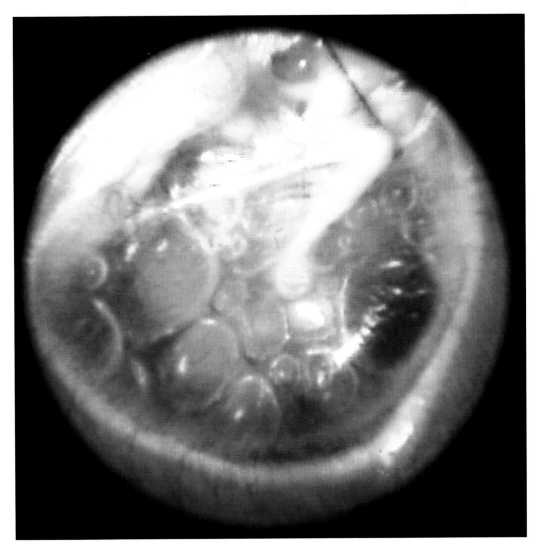

An example of an eardrum showing air bubbles in the middle ear related to otitis media. Reproduced with permission from Touma, J., and Touma, B., (2006), Atlas of otoscopy, *p. 12. Copyright ©️ 2006 Plural Publishing, Inc.*

Appendix 4D

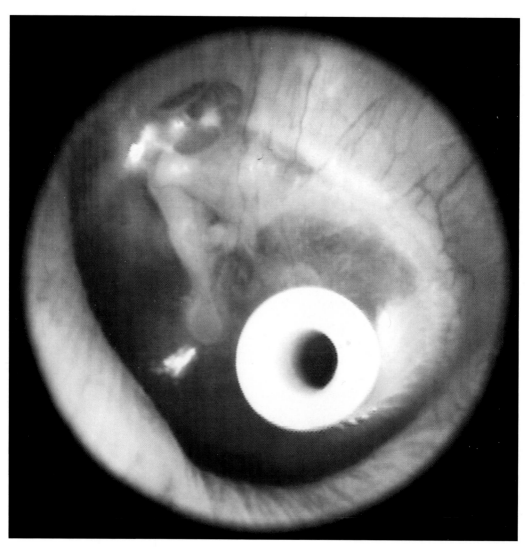

An eardrum with a Shepard-Grommet tube for ventilation of the middle ear space. Reproduced with permission from Touma, J., and Touma, B., (2006), Atlas of otoscopy, p. 35. Copyright © 2006 *Plural Publishing, Inc.*

Appendix 4E

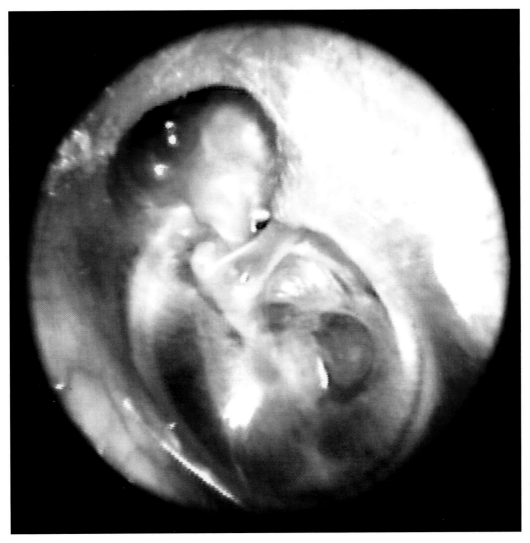

An example of a tympanic membrane with cholesteatoma. Reproduced with permission from Touma, J., and Touma, B., (2006), Atlas of otoscopy, *p. 102. Copyright © 2006 Plural Publishing, Inc.*

Appendix 4F

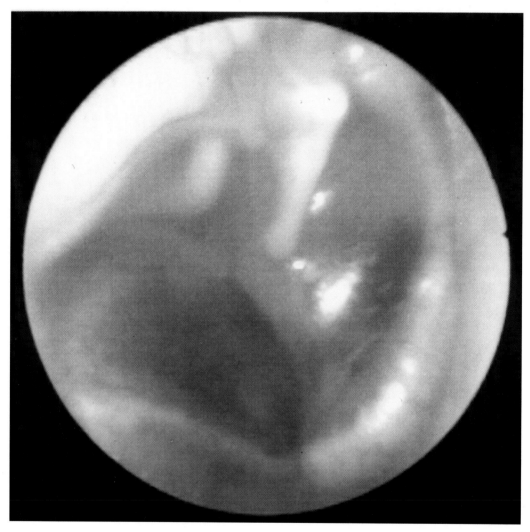

An example of a glomus tumor (note bluish hue).Reproduced with permission from Touma, J., and Touma, B., (2006), Atlas of otoscopy, *p. 153. Copyright © 2006 Plural Publishing, Inc.*

Appendix 4G

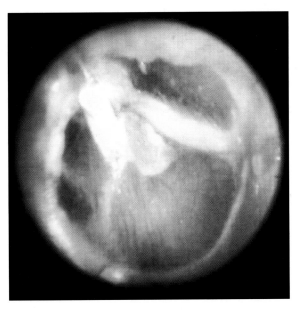

An example of ossicular discontinuity related to head trauma. Reproduced with permission from Touma, J., and Touma, B., (2006), Atlas of otoscopy, *p. 95. Copyright © 2006 Plural Publishing, Inc.*

Appendix 4H

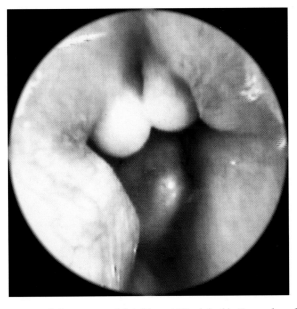

An example of exostoses of the ear canal (at 11 and 12 o'clock). Reproduced with permission from Touma, J., and Touma, B., (2006), Atlas of otoscopy, *p. 148. Copyright © 2006 Plural Publishing, Inc.*

Appendix 4I

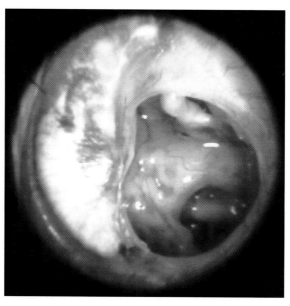

An example of a large perforation in the posterior tympanic membrane and tympanosclerosis in the anterior part of the eardrum. Reproduced with permission from Touma, J., and Touma, B., (2006), Atlas of otoscopy, *p. 64. Copyright © 2006 Plural Publishing, Inc.*

Appendix 4J

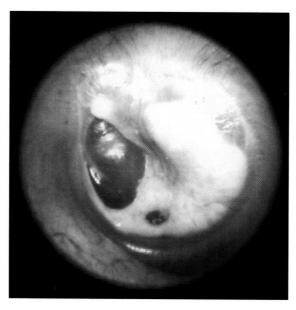

An example of tympanosclerosis covering most of the eardrum. Reproduced with permission from Touma, J., and Touma, B., (2006), Atlas of otoscopy, *p. 44. Copyright © 2006 Plural Publishing, Inc.*

5

Inner Ear Disorders

INTRODUCTION

This chapter covers a number of pathologic conditions that affect auditory function due to their effects on the inner ear. A brief overview of inner ear anatomy will orient the student of auditory sciences to the specific site of dysfunction, as well as to the treatment of these conditions. Recall from Chapter 2, Structure and Function of the Auditory and Vestibular Systems, that the cochlea is a sensory auditory organ encased in the dense bone of the petrous portion of the temporal bone. The bone surrounding the cochlea is formed via an endochondral ossification process and is referred to as the otic capsule. This bone is extremely dense compared with the surrounding temporal bone; however, it has poor reparative capacity. The cochlea is a bony canal that spirals 2½ times around the modiolus, which contains the spiral ganglion and myelinated and unmyelinated cochlear nerve fibers. This channel contains three distinct fluid-filled channels: the scala media, the scala tympani, and the scala vestibuli. The perilymph-filled flanking channels, which include the scala tympani and scala vestibuli, are confluent at the cochlear apex, the helicotrema. The central channel, referred

to as the scala media or cochlear duct, is filled with endolymph, a fluid that is secreted by the stria vascularis and contains the acoustic sensory apparatus called the organ of Corti. The organ of Corti rests on the basilar membrane, which separates the scala media and scala tympani. This structure is lined with one row of inner hair cells and three rows of outer hair cells along the entire length of the cochlea. A second membrane, Reissner's membrane, separates the scala media from the scala vestibuli and facilitates the translation of a cochlear fluid wave between the two compartments.

Sound waves within the external auditory canal are converted to vibratory mechanical energy by the tympanic membrane and the ossicles. This mechanical energy is conducted by the stapes into the scala vestibuli. A fluid wave is then propagated within the cochlea, which travels from the base to the apex. The fluid wave leads to deflection of the hair cells' stereocilia, which results in depolarization of the hair cells and neural transmission via the cochlear portion of the eighth cranial nerve. The cochlea is tonotopically organized so that the fluid wave within the cochlea transduces high-frequency acoustic information at the cochlear base and low-frequency information at the apex.

The otic capsule bone also encases the vestibular apparatus of the inner ear, which is composed of the utricle, the saccule, and the semicircular canals. These structures are filled with endolymph and are confluent with the scala media of the cochlea. Disease processes that affect the cochlea may also affect the vestibular system due to the close anatomic relationship of these structures and the confluence of endolymph, which may elicit vestibular symptoms along with auditory deficits. A wide variety of diseases, both acquired and congenital, can affect the inner ear and result in significant hearing and/or vestibular dysfunction.

TEMPORAL BONE TRAUMA

Introduction

The otic capsule is extremely dense and relatively resistant to fracture; however, injury to the cochlea may be related to blunt or penetrating trauma. Blunt trauma typically is due to automobile accidents, recreational vehicle accidents, falls, or assaults. Penetrating injuries are commonly related to gunshot injuries or stabbings and can carry a high mortality rate. Sudden changes in pressure within the external or middle ear can also lead to traumatic perilymph fistulas as discussed later in this chapter. This section deals with direct and indirect trauma to the otic capsule structures and the resulting effects on audiologic function.

Symptoms

Temporal bone injury typically is a small part of a multisystem trauma that often affects patients. Patients with temporal

bone trauma frequently suffer concomitant intracranial injuries with severe mental status changes and neurologic deficits, which may delay accurate audiologic assessment. Violation of the otic capsule bone results in sensorineural hearing loss, which usually is profound and irreversible. Vertigo, which often accompanies hearing loss, may be severe in the acute stages and may require weeks to months to abate. Bone fragmentation also may lead to facial nerve injury or even transection, and facial weakness may present in a delayed fashion due to hematoma or edema of the facial nerve. The external auditory canal and the tympanic cavity structures can also be damaged, but these sites of damage are not discussed in this chapter as they are outer and middle ear structures, which were discussed in Chapter 4. Damage to major blood vessels that traverse the temporal bone may present with massive hemorrhage from the ear and represents a true emergency requiring immediate medical attention.

Incidence and Prevalence

Automobile accidents are the leading cause of head trauma, representing up to 75% of all cases of temporal bone fractures. Other common causes include assaults, falls, motorcycle accidents, bicycle accidents, and gunshot wounds. These types of fractures are more common in men than in women, with a peak incidence in the third and fourth decades of life (Saraiya & Aygun, 2009).

Etiology and Pathology

A temporal bone fracture is the result of significant force to the skull. Fractures that are oriented longitudinally to the long axis of the petrous temporal bone are due to blunt force to the lateral skull and are more prevalent than other types of fractures, accounting for over 70 to 80% of all temporal bone fractures. Fractures transverse to the petrous bone are less common, but facial nerve injury occurs approximately 50% of the time in this type of fracture. Often, fractures involve both longitudinal and transverse fracture lines. Penetrating trauma results in comminuted fractures and classic fracture patterns are not seen. The location of the fracture line in relationship to the otic capsule is clinically significant (Dahiya et al., 1999).

Site of Lesion

An otic capsule sparing fracture is similar to the longitudinal fracture line discussed above and the cochlea and vestibule typically remain intact. An otic capsule violating fracture has a fracture line extending into the cochlea or vestibule and is associated with a significantly higher incidence of hearing loss and/or vertigo. This latter type of fracture line typically disrupts the delicate membranous labyrinth and results in profound, irreversible sensorineural hearing loss.

Fracture lines also may cause avulsion and separation of the spiral ganglion acoustic nerve fibers at the fundus of the internal auditory canal and blunt trauma to the temporal bone may open abnormal fistulae of the labyrinth in the area of the oval window or round window, resulting in what is referred to as a perilymph fistula. Hearing losses without discrete fracture lines also can be seen after blunt trauma due to concussive trauma; however, the exact mechanism for this type of insult is poorly understood.

As mentioned above, fractures of the temporal bone adjacent to the otic capsule may involve injury to the facial nerve and an abnormal fistula within the ear may

occur. Finally, major vascular injury to the sigmoid sinus, jugular bulb, or carotid artery can occur as a result of penetrating trauma or impinging bony fragments from blunt trauma.

Audiology

Audiologic testing of the patient who has sustained head trauma is performed following stabilization of the patient. Many approaches can be taken with respect to audiologic evaluation, but at a minimum comprehensive pure-tone and speech recognition testing along with tympanometry should be performed. Eventually, it may prove useful to determine both peripheral (cochlear and vestibular nerve) and central hearing status in these patients. Prior to any audiologic testing, however, otoscopy must be performed and often the external auditory meatus will need to be cleaned due to fluid and blood accumulation before any audiologic testing can be done. Clinicians must take extra caution when performing an audiologic evaluation on a patient with temporal bone trauma as these patients often are in an altered state and have significant pain. In some cases, it will be difficult, if not impossible, to perform bone conduction testing due to the presence of the fracture.

Results from the audiologic evaluation may present as a conductive hearing loss, a sensorineural hearing loss, or as a mixed hearing loss, with both conductive and sensorineural components. The type of loss often is correlated with the fracture characteristic. Fractures that are longitudinal in nature often result in more conductive involvement as those fractures run through the petrous pyramid and may extend as far as the mastoid bone, whereas sensorineural hearing loss tends to be more common in cases with transverse fractures (Jerger & Jerger, 1981).

It should be noted that approximately 10 to 20% of patients presenting with longitudinal fractures and nearly 50% of patients with transverse fractures will present with facial paralysis. If this occurs, electroneurography (ENoG) would be an appropriate test to administer so that a determination of the extent of facial nerve involvement can be made. This becomes a critical tool in determining if surgical intervention to debulk the nerve is needed. Due to the close proximity of the auditory and vestibular nerves to the facial nerve (i.e., both the facial nerve and the auditory and vestibular branches of the eighth cranial nerve course through the internal auditory canal), there is a high probability that auditory and vestibular nerve disruption will coexist with facial nerve involvement. In these cases, additional audiologic and vestibular testing for potential auditory and/or vestibular nerve involvement would be indicated.

Medical Examination

Temporal bone trauma is rarely isolated and patients typically experience compromise of other systems in addition to the auditory system. These patients frequently require stabilization and evaluation according to cardiopulmonary resuscitation protocols. Many may be intubated and mechanically ventilated due to their neurologic status and/or other injuries. This may delay an accurate and thorough examination for days; however, efforts should be taken to perform an initial assessment as close in time to the insult as is possible. This assessment should include examination of the pinna and ear canal. Periauricular bruising may indicate temporal bone fracture and extravasation of blood in subcutaneous tissue planes. Bony fragments, blood, and/or debris may hinder inspection of the ear canal. Blood also may fill the middle ear space, giving the tympanic membrane a bluish hue. If the tympanic membrane can be visualized, one should inspect for a bluish bulge of the membrane, which results from blood filling the middle ear space, a condition referred to as a hemotympanum. Pneumatic otoscopy should also be performed as this can evaluate the integrity of the tympanic membrane and also test for a perilymph fistula. Positive and negative pressure within the external canal can elicit nystagmus and support the diagnosis of a fistula. Cerebral spinal fluid may be found leaking from the ear, which will appear as clear watery otorrhea or rhinorrhea. A thorough cranial nerve exam as a part of the head and neck exam may reveal focal cranial neuropathies. Facial nerve function and the onset of facial weakness should be documented. Other injuries may postpone a thorough audiometric evaluation, thus a tuning fork evaluation (Weber and Rinne tests), which can give information regarding the conductive and sensorineural function of the ear, should be included with every temporal bone trauma evaluation. Typically, radiographic imaging is performed via a high-resolution computed tomography (CT) of the temporal bone with thin slices. This type of scan provides the information necessary to guide clinical decisions and predict outcomes. The fracture pattern can be identified and surrounding anatomy can be delineated with careful inspection of the CT scan (Saraiya & Aygun, 2009).

Audiologic Management

Recovery of auditory function typically ranges from 3 weeks to 6 months (Schulman, 1979). Due to the likelihood of fluctuations in hearing sensitivity, it is important to continually monitor hearing thresholds. Obtaining stable audiologic results is essential. If the patient presents with sustained hearing loss, appropriate audiologic management, including the fitting of hearing aids, would be warranted.

At times, the hearing loss may be so severe that amplification will not be useful. A profoundly deafened ear may utilize a contralateral routing of signal (CROS) aid (with a microphone on the involved ear and the receiver on the contralateral ear) or a bone-anchored hearing aid to improve help improve localization abilities. If bilateral sensorineural hearing loss is present, cochlear implantation may be considered (Morgan, Coker, & Jenkins, 1994); however, these patients represent a special challenge for cochlear implants due to the possibility of intracochlear fibrosis and the remote possibility that the cochlear nerve itself could have been injured medial to the cochlea.

Vertigo following temporal bone trauma should be evaluated by videonystagmography (VNG). Patients may have a concussive membranous labyrinth injury that presents with positional vertigo with an otherwise normal VNG. Traumatic cupulolithiasis can be managed by an Epley maneuver. A VNG test administered with the insertion of positive and negative pressure within the ear canal via a tympanometer may also identify a positive fistula test and may support a middle ear exploration with closure of the fistula.

Medical Management

The role of medical and surgical intervention is to manage complications caused by temporal bone fractures. Some cases may only involve concussive injuries to the inner ear structures and these patients may regain function spontaneously over time. Injury to the otic capsule, however, is unfortunately permanent. Vertigo that may be present due to vestibular injury can be effectively suppressed with benzodiazepines and antiemetics. Compensation of the vestibular system typically occurs in patients with temporal bone fractures affecting the vestibular structures. This compensation usually evolves over the first few weeks and is expedited by physical activity and limiting CNS-depressing medications. There is currently no role for medical or surgical intervention for sensorineural hearing loss related to temporal bone trauma.

Case 5–1:
Temporal Bone Trauma

History

A 33-year-old female was seen for a hearing evaluation due to complaints regarding hearing sensitivity, particularly in the presence of background noise, following a head injury. She was a horse trainer who in December of 2003 was thrown from a horse and subsequently kicked in the head by the horse resulting in a basilar skull fracture on the right side. Following her head injury, she experienced a general decrease in her hearing sensitivity and reported a number of concerns regarding her hearing sensitivity. She also experienced constant tinnitus, which she described as being centralized in her head, and significant imbalance, particularly when riding. The patient additionally reported that she often found herself asking for repetition and relying heavily on visual cues to aid in comprehension of spoken messages. Prior to her accident, she noted that she had no difficulties with her hearing. Although she has consistently reported a loss of balance when riding horses since the time of her accident, her "balance" deficit was recently made very clear to her when exiting a boat and returning to land following a boat trip. During this event, she reported that she was unable to move due to fear of falling. She also reported deficits in short-term memory, which she attributed to her head trauma. No other significant audiologic or otologic history was reported at the time of this patient's evaluation.

Audiology

An otoscopic check was unremarkable bilaterally. Tympanometry revealed normal pressure, volume, and compliance bilaterally (Figure 5–1A). Responses to pure-tone audiometry indicated normal peripheral hearing sensitivity for the left ear. Hearing sensitivity in the right ear was within normal limits through 1000 Hz and sloped to a mild sensorineural hearing loss for the remaining frequencies. Speech recognition thresholds were in good agreement with the pure-tone averages for both ears and word recognition ability was excellent bilaterally (see Figure 5–1A). Reliability was considered to be good. As the traditional audiologic evaluation did not fully explain the patient's complaints, a central auditory processing evaluation was initiated.

A central auditory processing (CAP) evaluation was completed and behavioral test results revealed a right ear deficit in temporal resolution and a bilateral deficit for temporally degraded speech (Figure 5–1B). Although it is possible that the right ear hearing loss may have played a role in the decreased performance noted on these central tests, it is unlikely given the extent of the hearing loss in the right ear (i.e., a very mild hearing loss in the high frequencies) and the finding of a bilateral deficit on the temporally degraded speech test. In addition, a combined auditory brainstem (ABR) and middle latency response (MLR) evaluation was completed to assess the physiologic status of the central auditory nervous system (CANS) from the brainstem to the level of primary auditory cortex (Figure 5–1C). Waveform morphology and repeatability were relatively good. The MLR testing revealed an abnormal asymmetry (ear effect), with a stronger right ear response. This can be interpreted as an abnormal MLR, but it does not lateralize the problem.

A vestibular evaluation also was performed. Computerized dynamic posturography (CDP) was performed in order to further assess the balance and vestibular complaints reported by the patient. Results from the CDP indicated a vision preference pattern. This pattern is often observed in patients who have experienced central insult resulting in balance problems (Black & Nashner, 1984). Patients with this type of pattern are more likely to demonstrate normal VNGs or only subtle deficits on VNG testing. In the current patient, the VNG testing demonstrated subtle abnormalities on ocular motor testing. This was likely the reason why this patient was having difficulty training and riding horses following her accident. This type of problem may be improved through the use of physical therapy designed to reduce the abnormal reliance on visual information.

DISORDER: Temporal Bone Trauma

PURE-TONE AUDIOMETRY

FREQUENCY in Hertz (Hz)

LEGEND		RIGHT (Red)	LEFT (Blue)
	UNMASKED	○	X
	UNMASKED NR	○	X
Air (AC)	MASKED	△	▢
	MASKED NR	△	▢
	SOUNDFIELD	$	$
	SOUNDFIELD NR		$
	UNMASKED		⌐
Bone (BC)	UNMASKED NR		L
	MASKED	[	]
	MASKED NR	L	L

NOTES:

Hearing Thresholds (HL) in Decibels (dB)

SPEECH AUDIOMETRY

Ear	PTA	SRT	Word Rec (%)
Right	17 dB HL	20 dB HL	92%
Left	10 dB HL	15 dB HL	100%
Soundfield			

TYMPANOMETRY

RIGHT
Compliance 1.1 ml
Volume 1.0 ml
MEP - 90 daPa

LEFT
Compliance 1.0 ml
Volume 1.1 ml
MEP - 100 daPa

ACOUSTIC REFLEX

		500 Hz	1000 Hz	2000 Hz
RIGHT	I			
	C			
LEFT	I			
	C			

A

Figure 5–1. Pure-tone thresholds, speech audiometry, and tympanometry results (**A**), behavioral central auditory tests results (**B**), and ABR–MLR tracings (**C**) for a 33-year-old female who sustained trauma to the temporal bone (Case 5–1). continues

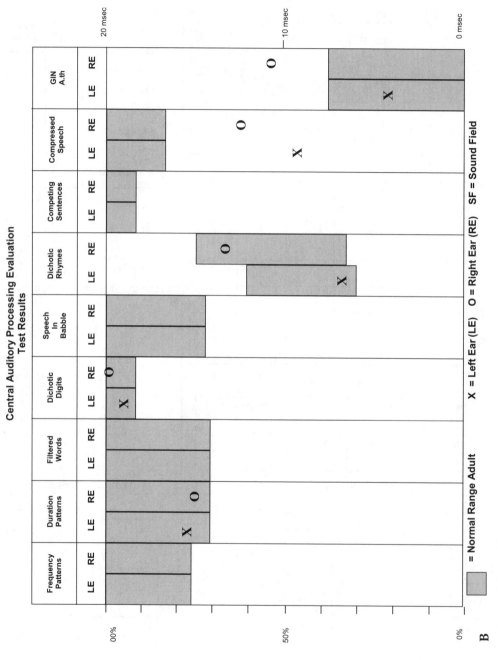

Figure 5–1. continues

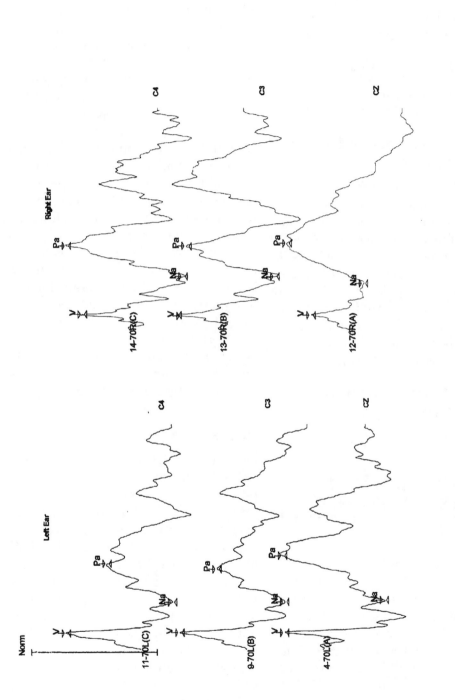

Figure 5–1. continued

177

Medical Examination Result

The patient presented with an essentially normal otolaryngologic examination.

Impression

Auditory processing and vestibular deficit secondary to head trauma.

Audiologic Recommendations and Management

It was recommended that the patient undergo both audiologic and vestibular rehabilitation. The aural rehabilitation procedures recommended included intense training exercises to build skills in the areas of temporal resolution and the processing of rapid and/or degraded speech. In addition, a mild gain hearing aid was recommended in order to assist with both the very mild peripheral hearing loss and auditory processing deficit.

Medical Recommendations and Management

None indicated.

NOISE-INDUCED HEARING LOSS

Introduction

Noise-induced hearing loss (NIHL) is a disorder that is ubiquitous and related to occupational or recreational noise exposure. Approximately 25% of the American work force is at risk for hearing loss due to significant occupational noise exposure (Suter & von Gierke, 1987). The Occupational Safety and Health Administration (OSHA) of the U.S. Department of Labor has developed standards for noise exposure in the workplace in order to decrease NIHL (OSHA, 1983). Both the intensity and duration of noise exposure can have an impact on audiologic function. Hearing loss related to noise exposure may be related to exposure to an isolated sudden high-intensity acoustic signal and is referred to as acoustic trauma or to exposure to elevated noise levels over time causing a more gradual onset of hearing loss (Daniel, 2007).

OSHA (1983) has provided regulations regarding occupational noise exposure and has determined that habitual exposure to high noise levels can cause a gradual hearing loss. Thus, unprotected noise exposure to (steady state) is limited to 8 hours per day at 90 dBA. However, exposure levels of 85 dBA for 8 hours can cause hearing loss and it is at this level that the employer must institute a hearing conservation program including yearly audiograms and the provision of ear protection. No unprotected steady-state exposure above 115 dBA is permitted. Also, unprotected exposure to impulse noise levels above 140 dB SPL is not allowed by these regulations.

Symptoms

Patients with a history of NIHL frequently present with tinnitus, typically a high-pitched constant tinnitus that is nonpulsatile in nature and develops gradually over time (Eggermont & Roberts, 2004). In addition, the development of hyperacsis may occur due to the presence of a reduced dynamic range secondary to hearing loss (Katzenell & Segal, 2001). The hearing loss in the majority of cases with NIHL is gradual in onset and typically involves primarily the high frequencies. Patients exposed to high-intensity noise may experience a temporary threshold shift (TTS) in hearing that may last 12 to 36 hours. This shift can be profound and more significant injury will lead to the loss of hair cells and neural fibers producing a permanent threshold shift (PTS). A threshold shift also is associated with a sensation of aural fullness or pressure. Vestibular symptoms are notably absent in NIHL, but may be present in cases of acoustic trauma.

Clinicians should be keenly aware of the rising trend toward blast-related injuries comorbid with noise exposure. There has been a significant increase in blast-related injuries by military personnel during deployments, which have resulted in both peripheral and central auditory and vestibular dysfunction (Fausti, Wilmington, Gallun, Meyers, & Henry, 2009).

Incidence and Prevalence

Noise-induced hearing loss is the second most common cause of sensorineural hearing loss. Ten million Americans are reported to have hearing loss related to excessive noise exposure (Brookhouser, 1994). Hearing loss of this scale carries a cost of billions in health care dollars for coverage of diagnostic services and therapeutic management (Daniell, Fulton-Kehoe, Smith-Weller, & Franklin, 1998). OSHA instituted workplace restrictions and regulations of noise exposure in the Hearing Conservation Amendment of 1983. However, a generation of workers who were employed prior to this amendment is at significant risk for NIHL. In addition, recreational exposure to noise with music concerts and portable music players has placed young adults at significant risk for NIHL. In fact, in a recent study, some degree of high-frequency hearing loss was found in nearly one-third of a cohort of college students (Mostafapour, Lahargoue, & Gates, 1998).

Etiology and Pathology

Although no specific gene locus has been identified, genetic factors are believed to play a role in development of NIHL (Davis, Kozel, & Erway, 2003). Risk factors related to NIHL include smoking (Palmer, Griffin, Syddall, & Coggon, 2004), male gender, diabetes mellitus, cardiovascular disease (Daniel, 2007), and exposure to toxins such as carbon monoxide or hydrogen cyanide (Fechter, 2004). The mechanisms by which acoustic energy damages the cochlea is via excessive stimulation of inner ear tissues, which leads to the generation of toxic metabolic by-products known as reactive oxygen species and free radicals (Prasher, 1998). These free radicals can overwhelm the inner ear defenses damaging hair cells and cochlear nerve fibers (Huang et al., 2000; Kopke et al., 1999; Kopke, Coleman, Liu, Campbell, & Riffenburgh, 2002). The mechanism whereby cells are destroyed by reactive oxygen species involves damage to the mitochondria of the cell and the initiation of a "programmed cell death pathway," referred to as apoptosis. The damage caused by exposure to high noise levels is dependent on a number of factors including the intensity of the noise, the frequency of the noise (higher frequencies result in more damage), the period of time the individual is exposed to noise, the amount of hearing protection worn by the individual, the time spent away from noise, and genetic factors. It has been postulated many times that, under high-intensity noise, capillaries in the inner ear constrict and a reduced blood supply results. This leads to metabolic exhaustion, which is related to the free radical action mentioned earlier (Møller, 2000). Bohne and Harding (2000) also report that high-intensity sound can damage the reticular lamina, which results in the intermixing of cochlear fluids creating metabolic dysfunction and hearing loss. The effects of noise exposure are additive over time. This is likely a result of the fact that stereocilia can either collapse or become fused over time, resulting in nonoperational tip-links (Harrison, 2001). If this occurs, the pores cannot open and the neural firing of the hair cell is not triggered due to the lack of the necessary ionic exchange, which in turn results in hearing loss. Additionally, significant damage can arise from compromise of the supporting cells (Bohne & Harding, 2000), which also leads to hearing deficits over time.

Site of Lesion

The primary cochlear structure affected by noise exposure is the organ of Corti. Specifically, the outer hair cells are damaged by oxidative stress from free radical formation, as well as from the direct shearing trauma caused by the movement of the high-intensity fluid waves through the cochlea. As the intensity of noise exposure increases, inner hair cells also become involved, and at high intensities, there may be excessive neurotransmitter release that could damage nerve cells on the receiving end of this action (Bohne & Harding, 2000). Sound transmission into the inner ear creates a cochlear fluid wave, which causes a shearing force on the stereocilia of the hair cells. Interestingly, for high-intensity sound, there is a one-half-octave shift of the main damage site on the basilar membrane in reference to the specific frequency of the stimulus (Møller, 2000). This shift is a result of the maximum point of displacement of the traveling wave on the cochlea moving in a more basal direction than for lower intensity stimuli. As Møller (2000) summarized in his review, most NIHL is greatest at approximately 4000 Hz. This commonly observed finding usually occurs from exposure to broad spectrum and/or impulse noise stimuli. This finding is likely related to the fact that the resonant frequency of the ear canal,

which typically occurs around 3000 Hz in the adult, augments the intensity of the stimulus at this frequency. If one considers this frequency and adds the one-half-octave shift, the resultant frequency of peak damage is 4000 Hz, where the greatest amount of hearing loss occurs. Exposure to ototoxic substances, such as solvents and heavy metals, may increase the injury caused by noise (Morata, Dunn, Kretschmer, Lemasters, & Keith, 1993). It should also be noted that there is significant evidence that insult at the level of the cochlea will result in transynaptic retrocochlear degeneration resulting in CANS involvement (Fabiani, Mattioni, Saponara, & Cordier, 1998). This should be kept in mind when evaluating these patients.

Noise-induced hearing loss is becoming an ever increasing and widespread hearing health problem. Noise exposure traditionally has been linked to occupational exposure to high noise levels, but an increasing number of patients are being seen today for NIHL related to recreational activities. In particular, the use of personal listening devices has become even more problematic today than it ever has in the past. Recently, it was estimated that nearly half of adolescents exceed safety standards with respect to acceptable levels of noise exposure (Vogel, Verschuure, van der Ploeg, Brug, & Raat, 2010). As a result, patient populations once believed not to be at risk for noise exposure have become target populations. Therefore, prior to any audiologic evaluation, a carefully elicited patient history becomes critical in determining if the patient may be at risk for NIHL.

Audiology

Audiologic evaluation of patients with noise exposure is essential for the identification and monitoring of NIHL. It is important to be sure the patient has recovered completely from any noise exposure that may have resulted in TTS before testing for permanent hearing loss. Usually, there is recovery from TTS within approximately 16 hours after last exposure to noise (i.e., assuming the TTS was not more than 40 dB) (Gelfand, 2001). The traditional evaluation should include, but not be limited to, otoscopy, comprehensive audiometry, and immittance testing. However, it is also recommended that the use of ultra-high-frequency audiometry be considered as part of the battery (Korres, Balasouras, Tzagaroulakis, Kandiloros, & Ferekidis, 2008) as it has been demonstrated that these patients will present with greater degrees of involvement in the high-frequency range when compared to patients who are not exposed to significant noise levels. In addition, it also has been recommended that patients with histories of noise exposure undergo otoacoustic emissions testing as this measure often demonstrates increased sensitivity to NIHL over the pure-tone audiogram (Helleman, Jansen, & Dreschler, 2010). The administration of otoacoustic emission testing therefore may allow earlier detection of ears at risk for NIHL; however, the improved sensitivity of otoacoustic emissions over the pure-tone audiogram has not been convincingly demonstrated and further research is needed in this area. The typical configuration of hearing loss is high frequency in nature with a "noise notch" observed in most cases. This notch typically occurs around 4000 Hz and will spread as the degree of hearing loss increases. This is believed to occur because the maximum damage occurs at approximately 5 to 15 mm from the oval window, which corresponds to this particular frequency range (Jerger & Jerger, 1981). Noise-induced

hearing loss also can affect neighboring frequencies; therefore, the interoctaves of 3000 and 6000 Hz should be tested. It should be remembered that 4000 Hz may not be the main frequency to reflect the maximum loss in NIHL. If the stimulation frequency is relatively narrow in spectrum and centered in the mid-frequencies, the maximum loss will likely not be at 4000 Hz, but at a lower frequency (recall the one-half-octave shift) (Lim, Dunn, Ferraro, & Lempert, 1982). The hearing loss in patients with NIHL is typically symmetrical unless there is a history of unilateral exposure through such activities as shooting in which unpredictable patterns may occur (Sataloff, Hawkshaw, & Sataloff, 2010). At times, individuals with long-standing conductive loss actually can preserve their hearing as the conductive loss attenuates the intensity of noise exposure. This sometimes happens in only one ear resulting in asymmetrical sensory levels.

Another factor to consider (alluded to earlier) in the evaluation of those with a history of noise exposure is the longer the exposure, the greater the degree of hearing loss, and the greater the number of frequencies that are affected (see Gelfand, 2001). However, it is important to know that there is considerable variability in humans in regard to the degree of hearing loss related to noise exposure (Gelfand, 2001). Susceptibility to NIHL may be genetically determined, at least in part, in that some auditory systems are simply more or less resistant to the damaging effects of noise. Factors related to this could be how well the acoustic reflex and efferent auditory systems function, the noise expose history (type, intensity, frequency, duration, etc.), the presence or absence of any comorbid toxic exposures, and the patient's age and general well being.

Medical Examination

Any patient with hearing loss should undergo a thorough head and neck history and physical examination. The clinician must carefully document the type and duration of occupational and recreational noise that the patient is exposed to, along with any protective measures the patient has utilized. Inspection of the external ear and tympanic membrane is typically unremarkable; however, acoustic trauma can cause spontaneous tympanic membrane perforation. Tuning fork evaluation should be performed. If asymmetry in pure-tone audiometry, tuning fork evaluation, or word recognition testing is identified, then further testing such as ABR or magnetic resonance imaging (MRI) should be performed to rule out retrocochlear pathology.

Audiologic Management

The management of patients with noise exposure typically involves both counseling and amplification (depending on the degree of severity). Hearing loss prevention and conservation practices are critical for any audiologist who sees patients with noise exposure. Prevention and conservation of hearing using appropriate tools such as ear plugs, muffs, or a combination of these devices is always recommended for patients with significant histories of noise exposure. In counseling and testing, it is important to consider the concept of damage risk criteria and the recommendations offered by OSHA (1983) and the National Institute of Occupational Safety and Health (NIOSH, 1998) for noise exposure criteria. Although a comprehensive discussion of damage risk criteria is beyond the scope of this section, a few comments will be made regarding the

NIOSH (1998) and OSHA (1983) recommendations. NIOSH has a 3 dB exchange rate for its maximum noise exposure recommendation of 85 dBA for 8 hours. This exchange rate means that for every increase of 3 dB in the noise level, the time of permissible exposure is halved. For example, using this exchange rate, the maximum exposure would be 4 hours at 88 dBA, 2 hours at 92 dBA, and only 28 seconds at 115 dBA. The OSHA regulations have a 5 dB exchange rate starting at 90 dBA for 8 hours. Applying the exchange rate specified in the OSHA regulations, the maximum exposure would be 4 hours at 95 dBA, 2 hours at 100 dBA, and 15 minutes at 115 dBA (see Gelfand, 2001). All employees are required to wear ear protection supplied by the employer when steady-state noise levels exceed these permissible exposure levels. However, for some employees (e.g., those who demonstrate significant changes in their hearing thresholds during their annual audiometric testing—see discussion below), the threshold for action is 85 dBA for 8 hours of exposure (or its equivalent time-weighted average for higher intensities). The same 5 dB exchange rate begins at 85 dBA exposure for 8 hours, so that the permissible noise exposure at 90 dBA would be 4 hours, etc. (OSHA, 1983).

Criteria are also suggested for the degree of permanent threshold shift. There have been several approaches over the years. These approaches account for aging and permanent threshold shift. In testing individuals' who have had noise exposure, NIOSH (1998) defined a significant threshold shift as equal to or greater than a 15 dB shift at 500, 1000, 2000, 3000, 4000, or 6000 Hz in either ear. This criterion is not employed as much as the OSHA criteria for pure-tone average (PTA), which is an average of 10 dB or more at 2000, 3000, and 4000 Hz in either ear. Counseling should include information on hearing protection which should be recommended for individuals working in 85 dBA or greater of noise. Protection commonly consists of ear plugs or muffs or a combination of the two. Earmuffs (especially those that are fluid-filled) generally provide a better noise reduction rating than earplugs in the field, but this is not necessarily the case in the laboratory. It is important to know that noise attenuation measured for both plugs and muffs are greater in the lab than in the field. For example E-A-R foam plugs provide a noise reduction rating of 14 dB in the field and 30 dB in the lab (Berger, 1993). This obviously reflects (among other things) the difference between ideal fitting and a less than ideal fitting in the workplace.

For patients who demonstrate hearing loss severe enough to warrant intervention, typically traditional amplification is appropriate. However, in extreme cases of hearing loss where hearing loss is too severe for traditional amplification, cochlear implantation should be considered.

Medical Management

At the current time, there is no known treatment for NIHL other than better hearing protection and better attention to good aural health. Because the injury caused by noise is oxidative in nature, some researchers have suggested the use of antioxidants, such as N-acetylcyteine, magnesium, salicylate, and vitamins B and E (Kopke et al., 2007; Kramer et al., 2006; Le Prell, Yamashita, Minami, Yamasoba, & Miller, 2007; Lynch & Kil, 2005; Sendowski, 2006; Suckfuell, Canis, Strieth, Scherer, & Haisch, 2007). A variety of antioxidants have been shown to reduce cell death in laboratory trials and are being investigated in preclinical trials. This work holds promise and in the future it is possible that medications may be available to combat NIHL.

Case 5–2: Noise-Induced Hearing Loss

History

A 46-year-old male was seen for evaluation of work-related hearing loss. He reported a 28-year history of occupational noise exposure from working as a heavy equipment operator in deep mines and noted a gradual decrease in hearing sensitivity with particular difficulty hearing in the presence of background noise. He denied the routine use of hearing protection, as well as any history of recreational noise exposure, family history of hearing loss, or ototoxic medicine exposure, but reported constant tinnitus bilaterally with no other significant history reported.

Audiology

A comprehensive audiologic evaluation indicated a mild sloping to severe sensorineural hearing loss bilaterally (Figure 5–2). The configuration of the hearing loss was consistent with noise exposure with a "noise notch" observed at 4000 Hz for both ears. Speech recognition thresholds were in good agreement with pure-tone averages bilaterally and word recognition was excellent for the right ear and good for the left ear. Tympanometry indicated normal pressure, volume, and compliance bilaterally suggesting normal middle ear status (see Figure 5–2). Acoustic reflex thresholds were consistent with audiologic test results bilaterally.

DISORDER: Noise-Induced Hearing Loss

PURE-TONE AUDIOMETRY

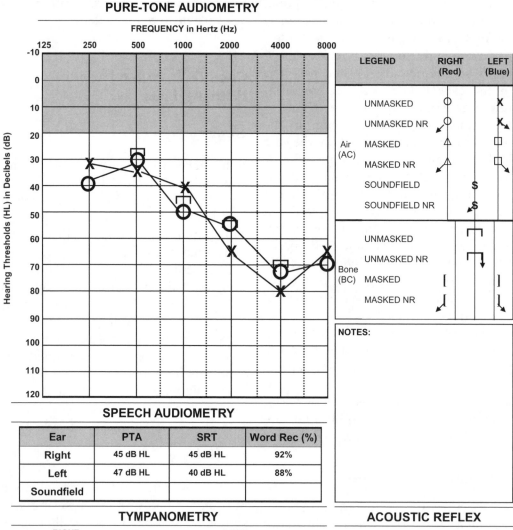

SPEECH AUDIOMETRY

Ear	PTA	SRT	Word Rec (%)
Right	45 dB HL	45 dB HL	92%
Left	47 dB HL	40 dB HL	88%
Soundfield			

TYMPANOMETRY

ACOUSTIC REFLEX

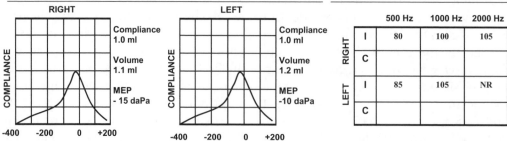

	500 Hz	1000 Hz	2000 Hz
RIGHT I	80	100	105
RIGHT C			
LEFT I	85	105	NR
LEFT C			

Figure 5–2. Pure-tone thresholds, speech audiometry, and tympanometry results for a 46-year-old male who had sustained a work-related noise-induced hearing loss (Case 5–2).

Medical Examination Result

The patient presented with an essentially normal otolaryngologic examination.

Impression

Bilateral noise-induced hearing loss.

Audiologic/Medical Recommendations and Management

It was recommended that the patient obtain binaural amplification to assist with hearing loss and difficulties. In addition, the patient was counseled regarding the importance of using hearing protection both occupationally and recreationally.

Case 5–3: Noise-Induced Hearing Loss

History

An 11-year-old female was seen following a recent failure on a school hearing screening test. The child's mother provided background information and reported significant concerns regarding her daughter's hearing health, indicating that her daughter had failed the school hearing screening for 2 consecutive years. However, the mother's most significant concern was the level at which her daughter listened to her MP3 player, stating that both she and her husband could hear it easily from across the room. No other significant audiologic or otologic history was reported.

Audiology

An otoscopic check was unremarkable bilaterally. Tympanograms indicated normal pressure, volume, and compliance suggesting normal middle ear function

(Figure 5–3A). Results from the audiologic examination revealed essentially normal peripheral hearing sensitivity in the low to mid frequencies with a characteristic "noise notch" in the higher frequencies with a maximum hearing loss of 30 dB HL observed for 4000 Hz in both ears. Word recognition scores were excellent bilaterally and speech recognition thresholds were in good agreement with the pure-tone averages. Distortion product otoacoustic emissions were performed and demonstrated present responses through 2000 Hz with absent responses for the remaining frequencies bilaterally (see Figure 5–3B).

Medical Examination Result

The patient presented with a normal otolaryngologic examination.

Impression

Bilateral noise-induced hearing loss.

Audiologic/Medical Recommendations and Management

The patient and her parents were counseled regarding the importance of hearing protection both occupationally and recreationally. It also was recommended that the patient undergo routine monitoring of her hearing sensitivity given the pure-tone findings of a mild hearing loss at 4000 Hz in both ears coupled with the fact that changes in cochlear sensitivity were seen on the otoacoustic emissions test at frequencies not reflected on the audiogram. The otoacoustic emissions test results implicated a decrease in cochlear function that eventually may appear on the audiogram; therefore, these findings were given serious consideration

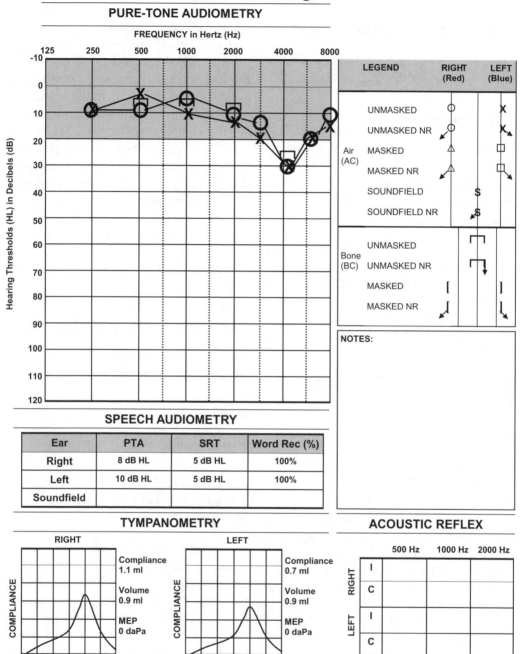

Figure 5–3. *Pure-tone thresholds, speech audiometry, and tympanometry results (A) and distortion product otoacoustic emissions (DPOAEs) (B) for an 11-year-old female with noise-induced hearing loss (Case 5–3). Note: The heavier (upper) solid line on the DPgram indicates the cutoff criteria for normal DPOAE values and the thinner (lower) solid line represent the average noise floors (see text for further explanation). Key: X = left ear response, O = right ear response, △ = recorded noise floor response.* continues

Distortion Product Otoacoustic Emissions

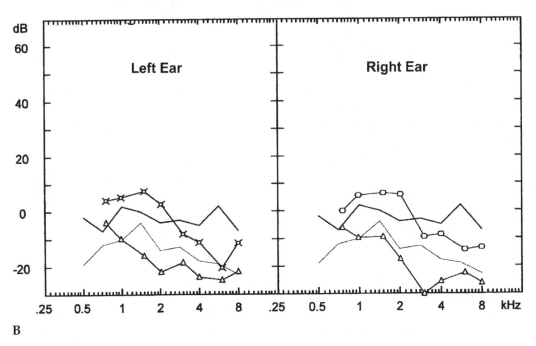

B

Figure 5–3. continued

OTOTOXICITY

Introduction

Ototoxicity has been defined as the effects of certain therapeutic agents and other chemical substances on inner ear structures, which result in cellular degeneration of the tissues of the inner ear, with a particular propensity for damage to the end-organs and neurons of the cochlear and vestibular branches of the eighth cranial nerve (Hawkins, 1976). The ototoxic side effects of medications have been known for over a century and were first noticed with the use of the antimalarial medication, quinine (Roosa & John, 1875). Since then many medicines have been implicated as being ototoxic; however, the majority of the ototoxic medications fall into five categories and include antibiotics, analgesics, antimalarials, antineoplastics, and diuretics. This segment of this chapter is limited to an overview of toxicity caused by drugs in these categories; however, a more exhaustive list of other agents/medications can be found elsewhere (Walker, Fazekas-May, & Brown, 1990). The term, ototoxicity, refers to a general toxic effect on the inner ear, but certain medications can be specifically cochleotoxic or vestibulotoxic. In addition, the effects of ototoxic agents may either be temporarily ototoxic (i.e., the damage is reversible) or largely irreversible, depending on the specific agent or medication. Some medications that are used represent the standard of care for treating life-threatening conditions (i.e., infections or cancer); thus, the potential benefit of using these medications outweighs the potential toxicity. Other commonly used medications may also carry the risk of ototoxicity, but that risk is lowered when careful prescription and monitoring practices are observed. Although the majority of ototoxic medications are administered orally or intraveneously, some are used in ototopic preparations and the potential exists for ototoxicity to develop if the drugs should enter the middle ear through a perforation of the tympanic membrane and be absorbed through the round window into the inner ear.

The primary antibiotic class implicated in ototoxicity are the aminoglycosides, which include gentamicin (Moffat & Ramsden, 1977), tobramycin (Walker et al., 1990), amikacin (Beaubien et al., 1990), neomycin (Murphy, 1970), kanamycin (Edson & Terrell 1987), and streptomycin (Hinshaw & Feldman, 1945). These medications have been used systemically in the treatment of bacterial sepsis and resistant infections. Topical preparations have been utilized in otologic and ophthalmologic infections as well. Some aminoglycosides, such as gentamicin and streptomycin, have a predilection to selectively ablate the vestibular system, which can be used therapeutically in cases of vestibulopathy. Other ototoxic antibiotics include erythromycin and vancomycin.

The primary ototoxic analgesics are salicylates, which include such agents as aspirin (Schwabach, 1884). The hearing loss associated with high doses of aspirin is often reversible. Quinine is an ototoxic naturally occurring compound derived from the bark of the cinchona tree that has been used for centuries as an analgesic, but it also has been utilized to treat and prevent malaria as well as leg cramps.

Antineoplastic drugs typically have an unfavorable side effect profile and can be toxic to multiple systems. Cisplatinum is a chemotherapeutic agent used to treat a variety of solid tumors but it carries significant ototoxicity. Other ototoxic antineoplastics include 5-fluorouracil, bleomycin, and vincristine (Walker et al., 1990).

Loop diuretics, such as furosemide, produce diuresis of excess body fluid to treat a variety of conditions ranging from pulmonary edema to hypertension; however, they also carry significant ototoxicity.

Symptoms

The clinical presentation of ototoxicity generally involves sensorineural hearing loss and tinnitus, and may also include vestibular dysfunction. The hearing loss is typically bilateral, involving primarily the high frequencies in the early stages of the ototoxic damage, with potential involvement of the mid and low frequencies if the ototoxic medication is continued. The tinnitus also tends to be high-pitched and is typically constant in nature. Patients may present with vertigo and nystagmus or may have global disequilibrium and poor balance when the vestibular system is affected. Salicylates and quinine present with reversible tinnitus and hearing loss that is dose dependent and abates when the medication is discontinued. Cochlear toxicity of aminoglycosides is more common with kanamycin, tobramycin, and neomycin, whereas vestibulotoxicity is more common with streptomycin and gentamicin; however, all of these drugs will have some toxic effects on cochlear and vestibular function. Antineoplastics, such as cisplatinum, initially result in a mild reversible high-frequency hearing loss, but as the total drug dose increases, the loss may progress to involve all frequencies and become permanent. Hearing loss due to loop diuretic use typically is in the middle frequencies and it tends to be accompanied by tinnitus, with both of these symptoms being reversible with discontinued use of the medication (Rybak, 1993).

Incidence and Prevalence

The incidence of ototoxicity due to aminoglycosides is reported to range from 2 to 15% (Kahlmeter & Dahlager, 1984) and may be related to concomitant use of other ototoxic drugs, total dose and duration of treatment, liver and renal function, and age. Loop diuretics have an ototoxicity incidence of 1 to 6% (Tuzel, 1981), with incidence and the extent of the hearing loss typically related to the medication dosage, and in the case of intravenous administration, to the rate of infusion. Cisplatinum causes ototoxicity in 25 to 90% of patients receiving the drug. The incidence of ototoxicity of salicylates and antimalarials is likely very low; however, considering the widespread worldwide use of these medications, inconsistent reporting leads to difficulty in prediction of toxicity.

Etiology and Pathology

A variety of mechanisms are involved in ototoxicity as these drugs affect a variety of inner ear structures. Aminoglycosides cause a disruption of neural function by causing degeneration of cochlear hair cells (Huizing & de Groot, 1987), endolymph electrolyte alteration (Mendelsohn & Katzenberg, 1972), and free radical formation (Forge & Schacht, 2000). As described previously, free radical forma-

tion can lead to cell death. Loop diuretics alter electrolyte composition in the inner ear fluids leading to sensory dysfunction of the organ of Corti (Arnold, Nadol, & Weidauer, 1981), and medications in the antineoplastic, analgesic, and antimalarial categories affect multiple cochlear structures; however, the mechanisms by which they cause hearing loss are unknown.

Site of Lesion

There is significant overlap in the site of toxicity for many of these medications; therefore, they may act synergistically to damage the cochlea. Aminoglycosides have been shown to deplete hair cells both in the vestibule and in the organ of Corti (McGee & Olszewski, 1962). Initially, the cochlear hair cells are lost at the basal cochlea, with subsequent involvement of the hair cells toward the apex with continued use of the agent/medication. Platinum-containing chemotherapeutics cause degeneration of the outer hair cells of the cochlear basal turn (Strauss et al., 1983). Loop diuretics cause injury to the stria vascularis, which regulates electrolyte balance of the fluids within the cochlear duct (Quick & Duvall, 1970). Outer hair cell function is likely affected by analgesics and antimalarials; however, the exact location of injury has yet to be elucidated.

Audiology

The prevalence of hearing loss among patients undergoing ototoxic treatment is high, but it is particularly detrimental to pediatric patients. In fact, in children and adolescents undergoing treatments using ototoxic agents the prevalence is estimated to be nearly 42% (da Silva, Latorre Mdo, Cristofani, & Odone Filho, 2007).

As a result, it is critical that these patients have careful monitoring of audiologic status pre-, peri- and post-treatment.

Ototoxicity typically yields an audiometric configuration of high-frequency hearing loss that affects both ears. In advanced cases, the mid to low frequencies can become involved. As with NIHL, otoacoustic emissions may be useful in heralding hearing loss before audiometric evidence of the hearing loss can be documented.

The evaluation of these patients is entirely dependent on a number of factors, which include the age of the patient, his or her ability to respond to testing, and the medication itself. The authors suggest using the model recommended by Jacob, Aquiar, Tomiasi, Tschoeke, and Bitencourt (2006) for initial evaluation, as outlined below. The subsequent schedule for audiologic monitoring typically is decided by the team of individuals managing the patient, and is based on a consideration of the variables mentioned above.

I. For patients who cannot respond behaviorally
  a. OAEs
  b. Immittance audiometry
  c. ABR
II. For patients who can respond behaviorally
  a. Threshold audiometry (including ultra-high-frequency testing)
  b. Immittance audiometry
  c. OAEs
  d. ABR

Medical Examination

Patients who are taking medications that are known to be ototoxic may be doing so to treat significant medical disease, thus thorough evaluation may not be possible on all patients. Care must be taken with all patients with hearing loss to document the use of all medications being taken as these medications may act synergistically to affect inner ear function. Also, the type and duration of occupational and recreational noise exposure should be documented. Inspection of the external ear and tympanic membrane typically is unremarkable. Tuning fork evaluation should be performed. If the vestibule has been compromised, spontaneous or gaze-evoked nystagmus may be present. Tests of central balance function, such as the head-shake maneuver or the Romberg test may indicate global balance dysfunction. The head-shake maneuver is performed by having the patient vigorously shake his/her head back and forth for approximately 20 to 30 seconds. The patient then abruptly stops shaking his/her head. A positive head-shake occurs when a nystagmic response is observed even after the head-shake has stopped, indicating an uncompensated imbalance of the vestibulo-ocular system. Videonystagmography may further be used to confirm clinical findings of vestibulopathy. If asymmetry in pure-tone audiometry, tuning fork evaluation, or word recognition testing is identified, then further testing such as imaging (MRI) and/or ABR should be performed to rule out retrocochlear pathology.

Audiologic Management

The clinical course for the progression of hearing loss varies significantly among patients with ototoxic exposure. Certainly periodic testing when patients are receiving ototoxic agents for either treatment or ablation is necessary. The interval at which this occurs varies from individual to individual. As discussed earlier, the hearing loss in patients with ototoxic exposure typically begins as a high-frequency sensorineural hearing loss that progresses to varying degrees, often spreading to involve the mid to low audiometric frequency range. Tympanometry typically is normal unless comorbid otitis media or some other middle ear condition occurs. The primary treatment for patients with sensorineural hearing loss following treatment involving ototoxic agents is amplification. However, in extreme cases of hearing loss where the hearing loss is too severe for traditional amplification, cochlear implantation can be considered.

Medical Management

The primary treatment of ototoxicity is discontinued use of the offending agent. As stated above, this may not be possible if the medication is the primary treatment for serious disease. However, prevention of ototoxicity for many patients without life-threatening disease is a realistic goal for clinicians; therefore, health care providers in all disciplines should be aware of steps that can be taken to minimize inner ear injury. Aminoglycoside blood serum levels have been used to measure peaks and troughs in the amount of medication present in the patient's blood; however, ototoxicity can be most accurately predicted by the total dose of drug given over the course of treatment (Beaubien et al., 1991). The dose can be corrected based on kidney function (Cronberg, 1994). Generally, loop diuretics and antineoplastics should be administered slowly and rapid intravenous push administration should be avoided. Often, salicylate and quinine toxicity can be reversed by stopping usage of the drugs. Patients who are able to be tested audiologically and in whom a prolonged course of treatment is anticipated are often evaluated with a baseline audiogram and renal function tests and then these are repeated during therapy to identify toxicity at its early stages. This pretreatment assessment and then monitoring with regular audiograms during therapy often is done for certain chemotherapeutic agents, such as cisplatinum. The administration of fosfomycin, an antibiotic, has been shown to protect the cochlea during cisplatinum administration (Schweitzer, Dolan, Abrams, Davidson, & Synder, 1986). The use of antioxidants also may have a role in preventing hearing loss in some patients receiving ototoxic medications, but application of antioxidants as a preventive intervention for ototoxic hearing loss has not yet reached clinical practice.

Case 5–4: Ototoxicity

History

A 36-year-old female was seen for an audiologic evaluation prior to beginning chemotherapy for tonsilar cancer. The patient presented with no reported history of audiologic or otologic involvement.

Audiology

An otoscopic check was unremarkable bilaterally. Prechemotherapy responses to pure-tone audiometry indicated normal peripheral hearing sensitivity bilaterally and excellent word recognition scores for both ears (Figure 5–4A). Test reliability was considered to be good. Postchemotherapy results demonstrated normal peripheral hearing sensitivity sloping to a mild sensorineural hearing loss for the high frequencies in both ears (Figure 5–4B).

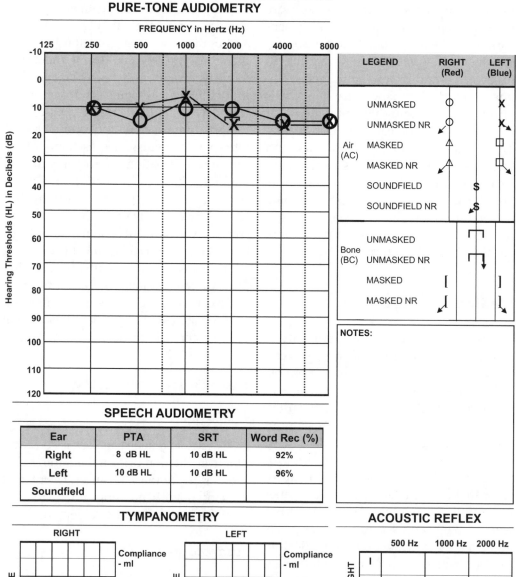

DISORDER: Ototoxicity (Prechemotherapy)

PURE-TONE AUDIOMETRY

SPEECH AUDIOMETRY

Ear	PTA	SRT	Word Rec (%)
Right	8 dB HL	10 dB HL	92%
Left	10 dB HL	10 dB HL	96%
Soundfield			

TYMPANOMETRY

ACOUSTIC REFLEX

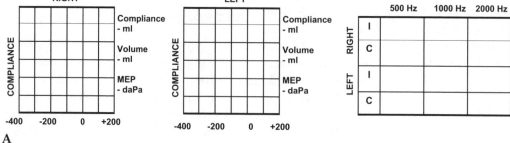

A

Figure 5–4. Pure-tone thresholds and speech audiometry prior to (*A*) and after chemotherapy (*B*) for a 36-year-old female with tonsillar cancer (Case 5–4). continues

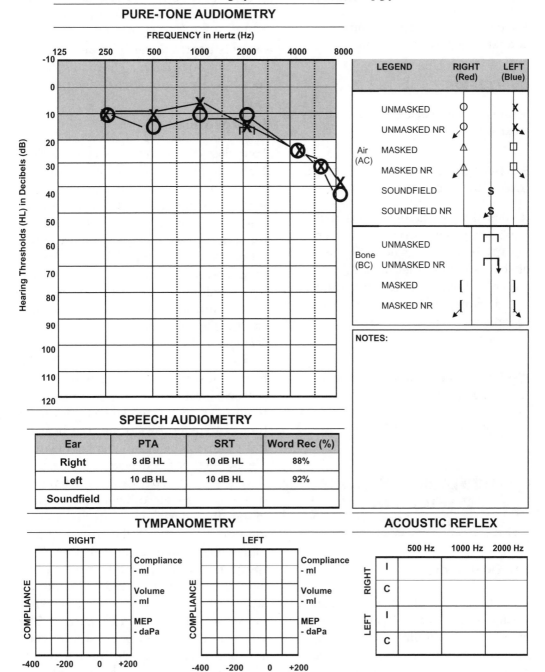

DISORDER: Ototoxicity (Postchemotherapy)

PURE-TONE AUDIOMETRY

SPEECH AUDIOMETRY

Ear	PTA	SRT	Word Rec (%)
Right	8 dB HL	10 dB HL	88%
Left	10 dB HL	10 dB HL	92%
Soundfield			

B

Figure 5–4. continued

Medical Examination Result

The patient presented with an essentially normal otologic examination.

Impression

Sensorineural hearing loss secondary to otoxicity.

Audiologic Recommendations and Management

Results of the audiologic evaluation were reported to the oncologist. The chemotherapy regimen was adjusted given the ototoxic effects of the chemotherapy. The patient's hearing stabilized following the adjustment to her medication and she continues to be monitored throughout her treatment.

Medical Recommendations and Management

Continue to monitor hearing.

MÉNIÈRE'S DISEASE (ENDOLYMPHATIC HYDROPS)

Introduction

The clinical constellation of episodic vertigo with unilateral hearing loss, tinnitus, and aural fullness is referred to as Ménière's syndrome. This may be caused by infectious, immunologic, or traumatic insults to the inner ear, which result in increased endolymphatic fluid pressure. The idiopathic form of this syndrome is referred to as Ménière's disease. The French otologist, Prosper Ménière, first described this disorder in 1861 (Ménière,

1861a, 1861b) and this disease bears his name. Although the clinical presentation of this disease has been described, the etiology is poorly understood and this disease continues to be a clinical challenge for physicians, audiologists, and patients.

Symptoms

Four classic symptoms are seen as a cluster in patients with Ménière's disease. These include intermittent attacks of vertigo lasting 20 minutes to 2 hours in duration along with the sensation of aural fullness or pressure, the experience of tinnitus, and sensorineural hearing loss in the involved ear (Gates, 2006). Clinically, these symptoms can exist independently of each other and can present at different times; however, for a diagnosis of Ménière's disease to be made all of these symptoms must be present. Initially, the hearing loss presents as a low-frequency sensorineural hearing loss that may fluctuate over an unpredictable amount of time. However, over time, the hearing loss gradually beings to involve the middle and higher frequencies, often leaving the patient with a permanent moderately-severe to severe sensorineural hearing loss in the affected ear. Severe, even debilitating, episodic vertigo is the primary symptom that leads to medical evaluation. This spinning sensation is accompanied by nausea and vomiting and following an attack patients experience an overwhelming sense of fatigue and exhaustion. The interval between episodes is quite variable and may change during the course of the disease. Around the time of each attack, a sensation of aural fullness is often experienced and the severity of the tinnitus is typically amplified. These episodes may vary from as frequently as several times a week to as rarely as once or twice in a lifetime. A significant number of patients with Ménière's disease will experience a phenomenon known as "burnout" in which they no longer experience attacks of vertigo but are left with a stable hearing loss, tinnitus, and varying degrees of aural fullness. Patients also may experience a sudden drop attack, also referred to as a crisis of Tumarkin, in which they fall suddenly without provocation or warning but maintain consciousness. These drop attacks may be related to otolithic stimulation by the increased inner ear fluid pressure (Baloh, Jacobson, & Winder, 1990). Lermoyez variant of Ménière's disease is characterized by a hearing loss that briefly improves around the time of a vertigo attack (Xenellis, Linthicum, & Galey, 1990). Ménière's disease initially affects one ear, but may involve both ears in 17 to 50% of patients (Silverstein & Rosenberg, 1992; Stahle, Friberg, & Svedberg, 1991).

As diagnosis of Ménière's disease is made based primarily on reported symptoms, it is important for the clinician to understand the diagnostic criteria set forth by the American Academy of Otolaryngology-Head and Neck Surgery's Committee of Hearing and Equilibrium, which were designed to aid in the diagnosis of this particular inner ear disorder. The criteria are based on the following major symptoms: (1) vertigo, (2) deafness [hearing loss], and (3) tinnitus. The vertigo must include recurrent, well-defined episodes of spinning lasting from 20 minutes to 24 hours. In addition, nystagmus associated with the vertiginous attacks must be observed, resulting in possible nausea and vomiting during the spells when the neurologic symptoms are experienced. The deafness (hearing loss) typically reveals a unilateral fluctuating sensorineural hearing loss. And finally, tinnitus as a symptom is often unilateral, subjective, variable, and low-pitched in nature. There are four categorizations of Ménière's disease and patients are categorized based on their reported symptoms and test findings as detailed in Table 5–1 from the American Academy of Otolaryngology (AAO, 1995).

Table 5–1. Categorization of Ménière's Disease Based on Reported Symptoms (AAO, 1995)

Possible	• Episodic vertigo of the Ménière's type without documented hearing loss or sensorineural hearing loss, fluctuating or fixed with disequilibrium but without definitive episodes • Other causes excluded
Probable	• One definitive episode of vertigo • Audiometrically documented hearing loss on at least one occasion • Tinnitus or aural fullness in the treated ear • Other causes excluded
Definite	• Two or more definitive spontaneous episodes of vertigo 20 minutes or longer in duration • Audiometrically documented hearing loss on at least once occasion • Tinnitus or aural fullness in the treated ear • Other causes excluded
Certain	• Definite Ménière's disease, plus histopathologic confirmation of hydrops

Incidence and Prevalence

The majority of people with Ménière's disease are over 40 years of age, with equal distribution between males and females. Ménière's disease occurs in anywhere from 15 to 157 people per 100,000 (Wladislavosky-Waserman, Facer, Mokri, & Kurland, 1984), and it appears to be more common in Caucasians, with an incidence of about one in 2,000 (Morrison, Bailey, & Morrison, 2009). There may be a genetic predilection; however, no specific gene loci have been associated with Ménière's disease.

Etiology and Pathology

The exact mechanism by which Ménière's disease occurs is unclear, but it is related to excess endolymph fluid pressure, also known as endolymphatic hydrops. Typically, the disease is unilateral in nature, but will increase to a bilateral condition in up to 35% of the population at 10 years and up to 47% of the population within 20 years of onset of the disease (Huppert, Strupp, & Brandt, 2010). Some suggest that this increased pressure, whether from overproduction or under absorption of endolymph, results in the cochlear and vestibular symptoms (Horner, 1995; Zenner et al., 1994). Increased fluid pressure leads to the sensation of aural fullness and results in dysfunction of the organ of Corti with resulting hearing loss and tinnitus. As pressure increases, the cochlear duct membranes are distended and eventually rupture causing a dysfunction of the vestibular system and a vertiginous attack. The stria vacularis may possibly be implicated in the process because it is responsible for the overproduction of endolymph. Following this rupture and pressure release, the membranes relax

leading to a resolution of the vertigo. The observed pathophysiology, although it correlates well with disease activity, provides little insight into the periodicity of the disorder or the basic underlying etiologic agent. Others propose that electrolyte imbalance and altered fluid composition result in the cochlear and vestibular dysfunction (Juhn, Ikeda, Morizono, & Murphy, 1991; Kitahara, Takeda, Yazawa, Matsubara, & Kitano, 1984). As mentioned before, most reports indicate that this disease generally manifests itself in the fourth decade of life, with the onset of symptoms occurring between the ages of 20 and 60 years (Mancini, Catalani, Carru, & Monti, 2002). This disease is most likely multifactorial in etiology in that, immunologic, infections, and genetic elements potentially play a role.

Site of Lesion

Histopathologic evaluation of temporal bones has revealed distention of the cochlear duct (scala media) and the saccule in patients with Ménière's disease (Hallpike & Cairns, 1938). The etiology of the excess fluid within these compartments is not clear, but the endolymphatic duct and sac are thought to play a role (Arenberg, Marovitz, & Shambaugh, 1970). Fibrosis or bony compression of the duct or sac may lead to an increase in the endolymphatic fluid pressure. Histopathology studies demonstrate that there is significant degeneration of the spiral ligament, hair cells, dendrites, and apical spiral ganglion cells, which are believed to result in the typical low-frequency hearing loss observed in patients during the early stages of the disease (Vasama & Linthicum, 1999). As the disease progresses, nearly all of the audiometric frequencies will become involved. This involvement is likely secondary to the permanent and extensive morphological changes that occur in the cochlea during the disease process.

Audiology

The evaluation of patients with Ménière's disease should include a comprehensive audiologic evaluation including both pure-tone and speech audiometry. In addition, some clinicians advocate the use of electrocochleography (ECochG) for evaluation of Ménière's disease. Audiologic results in patients with Ménière's disease, although varied, often demonstrate a unilateral (as cases of bilateral Ménière's disease are rare, at least in early stages of the disease), fluctuating, low-frequency, sensorineural hearing loss. Although the hearing loss may start out as a mild degree of impairment, it often progresses to a moderate to severe hearing loss with more involvement of the high-frequency regions of hearing throughout the course of the disease, and bilateral involvement may evolve in many cases. Finally, it is not unusual for patients with Ménière's disease to also demonstrate poor word recognition abilities, which often makes aiding such hearing losses difficult (Jerger & Jerger, 1981).

Videonystagmography may further be used to confirm clinical findings of vestibulopathy; however, this test is normal in many patients with Ménière's disease, particularly in the early stages of the disease. Electrocochleography is a test that measures evoked potentials from the cochlea and the cochlear nerve, which has been used to assist in the diagnosis of Ménière's disease. Summating potentials (SP) and action potentials (AP) are recorded and a SP/AP amplitude ratio above 0.40 is associated with endolymphatic hydrops (Schwaber, Hall, & Zealear, 1991). If asymmetry in pure-tone audiometry, tuning fork evaluation, or word recognition testing is identified, then radiologic testing, such as MRI, or tests such as ABR should be performed to rule out retrocochlear pathology.

Two other procedures related to audiologic evaluation of the Ménière's patient need to be mentioned. One is glycerol testing and the other is the traveling wave velocity test (TWV), also referred to as the cochlear hydrops masking procedure (CHAMP). The former is an older procedure, the latter is just emerging, and both have their advantages and disadvantages. The glycerol test requires the ingestion of glycerol (a diuretic) by the patient, which supposedly increases osmolarity and reduces the amount of endolymph in the inner ear. This results in the lessening of symptoms, including the improvement of hearing, which is tested usually at 1, 2, and 3 hours after ingestion. If pure-tone hearing improves significantly, then the interpretation is that the patient has Ménière's disease. If there is no significant improvement in the patient's hearing thresholds, then the presence of Ménière's disease is unlikely. Recently, glycerol testing has grown into disfavor; however, it still is used and has its proponents—especially those who claim vestibular testing enhances its accuracy (see Di Girolamo, Picciotti, Sergi, D'Ecclesia, & Di Nardo, 2001). Recent reviews of the clinical value of glycerol testing indicate its continued use in atypical cases of Ménière's disease (Aetna, 2011).

The TWV or CHAMP procedure was introduced by Don and colleagues (Don, Kwong, & Tanaka, 2005). It uses ABR and high-band pass masking to derive waveforms by masking bands of high-frequency energy that contribute to the ABR waveform. By doing this in a sequential manner, more high frequencies are masked and the latency of the waveform increases because the low-frequency energy becomes the key component. This increase in latency does not evolve in patients with Ménière's disease — hence the diagnostic differential. The rationale for this lack of increase in latency despite the presence of more low-frequency energy components in the stimulus is related to an increase in stiffness primarily in the apical end of the basilar membrane secondary to the increased pressure in the scala media from the hydrops (Donaldson & Ruth, 1996). However, Don and colleagues relate that antimasking (less effective masking) at the basal end of the cochlea also plays a key role in the lack of latency change in hydrops. The theory is that this increased stiffness allows the traveling wave velocity to increase; hence less latency delay is observed for wave V of the ABR. This explanation has been championed by others and the rationale is solid and consistent with the hydromechanics of Ménière's disease (Donaldson & Ruth, 1996). Although Don et al.'s original study yielded compelling results, the results of a subsequent study have not been as favorable toward the use of the technique (Claes et al., 2008). The authors feel the TWV test holds promise for the diagnosis of Ménière's disease and encourage further clinical research into its application as a diagnostic measure for this disorder.

Medical Examination

The diagnosis of Ménière's disease is made primarily by a thorough medical history and not necessarily by an exam or diagnostic test. Specific questions should be asked to rule out other potential diagnoses, such as perilymph fistula, ototoxicity, autoimmune disease, infectious etiologies, and retrocochlear pathology. A thorough head and neck examination augments the medical history and is typically unremarkable. In the midst of a vestibular attack, patients will exhibit spontaneous nystagmus. Neurotologic examination of vestibular function may indicate the side of vestibulopathy.

Audiologic Management

Management of patients with Ménière's disease often is difficult from both a medical and an audiologic standpoint. This is because the fluctuations in the disease process make it hard to predict audiologic sensitivity and word recognition ability from day to day. In addition, although many patients' hearing sensitivity warrants amplification, their word recognition abilities are often so poor that they may receive little to no benefit from amplification. Moreover, most patients with Ménière's disease are not candidates for cochlear implants because their non-involved ear does not meet candidacy criteria. However, there are occasions in which the patient presents with bilateral involvement severe enough to warrant cochlear implantation. As outlined by Valente and colleagues, it is recommended that for those patients with serviceable hearing that hearing aids with digital processing be employed along with directional microphones and assistive listening devices to aid in hearing in the presence of noise (Valente, Mispagel, Valente, & Hullar, 2006). Most patients with Ménière's disease who are to be fitted with amplification will be managed most effectively with programmable hearing aid devices that allow them the flexibility to have multiple programs that can accommodate their changing hearing needs. And finally, counseling regarding the use of such programs and the establishment of reasonable expectations of hearing aid benefit in various listening conditions is also a critical component of any hearing aid fitting.

Medical Management

Acute episodes of vertigo are treated with vestibular suppressants and antiemetics, but long-term medical treatment of this disease is directed primarily at preventing vertigo attacks. The uncertainty in the etiology of this disease is reflected in the types of management that are offered to patients. No medical treatment has been proven to be effective in improving hearing or decreasing tinnitus and aural fullness in all patients; however, some patients experience some relief in all of these symptoms with treatment. Although this disease is not fatal and does not require treatment, most patients suffering from recurrent vertigo desire intervention. Hearing loss related to Ménière's disease is treated with amplification. Prior to initiation of treatment, the degree of usable hearing must be taken into account. Generally, patients with word recognition testing scores of greater than 30 to 50% are treated with hearing preservation options; although all patients may be treated conservatively initially. In order to decrease the endolymphatic fluid pressure, conservative medical therapy involves the use of a low-salt diet and diuretics (Bojrab, Bhansali, & Battista, 1994). Such an approach has been shown

to be successful at vertigo control in 50 to 70% of patients so treated (Ruckenstein, Rutka, & Hawke, 1991). The use of steroids, either through a systemic or transtympanic route, can also relieve recurrent vertigo (Bojrab et al., 1994).

When the vertigo is not reasonably controlled by these measures, further intervention is indicated, which involves ablating vestibular function on the affected side. It is counterintuitive to purposely destroy vestibular function in patients with vestibulopathy; however, removal of residual vestibular function in the diseased ear will allow the central vestibular centers to compensate for the unilateral involvement and prevent further vertigo. Most of the ablative options have efficacy measures that range from 70 to 95% but they carry a risk of hearing loss. The transtympanic administration of the vestibulotoxic antibiotic, gentamicin, can be used to ablate vestibular function if functional hearing is present and typically can be performed in an office setting. These types of nonsurgical ablative procedures should be supported with periodic audiologic and vestibular monitoring.

A first-line surgical procedure in the treatment of Ménière's vertigo is a decompression of the endolymphatic sac and duct and placement of a shunt into the sac that allows for egress of excess endolymph into the mastoid, although the efficacy of this procedure has been debated. This surgical procedure is performed using a transmastoid surgical approach and typically is completed as an outpatient procedure. The vestibular nerve also can be sectioned surgically through an intracranial retrosigmoid approach and carries a high success rate of vertigo relief, but requires a craniotomy and a significant postoperative recovery period. In cases where hearing is nonfunctional, a transmastoid labyrinthectomy can be performed by drilling away the semicircular canals and removing of all the neuroepithelium from the vestibule. This procedure removes the remainder of hearing, but is over 95% successful at vertigo control (Schwaber, 2007).

Case 5–5: Bilateral Ménière's Disease

History

This 53-year-old male presented with chronic and debilitating vertigo for a year prior to his evaluation. He reportedly experienced several episodes per week lasting from a few minutes to hours. He also presented with aural fullness and low-frequency tinnitus bilaterally, and mentioned that these symptoms were more severe in his left ear than in his right ear. Hearing was reported to be significantly decreased with daily fluctuations.

Audiology

An otoscopic check was unremarkable bilaterally. The results of a comprehensive audiologic evaluation indicated a moderate rising to mild sensorineural hearing loss bilaterally with asymmetry between the ears noted (Figure 5–5). Speech recognition thresholds were in good agreement with pure-tone averages and word recognition was poor in the right ear and good in the left ear.

Medical Examination Result

The patient presented with an essentially normal otolaryngologic examination. Imaging results revealed no retrocochlear involvement.

Impression

Probable bilateral Ménière's disease.

Audiologic Recommendations and Management

Binaural amplification was recommended to assist the patient with his significant hearing difficulties. The patient obtained hearing aids, which were programmed with multiple programs to help manage the daily fluctuations in his hearing.

Medical Recommendations and Management

The decision was made to treat the patient's left ear due to the fact that the symptoms (hearing loss, aural fullness, and tinnitus) were more severe on this side per patient report, and the patient underwent a course of prednisone and gentamicin treatments and demonstrated some improvements with this approach. The prednisone and gentamicin treatments were employed in an effort to control the vertigo by pharmacologic intervention. The prednisone was used to reduce inner ear inflammation, whereas the transtympanic gentamicin titration was employed to ablate labrynthine function, resulting in relief from the vestibular symptoms. A low sodium diet was also recommended to help control symptoms. In addition, vestibular rehabilitation to assist with the patient's imbalance was recommended.

Additional Information

The patient continues to struggle with bilateral Ménière's disease; however, he has demonstrated significant improvement in his vestibular systems since the initial onset of his symptoms.

DISORDER: Bilateral Ménière's Disease

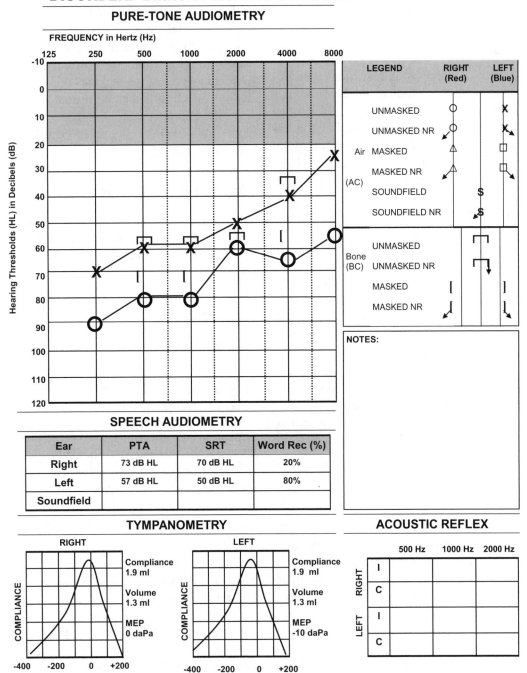

PURE-TONE AUDIOMETRY

SPEECH AUDIOMETRY

Ear	PTA	SRT	Word Rec (%)
Right	73 dB HL	70 dB HL	20%
Left	57 dB HL	50 dB HL	80%
Soundfield			

TYMPANOMETRY

RIGHT — Compliance 1.9 ml, Volume 1.3 ml, MEP 0 daPa

LEFT — Compliance 1.9 ml, Volume 1.3 ml, MEP -10 daPa

ACOUSTIC REFLEX

Figure 5–5. Pure-tone thresholds, speech audiometry, and tympanometry results for a 53-year-old male with bilateral Ménière's disease (Case 5–5).

Case 5–6: Unilateral Ménière's Disease

History

A 27-year-old graduate student was initially seen for medical evaluation of a long-standing hearing loss. At the time of her evaluation, she reported that she has had a hearing loss since birth and that her hearing loss originally was diagnosed as a mild sensorineural hearing loss. However, she additionally noted that her hearing loss had become progressively worse in recent years and that, over the last several months prior to her evaluation, she had developed some episodic vertigo. She denied any tinnitus or aural fullness. She initially thought that the change in her hearing loss and the origin of her episodic vertigo were caused by a mild carbon dioxide exposure, but these symptoms continued to persist following the exposure, with the severity of the symptoms becoming progressively worse, resulting in both nausea and vomiting. She also reported an unsuccessful attempt to use amplification.

Audiology

An otoscopic check was unremarkable bilaterally. Results of a comprehensive audiologic evaluation indicated a relatively flat, moderate sensorineural hearing loss in the right ear and normal peripheral hearing sensitivity for the left ear (Figure 5–6A). Speech recognition thresholds were in good agreement with pure-tone averages, and word recognition scores were excellent for both ears. Both VNG (including ocular motor, positional, and caloric evaluation) and vestibular evoked myogenic potentials (VEMP) examinations were found to be within normal limits. Due to presence of the congenital hearing loss and normal VNG findings, determining which ear was the involved ear was difficult. Electrocochleography testing was completed using a 90 dBnHL click stimulus. Results from the ECochG demonstrated a SP/AP ratio of about 60 to 70% on the right side (Figure 5–6B).

Medical Examination Result

The patient presented with an essentially normal otolaryngologic examination. Imaging results revealed no retrocochlear involvement.

Impression

Probable unilateral Ménière's disease.

Audiologic Recommendations and Management

Unilateral amplification was recommended to assist the patient with her significant hearing difficulties. The patient obtained a hearing aid, which was programmed with multiple programs to help manage the daily fluctuations in her hearing sensitivity.

Medical Recommendations and Management

The patient underwent a course of prednisone and gentamicin treatments and demonstrated some improvements with this approach. A low-sodium diet was recommended to help control her symptoms. In addition, vestibular rehabilitation to assist with the imbalance was recommended.

DISORDER: Unilateral Ménière's Disease

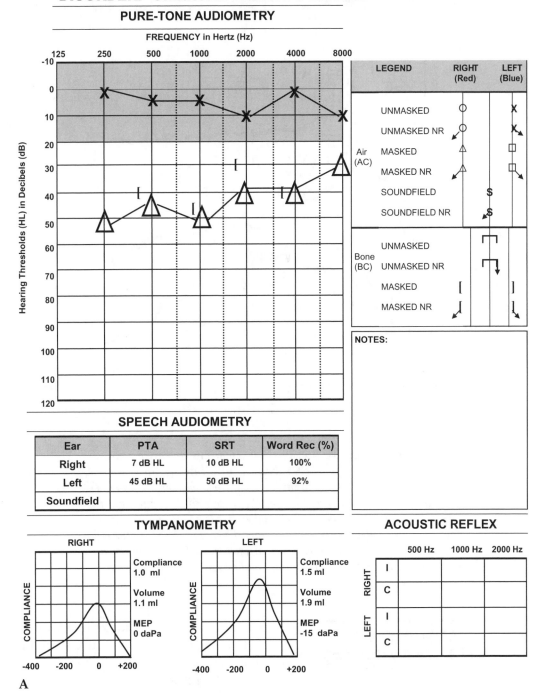

Figure 5–6. *Pure-tone thresholds, speech audiometry, and tympanometry results for a 27-year-old female with unilateral Ménière's disease (Case 5–6) (A) and electrocochleographic recordings from a second individual with Ménière's disease (B). The latter figure is included to demonstrate the application of EcochG in Ménière's disease.* continues

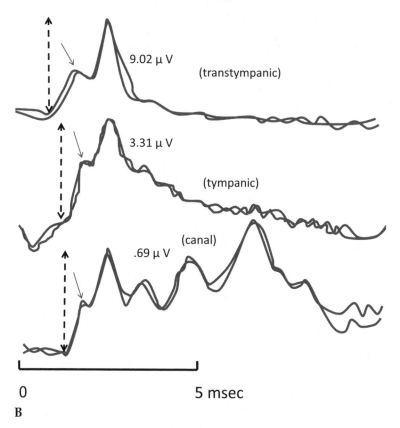

Figure 5–6. continued *Transtympanic, tympanic, and extra tympanic recordings are shown from top to bottom (inverting electrode was the ECochG electrode and the noninverting electrode was on the forehead). Note the differences in amplitude for the three recording sites and the presence of the ABR waves in the canal electrode recording. The amplitude measures reflect measurements from the base of the SP to the peak of the AP wave I as shown by dotted arrows. The SP/AP ratio remains about the same for all three recordings and exceeds 50% in each case.*

AUTOIMMUNE INNER EAR DISEASE

Introduction

Dysfunction of the immune system can involve the inner ear resulting in fluctuating hearing loss and potentially tinnitus and vestibular dysfunction. This disease may be caused by antibodies or activated immunologic cells that are directed at the inner ear. An autoimmune inner ear disease (AIED) classification system has been developed and consists of: (1) primary disease, which originates within the inner ear, and (2) secondary disease, which is characterized by systemic disease that affects the inner ear (Hughes, Barna, Calabrese, & Koo, 1993). Multiple systemic autoimmune diseases have been known to be related to AIED, several of which are Cogan's syndrome, rheumatoid arthritis, lupus, Hashimoto's thyroiditis, ulcerative colitis, and Wegener's granulomatosis (Hughes et al., 1993). Cogan's syndrome is of particular interest because it mimics Ménière's disease in its presentation, but it frequently is accompanied by ocular symptoms. A diagnosis of AIED is typically made by exclusion of other diseases that cause similar symptoms.

Symptoms

Autoimmune inner ear disease is characterized by bilateral fluctuating sensorineural hearing loss. The hearing loss typically occurs over a few months, unlike noise-induced or age-related hearing losses, which tend to have a much longer time course. In addition, tinnitus typically accompanies the hearing loss, whereas vertigo or imbalance may or may not accompany the cycles of hearing loss. Although the audiometric configuration in AIED may often mimic that of Ménière's disease, in many patients with AIED, hearing loss is not the primary symptom. In cases with secondary autoimmune disease, such as lupus or Wegener's, the external and middle ears may also be affected.

Incidence and Prevalence

The incidence of AIED is debated, but likely accounts for less than 1% of all cases of hearing loss. About 50% of patients with AIED have symptoms related to balance (dizziness or unsteadiness) and AIED is more common in patients with other forms of systemic autoimmune disease (Ruckenstein, 2004).

Etiology and Pathology

The dysfunction of the immune system that leads to inner ear disease is complex and has yet to be fully elucidated. T-cell lymphocytes have found to be reactive against inner ear structures (McCabe & McCormick, 1984). Antibodies that are directed at the human inner ear also have been identified (Arnold, Pfaltz, & Altermatt, 1985). The mechanism by which this autoimmune process occurs, however, is unknown.

Site of Lesion

Relatively little information is available regarding the site at which AIED-induced compromise occurs due to a paucity of temporal bone specimens from patients with active disease processes. It has been assumed to be a cochlear disorder. A 68 kilodalton protein has been identified from inner ear extracts, which would implicate the cochlea as the site of action for autoantibodies (Harris & Sharp, 1990).

Audiology

Audiologic evaluation of AIED typically involves a comprehensive audiologic evaluation along with immittance audiometry. As these patients often present with fluctuations in hearing sensitivity, serial audiograms are often necessary.

Medical Examination

The diagnosis of AIED is primarily made through careful review of a patient's history history and the exclusion of other common causes of hearing loss. Laboratory testing may be normal, especially in times of normal hearing. Specific questions should be asked to rule out other potential diagnoses, such as perilymph fistula, ototoxicity, Ménière's disease, infectious etiologies, and retrocochlear pathology. A thorough head and neck examination augments the medical history and typically is unremarkable. Other systemic autoimmune disease may cause other otologic manifestations, such as a middle ear effusion in Wegener's granulomatosis. Care should be taken to document other head and neck manifestations of disease, such as skin rashes or mucosal lesions. Neurotologic examination of vestibular function typically is normal. A panel of serologic blood tests are ordered to examine for markers of systemic inflammation and autoimmune antibodies. If asymmetry in pure-tone audiometry, tuning fork evaluation, or word recognition testing is identified, then further testing such as ABR or MRI, should be performed to rule out retrocochlear pathology.

Audiologic Management

Patients with AIED often present in a manner similar to patients with Ménière's disease. That is, they often have unpredictable fluctuations in their hearing sensitivity. Hearing aids may be utilized for hearing loss; however, significant fluctuations make appropriate programming more challenging. In patients who progress to severe or profound hearing loss, cochlear implants can be used successfully.

Medical Management

The mainstay of treatment for this disorder is systemic steroids, which may have to be titrated to manage acute changes in auditory function. Long-term steroid use is not without complication and typically is not recommended; thus, chemotherapeutic agents, such as cyclophosphamide or methotrexate, are utilized for long-term management. More recently, intratympanic injections have been utilized to achieve the same clinical effect without the systemic side effects.

Case 5–7: Autoimmune Inner Ear Disease

History

This is a 60-year-old female who has been followed for fluctuating hearing loss for 10 years. She was first evaluated for a sudden sensorineural hearing loss. Throughout her treatment, she has presented with issues of imbalance and intermittent vertigo. Since the onset of her sudden hearing loss, she has had significant fluctuations in her hearing sensitivity.

Audiology

This patient has undergone many serial audiograms over the years. Audiometric test results both prior to and following treatment with dexamethasone are presented in Figures 5–7A and 5-7B. Results obtained prior to transtympanic administration of dexamathasone demonstrated a severe sensorineural hearing loss and poor word recognition scores bilaterally (see Figure 5–7A), whereas postinjection results revealed significant improvement in both hearing sensitivity and word recognition ability with only a mild hearing loss being observed (see Figure 5–7B).

DISORDER: Autoimmune Inner Ear Disease (Pretreatment)

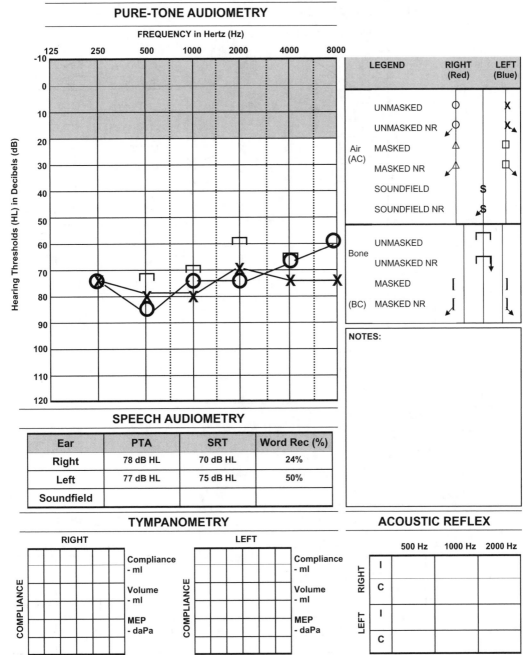

PURE-TONE AUDIOMETRY

SPEECH AUDIOMETRY

Ear	PTA	SRT	Word Rec (%)
Right	78 dB HL	70 dB HL	24%
Left	77 dB HL	75 dB HL	50%
Soundfield			

TYMPANOMETRY

ACOUSTIC REFLEX

A

Figure 5–7. Pure-tone thresholds and speech audiometry prior to treatment (**A**) and after treatment (**B**) for a 60-year-old female with probable autoimmune inner ear disease (Case 5–7). continues

DISORDER: Autoimmune Inner Ear Disease (Posttreatment)

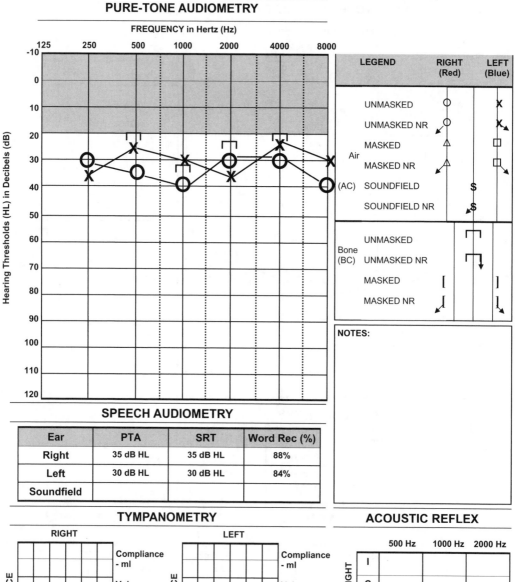

PURE-TONE AUDIOMETRY

SPEECH AUDIOMETRY

Ear	PTA	SRT	Word Rec (%)
Right	35 dB HL	35 dB HL	88%
Left	30 dB HL	30 dB HL	84%
Soundfield			

TYMPANOMETRY

ACOUSTIC REFLEX

B

Figure 5–7. continued

Medical Examination Result

This patient has undergone extensive medical evaluation by both rheumatology and otolaryngology. Imaging test results ruled out any retrocochlear involvement.

Impression

Probable autoimmune inner ear disease.

Audiologic Recommendations and Management

Given the significant fluctuations in hearing sensitivity, it was recommended that the patient obtain binaural amplification with multiple programs and close audiologic management in order to assist with the significant fluctuations in hearing sensitivity.

Medical Recommendations and Management

The patient continues to be treated with oral prednisone and dexamathsone as needed to manage the fluctuating hearing loss.

PRESBYCUSIS

Introduction

Presbycusis is the decrease of auditory function that occurs with aging. Although the severity ranges greatly, this type of auditory disease involves a decrease in acuity, understanding, and overall communication and cognitive function. Although nearly all adults experience a decrease in hearing sensitivity with time, some individuals are affected earlier in life and more severely. Unfortunately, the peripheral auditory system has very little reparative capacity, so insults to the auditory system are additive over time.

Symptoms

Presbycusis typically presents with a slowly progressive, bilateral hearing loss that is often accompanied by tinnitus (Rosenhall & Karlsson, 1991). Although vestibular function may be affected during the aging process, vertigo and imbalance typically do not accompany the hearing loss. However, word recognition performance may be disproportionally decreased compared to pure-tone auditory function. This reduction in word recognition ability is referred to as "phonemic regression" (Gaeth, 1948). The hearing loss from aging is sensorineural in nature, but can be divided into the following categories: sensory, neural, or strial (Schuknecht, 1974). These categories indicate that sensory structures such as hair cells, the stria vascularis, and the auditory nerve all can undergo changes with aging yielding a variety of hearing deficits.

Incidence and Prevalence

According to the National Institute on Deafness and Other Communication Disorders (NIDCD), "about 30-35 percent of adults between the ages of 65 and 75 years have a hearing loss." and "It is estimated that 40-50 percent of people 75 and older have a hearing loss" (NIDCD, 2010). There appears to be a genetic component in presbycusis in that, although nearly all individuals will show evidence of progressive hearing loss with age, some families demonstrate this loss at an earlier age and to a greater extent than other families.

Etiology and Pathology

The mechanism of injury involved in presbycusis is unknown. Patients with a genetic predisposition for this type of loss may be more susceptible to injury. Similar to other pathologies of the cochlea, this may involve oxidative damage or failure to scavenge free radicals. Other metabolic, noise, or toxic insults to the auditory system may lead to acceleration of the disease process.

Site of Lesion

The different categories of presbycusis provide information on the site of involvement. The sensory type of injury likely involves damage to the hair cells within the organ of Corti. Neural presbycusis involves adegeneration of first order neurons of the cochlear nerve. The strial pattern of loss is due to injury to the stria vacularis, which maintains endolymph production and composition. Although much of the literature on presbycusis addresses the involvement of the cochlea and the cochlear nerve, additional effects are noted throughout the auditory system, particularly in the central auditory system (see Chapter 7, Disorders Affecting the Central Auditory Nervous System).

Audiology

The presbycusic patient is the hallmark patient in any given audiologic clinic. Patients with presbycusis are evaluated by comprehensive audiometry, which generally reveals a bilateral sloping sensorineural hearing loss that gradually progresses over time. There is a significant variability among patients with respect to the degree of hearing loss as correlated with age. In addition, the word recognition ability of these patients can vary significantly, which will directly impact management approaches. It is well documented that age-related changes in auditory function are not only a result of peripheral involvement, but central auditory decline as well (Martin & Jerger, 2005; Pichora-Fuller & Souza, 2003). This may account for the significant variability among patients with respect to their word recognition abilities. Patients with a greater degree of central auditory involvement will likely demonstrate poor word recognition performance (see Chapter 7, Disorders Affecting the Central Auditory Nervous System). Gender effects also have been observed in the aging population with respect to degree of hearing impairment. It has been found that the average rate of change in audiometric thresholds is 1 dB per year over the age of 60 with gender a contributory variable (see Lee, Matthews, Dubno, & Mills, 2005). Specifically, Lee and colleagues found that the rate of change for females increased significantly with age for the low frequencies (250 to 300 Hz) and for high frequencies (10 and 11 kHz), whereas the rate of change in males increased more noticeably at 6 kHz. After adjusting for age, females had a significantly slower rate of change than males at 1 kHz, but a significantly faster rather of change at 6 to 12 kHz. Additionally, the ability to hear in noise has been well documented to be poorer as individuals age (Wiley et al., 1998) with greater difficulty exhibited by men when compared to women. Therefore, there is a need for tests of hearing in noise and central auditory function to be applied to the aging population.

Medical Examination

The diagnosis of presbycusis is made primarily through careful history and exclusion of other common causes of hearing loss. The history of a slowly progressive sensorineural loss is a key portion of the history. Specific questions should be asked to rule out other potential diagnoses, such as perilymph fistula, ototoxicity, Ménière's disease, infectious etiologies, and retrocochlear pathology. A thorough head and neck examination augments the medical history and typically is unremarkable. Neurotologic examination of vestibular function usually is also normal. If asymmetry in pure-tone audiometry, tuning fork evaluation, or word recognition testing is identified, then further testing, such as MRI and/or ABR, should be performed to rule out retrocochlear pathology.

Audiologic Management

Treatment of hearing loss in the elderly involves many considerations and variables. According to the World Health Organization (WHO, 2005), within the next 15 years, there will be approximately 1.2 billion people over the age of 60 with 70 to 80% of them suffering from hearing loss. The hallmark management of patients with presbycusis is hearing aids; however, for those demonstrating no benefit from traditional amplification, cochlear implants may be an appropriate option to consider. Many other treatment options should also be considered when managing the elderly patient, such as assistive listening devices as well as aural rehabilitation and support groups. Support groups and appropriate counseling are an important part of audiologic management of these patients because there is a direct correlation between a decreased quality of life and depression (Sprinzl & Riechelmann, 2010).

Medical Management

The mainstay of treatment for this disorder is hearing aids; however, care must be taken to avoid over amplification, as this may accelerate the loss of functional hearing. Currently, there are no proven antioxidants that prevent progression of the disease. In those patients who progress to severe or profound hearing loss, cochlear implants can be used successfully.

Case 5–8: Presbycusis

History

A 64-year-old female presented with a report of a gradual decrease in hearing sensitivity over the past 5 years. Specifically, she reported having difficulty hearing her grandchildren as well as hearing difficulties in the presence of background noise. She noted only occasional intermittent tinnitus bilaterally. No other significant audiologic history was reported.

Audiology

An otoscopic check was unremarkable bilaterally. A comprehensive audiologic evaluation indicated a mild sloping to moderate sensorineural hearing loss bilaterally (Figure 5–8). Speech recognition thresholds were in good agreement with the pure-tone averages and word recognition was good in both ears.

DISORDER: Presbycusis

PURE-TONE AUDIOMETRY

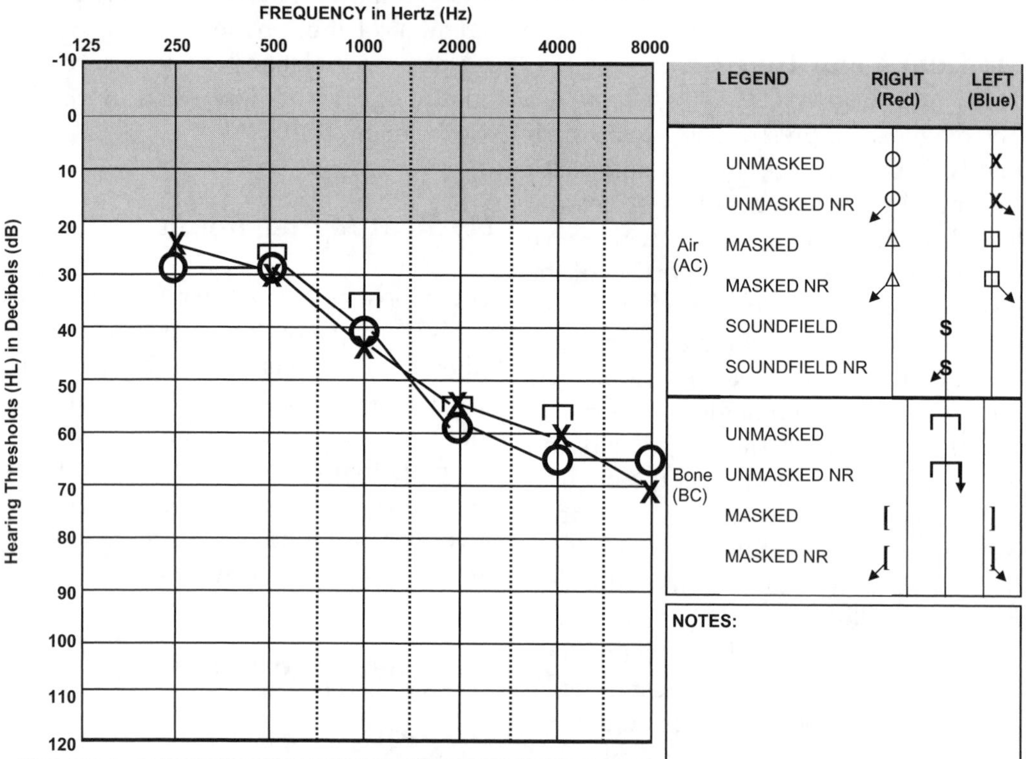

FREQUENCY in Hertz (Hz)

LEGEND		RIGHT (Red)	LEFT (Blue)
Air (AC)	UNMASKED	○	X
	UNMASKED NR	○	X
	MASKED	△	□
	MASKED NR	△	□
	SOUNDFIELD		S
	SOUNDFIELD NR		S
Bone (BC)	UNMASKED		
	UNMASKED NR		
	MASKED	[	]
	MASKED NR	[	]

NOTES:

SPEECH AUDIOMETRY

Ear	PTA	SRT	Word Rec (%)
Right	43 dB HL	40 dB HL	88%
Left	43 dB HL	45 dB HL	84%
Soundfield			

TYMPANOMETRY

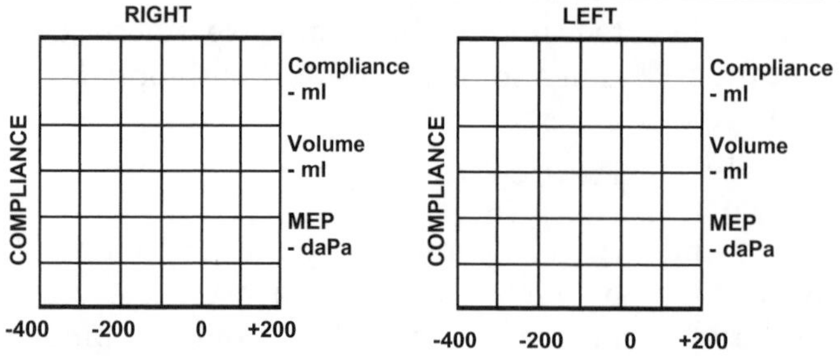

RIGHT

Compliance - ml

Volume - ml

MEP - daPa

LEFT

Compliance - ml

Volume - ml

MEP - daPa

ACOUSTIC REFLEX

		500 Hz	1000 Hz	2000 Hz
RIGHT	I			
	C			
LEFT	I			
	C			

Figure 5–8. Pure-tone thresholds and speech audiometry for a 64-year-old female diagnosed with presbycusis (Case 5–8).

Medical Examination Result

The patient presented with an essentially normal otolaryngologic examination.

Impression

Presbycusis.

Audiologic Recommendations and Management

Binaural amplification was recommended to assist the patient with her significant hearing difficulties.

Medical Recommendations and Management

Monitor hearing.

SUPERIOR CANAL DEHISCENCE SYNDROME

Introduction

Superior semicircular canal dehiscence (SSCD) is a relatively new clinical entity that was described in 1998 (Minor, Solomon, Zinreich, & Zee, 1998). The normal inner ear is fully encased by otic capsule bone with the exception of the oval and round windows. This syndrome involves an abnormal dehiscence of the bony covering of the superior semicircular canal that separates the canal from the middle fossa dura. Although typically there is no leakage of perilymph in SSCD, this entity represents a fistula of the labyrinth. Infectious or iatrogenic dehiscence of otic capsule bone has been known for years to cause auditory symptoms. The clinical use of high-resolution CT scans has made the identification of SSCD possible, and this radiographic finding has been linked to inner ear dysfunction.

Symptoms

Patients with SSCD typically experience vertigo that is elicited by loud noise (Tullio's phenomenon) and/or by straining (Valsalva maneuver). The imbalance also may be accompanied by instability of visual fields, known as oscillopsia. This vertigo is short in duration and may be accompanied by nausea and vomiting. Patients with SSCD present with various types of hearing loss, including sensorineural hearing loss, mixed hearing loss, conductive hearing loss, and normal hearing (Chi, Ren, & Dai, 2010). Although conductive hearing loss can be present in patients with SSCD, research has shown that the conductive hearing loss or component is not related to the presence of a middle ear compromise, but rather to the presence of a pathologic "third window" in the inner ear that results in an "inner ear" conductive loss. This type of conductive hearing loss results by the dual mechanism of worsening of air conduction thresholds and improvement of bone conduction thresholds (see Merchant & Rosowski, 2008). Some patients also experience an increased auditory sensitivity to their own voice (autophony), footsteps, heartbeat, and even eye movements (Chi, Ren, & Dai, 2010).

Incidence and Prevalence

The true incidence of this disease is unknown due to the fact that some patients with radiographic findings of SSCD lack the clinical symptoms. However, examination of temporal bones in cadavers has revealed SSCD in 0.4 to 0.5% of the temporal bones examined (Carey, Minor, & Nager, 2000; Watson, Halmagyi & Colebatch, 2000). This is a condition that has been diagnosed primarily in adults, although it appears to be the result of a congenital defect (see discussion below).

Etiology and Pathology

Superior semicircular canal dehiscence is likely a congenital defect, in which the bone overlying the semicircular canal fails to completely close (Carey et al., 2000; Watson et al., 2000). This typically is a bilateral condition, but both ears may not be affected equally. As noted above, SSCD typically is not identified until the patient with this condition is an adult as the symptoms associated with the condition tend to be delayed in terms of their presentation. It is not clear why the symptoms do not present until adulthood and what specific factors are involved in causing the symptoms. One possibility is that the bone covering the superior semicircular canal may be exceptionally thin, rendering it vulnerable to potential degradation later in life secondary to trauma or pulsation of cerebral spinal fluid.

Site of Lesion

The dehiscence of bone occurs in the thin rim of bone that separates the canal from the middle fossa dura. This opening creates a third window, similar to the oval or round window (Minor, 2000). Fluid wave transmission in the inner leads to aberrant movement of perilymph and loss of acoustic energy at the dehiscence site when sound is transmitted through the conventional conductive system into the oval window, resulting in elevated air conduction thresholds. However, the third window also acts to amplify sound that is transmitted through bone, which may result in improved or supernormal bone conduction thresholds (see Merchant & Rosowski, 2008). This is the proposed mechanism by which increased hearing thresholds and vertigo occurs. Clinical signs and symptoms also suggest that the utricle may be implicated in this disease process, although the mechanism by which this occurs is unclear (Tsunoda & Terasaki, 2002).

Audiology

Although not a new disease, SSCD is gaining more and more attention. And although not difficult, the audiologic examination of patients with dehiscence is slightly different than for patients with other types of inner ear disorders. Each patient with potential SSCD should undergo a comprehensive audiologic evaluation. There is a variety of findings in these patients, which may range from a conductive hearing loss to profound sensorineural involvement in those patients for whom hearing loss is documented (Chi et al., 2010). It should be noted, however, that the air-bone gap noted in patients with SSCD is actually believed to be nonconductive in nature (Songer & Rosowski, 2010). In addition, VEMPs can also be of benefit as patients with SSCD display responses at a decreased threshold (<70 dB nHL). Patients with SSCD can be divided into three distinct groups based upon their audiologic and vestibular complaints and findings. These groups include patients who present with: (1) vestibulocochlear signs and/or symptoms, (2) cochlear signs and/or symptoms, or (3) vestibular signs and/or symptoms. In addition, the size of the dehiscence can be positively correlated with the vestibulocochlear symptoms, lower VEMP thresholds, and more severe objective reports (Pfammatter et al., 2010).

Medical Examination

A careful and accurate medical history can raise suspicion of this disease process. A history of vertigo that is precipitated by loud noise or pressure changes in the ear is typical. A thorough head and neck examination augments the medical history. The external ear, tympanic membrane, and the middle ear typically are normal. The application of positive and negative pressure may evoke nystagmus and vertigo during pneumatic otoscopy procedures. Similarly, different Valsalva maneuvers can also elicit vestibular symptoms. Frenzel glasses should be used to identify nystagmus during these procedures because they prevent visual fixation and render the nystagmus more pronounced. The nystagmus related to SSCD is upward and torsional. Tuning fork examination is important in this disease process because of the suprathreshold bone conduction measures often noted. Patients can detect sound in the affected ear when a tuning fork is placed on the lateral malleolus of the foot. Videonystagmography testing also can confirm the presence of nystagmus with sound or pressure provocation. The gold standard diagnostic test in SSCD is high-resolution thin slice noncontrasted temporal bone CT scan in the plane of the superior canal. This study can clearly identify the absence of bone overlying the canal. In addition, MRI scanning may be necessary if there is significant asymmetry in pure-tone audiometry, tuning fork evaluation, or word recognition testing; however, it typically does not aid in the identification of SSCD.

Audiologic Management

Audiologic management is primarily dependent on surgical outcomes. As sensorineural hearing loss and disequilibrium are the most frequent complications encountered postoperatively, amplification, and vestibular exercises may be warranted in a handful of cases.

Medical Management

This disease may be self-treated by patients by the avoidance of loud noises and pressure changes. However, this may prove futile and unrealistic. Evoked vertigo may make driving and other common tasks difficult. Surgical management is the mainstay for treatment of SSCD. The objective in surgery is closure of the third window (i.e., the dehiscence). This can be performed by completely occluding the superior semicircular canal via a transmastoid or middle cranial fossa craniotomy approach (Minor et al., 1998; Minor et al., 2001; Minor et al., 2003). Plugging of the canal carries a risk of hearing loss but may effectively treat the symptoms of SSCD in 90% of patients (Minor, 2005). Vestibular evoked myogenic potentials have been shown to normalize following SSCD plugging. Another surgical technique for treatment of SSCD is the resurfacing of the canal, which maintains patency of the canal (Brantberg et al., 2001; Minor et al., 1998). This is performed through a middle cranial fossa approach and a variety of materials may be used to cover the dehiscent canal. This technique may have less risk of hearing loss, but the persistence of symptoms tends to be more common (Brantberg et al., 2001; Smullen, Andrist, & Gianoli, 1999). This disease entity is relatively new to clinical medicine; therefore, further research will need to be directed at the long-term natural history of the disease, as well as the surgical outcomes.

Case 5–9: Superior Semicircular Canal Dehiscence

History

A 54-year-old male was seen for consultation regarding a decrease in hearing sensitivity and aural fullness in his left ear and unusual complaints related to exposure to loud noises. The patient reported that for 9 months prior to his evaluation, he had noticed that when he was exposed to loud noises, he would experience brief "blacking out" episodes.

Audiology

A comprehensive audiologic exam demonstrated normal peripheral hearing sensitivity in the right ear and essentially normal peripheral hearing sensitivity in the left ear with the exception of a mild conductive hearing loss at 4000 Hz (Figure 5–9). Tympanograms revealed normal pressure, volume, and compliance bilaterally suggesting normal middle ear function. Speech recognition was excellent bilaterally.

Additionally, a VEMP examination was ordered to evaluate for possible SSCD. Results were normal and symmetrical at suprathreshold levels (100 dB nHL); however, the left ear (involved side) responses were present down to low levels (60 dB nHL), indicating involvement of the vestibular end organ in the left inner ear. This was not observed for the right ear. In addition, a VNG was performed for evaluation of the vestibular system, with the results of ocular motor, positional, and caloric testing all being unremarkable.

Medical Examination Result

The patient presented with a normal otolaryngologic examination. Based on the unusual patient presentation, a high resolution MRI was ordered to rule out retrocochlear involvement and a CT scan was ordered to evaluate for possible SSCD.

Impression

Superior canal dehiscence left side.

Audiologic Recommendations and Management

Continue to monitor hearing and vestibular status.

Medical Recommendations and Management

It was recommended that the patient have a collaborative otolaryngologic and neurosurgical consultation regarding repair of the dehiscent canal.

Additional Comments (i.e., surgical results, postaudiologic results)

The patient elected to undergo surgery. The surgical procedure involved exposing the dehiscence and grafting with a fast-setting cement. The patient has done well since the surgery with essentially no return of vertiginous symptoms and an essential closure of the conductive component observed prior to surgery (see Figure 5–9).

Case 5–10: Superior Semicircular Canal Dehiscence

History

A 41-year-old male was seen for consultation regarding a bilateral decrease in his hearing sensitivity and chronic vertigo. He had worn hearing aids for 12 years prior to the present evaluation, but was

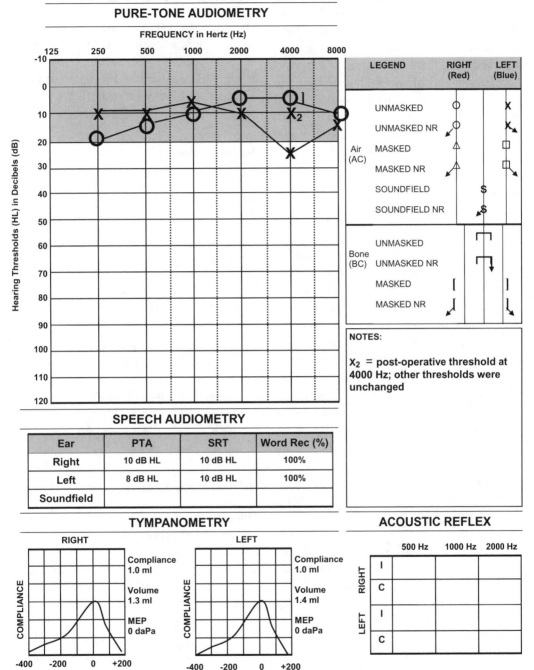

DISORDER: Superior Canal Dehiscence (Pre- & Post-Op)

PURE-TONE AUDIOMETRY

NOTES:

X_2 = post-operative threshold at 4000 Hz; other thresholds were unchanged

SPEECH AUDIOMETRY

Ear	PTA	SRT	Word Rec (%)
Right	10 dB HL	10 dB HL	100%
Left	8 dB HL	10 dB HL	100%
Soundfield			

TYMPANOMETRY

RIGHT
Compliance 1.0 ml
Volume 1.3 ml
MEP 0 daPa

LEFT
Compliance 1.0 ml
Volume 1.4 ml
MEP 0 daPa

ACOUSTIC REFLEX

Figure 5–9. Pure-tone thresholds and speech audiometry for a 54-year-old male diagnosed with a left-sided superior semicircular canal dehiscence (Case 5–9). Results are shown for both preoperative and postoperative testing. Note the postoperative improvement of the left ear at 4000 Hz (see X_2 on the audiogram).

seen for consultation due to a worsening of his symptoms. He reported the presence of a "whooshing" tinnitus in the left ear. He also experienced vertigo associated with loud noises, where he reported he experienced his eyes "bouncing." He did have a significant left-sided head injury to the temporal bone as a child; however, no other significant audiologic or otologic history was reported.

Audiology

An otoscopic check was unremarkable bilaterally. A comprehensive audiologic evaluation indicated a moderate to severe sensorineural hearing loss bilaterally (Figure 5–10A). Word recognition ability was considered fair for both ears. Tympanograms were performed and revealed normal pressure, volume, and compliance measures bilaterally, suggesting normal middle ear status for both ears. It should be noted that the patient did report vertigo while the tympanometric testing was being performed on the left ear; therefore, a fistula test was performed. The fistula test was subjectively positive for the left ear; however, the patient did not demonstrate a typical nystagmus pattern during the testing procedure.

Additionally a VNG was performed, which was abnormal, suggesting primarily central findings based on abnormal ocular motor findings, with the remainder of the positional and caloric exam being unremarkable. In addition, a VEMP examination was ordered to evaluate for possible SSCD. Test results were normal and symmetrical at suprathreshold levels (100 dB nHL); however, the left ear responses were present down to low levels (60 dB nHL) consistent with SSCD (Figure 5–10B).

Medical Examination Result

The patient presented with a normal otolaryngologic examination. Based on the unusual patient presentation, a high resolution MRI was ordered to rule out retrocochlear involvement and a CT scan was ordered to evaluate for possible SSCD.

Impression

Superior semicircular canal dehiscence left side.

Audiologic Recommendations and Management

Continued use of binaural amplification and further follow-up as needed.

Medical Recommendations and Management

It was recommended that the patient have a collaborative otolaryngologic and neurosurgical consultation regarding repair of the dehiscent canal.

Additional Comments

The patient elected to undergo surgery. The surgical procedure involved exposing the dehiscence and grafting with a fast-setting cement. The patient did present with complications during surgery, which included a hematoma. Although the patient reported significant improvement in his vertigo, he did present with a Grade 2–3 facial nerve weakness on the left side, a significantly unsteady gate, and changes in speech following surgery. Since that time, however, all of these symptoms essentially have resolved and his hearing has remained stable.

DISORDER: Superior Canal Dehiscence (Pre- & Post-Op)

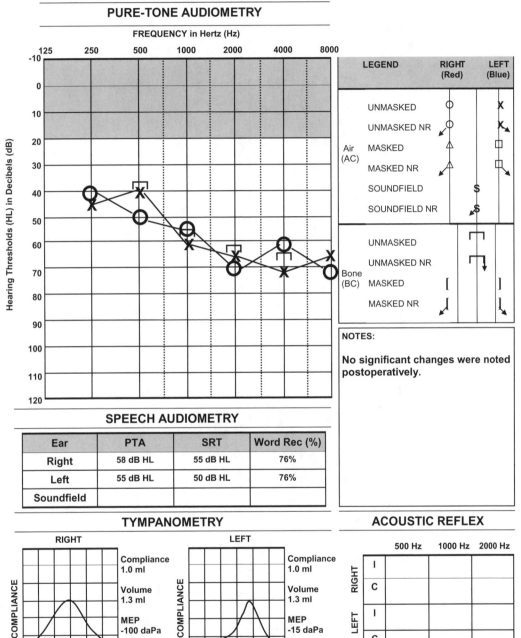

PURE-TONE AUDIOMETRY

SPEECH AUDIOMETRY

Ear	PTA	SRT	Word Rec (%)
Right	58 dB HL	55 dB HL	76%
Left	55 dB HL	50 dB HL	76%
Soundfield			

NOTES:

No significant changes were noted postoperatively.

TYMPANOMETRY

RIGHT — Compliance 1.0 ml; Volume 1.3 ml; MEP -100 daPa

LEFT — Compliance 1.0 ml; Volume 1.3 ml; MEP -15 daPa

ACOUSTIC REFLEX

A

Figure 5–10. Pure-tone thresholds, speech audiometry, and tympanometry results (A) and vestibular evoked myogenic potentials (B) for a 41-year-old male diagnosed with a left-sided superior semicircular canal dehiscence (Case 5–10). continues

219

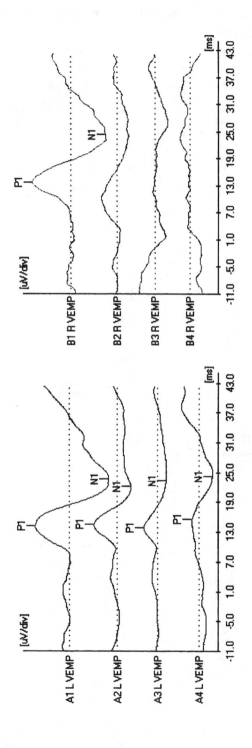

Intensity Levels:
1 = 100 dB nHL
2 = 80 dB nHL
3 = 70 dB nHL
4 = 60 dB nHL

B

Figure 5–10. continued

SUDDEN IDIOPATHIC SENSORINEURAL HEARING LOSS

Introduction

Sudden sensorineural hearing loss (SSHL) is a disease in which very little is known about the etiology or proper treatment, yet it is considered a medical emergency, which should be promptly evaluated. Although sudden hearing loss of any degree is significant, SSHL can formally be defined as sensorineural loss of at least 30 dB within a 72-hour time period (Whitaker, 1980; Wilson, Byl, & Laird, 1980). Although some of the diseases discussed in the text thus far may cause acute onset hearing loss, SSHL is idiopathic in nature.

Symptoms

Sudden sensorineural hearing loss presents with a rapid onset of unilateral hearing loss that is sensorineural in nature. Some patients may experience a popping sensation prior to the hearing loss; others notice hearing loss upon awakening from sleep. Vertigo and tinnitus may also accompany SSHL, and some patients may complain of aural fullness or pressure. An upper respiratory infection often precedes many cases of SSHL.

Incidence and Prevalence

Sudden sensorineural hearing loss accounts for 1% of all forms of sensorineural hearing loss, with 4000 new cases reported in the United States each year (Jaffe, 1973). Sudden sensorineural hearing loss is more common in the elderly (Byl, 1977) and may be bilateral in 4 to 17% of patients (Jaffe, 1973).

Etiology and Pathology

This disease is considered idiopathic, but is likely to be multifactorial. The history of the patient may provide some indication of a potential etiology; however, in most cases a clear etiologic factor cannot be identified. Vascular compromise to the inner ear due to microembolism or vasospasm may have a role in this disease and some historical therapies have been directed at improving cochlear blood supply. The relationship of infection preceding many cases of SSHL makes a viral etiology theory reasonable. Toxic, immunologic, and neurologic insults also are thought to be involved in the disease process. Approximately 10% of patients with vestibular schwannomas may present with SSHL (Berg, Cohen, Hammerschlag, & Waltzman, 1986). The etiology of SSHL can be placed into six broad categories that include: (1) viral and infectious (i.e., mumps, herpes viruses, rubella, toxoplasmosis), (2) autoimmune (i.e., Cogan's syndrome, AIED, lupus), (3) labyrinthine membrane rupture/trauma (i.e., perilymph fistula, barotrauma, temporal bone fracture, ear surgery complications), (4) vascular (i.e., vascular spasm, occlusion, rupture, sickle cell disease, vertebrobasilar disease), (5) neurologic (multiple sclerosis, focal pontine ischemia, migraine), and (6) neoplastic (acoustic neuroma and other tumors affecting the auditory system) (see Wynne, 2003).

Site of Lesion

The cause of this disease has yet to be elucidated, thus identifying the site in which damage occurs has also been difficult. Postmortem analysis of the temporal bones of a group of patients who suffered from SSHL revealed global degeneration of the cochlear duct structures near the basal turn of the cochlea (Beal, Hemenway, & Lindsay, 1967; Schuknecht, Kimura, & Naufal, 1973). Although the cochlea is often the site of this disorder, there also can be eighth nerve and central sites of involvement. As discussed in Chapter 6, Auditory Nerve Disorders, acoustic neuromas can present as a sudden sensorineural loss. It is also significant that multiple sclerosis has been linked to SSHL (Marangos, 1996).

Audiology

Patients who present with SSHL should have a comprehensive audiologic evaluation, OAEs, and immittance audiometry performed as soon as possible. The use of these measures may help to differentiate between cochlear versus retrocochlear involvement. Sudden hearing loss generally refers to hearing loss of sensorineural origin. It has been defined for research purposes and has been accepted by most authorities as 30 dB or more of sensorineural hearing loss over at least three contiguous audiometric frequencies occurring within 3 days or less (University of Texas Medical Branch Grand Rounds [UTMB], 2001). Because it is possible that SSHL can have a retrocochlear basis, it may be worthwhile to consider performing an ABR if there is sufficient residual hearing. This is usually a judgment call and dependent on history and otologic consultation. It is also important to discriminate between sudden hearing loss and suddenly noticed hearing loss.

Medical Examination

Sudden sensorineural hearing loss represents a medical emergency and all efforts should be taken to evaluate and initiate treatment as soon as possible. The diagnosis of SSHL is made primarily through careful history and exclusion of other common causes of hearing loss. The history of a rapid unilateral sensorineural loss is a key portion of the history. Specific questions should be asked to rule out other potential diagnoses, such as perilymph fistula, ototoxicity, Ménière's disease, infectious etiologies, and retrocochlear pathology. A thorough head and neck examination augments the medical history and typically is unremarkable. Neurotologic examination of vestibular function typically is normal. Laboratory tests may be performed to detect an autoimmune etiology, but if done, they typically are normal. An MRI should be performed to rule out retrocochlear pathology.

Audiologic Management

Serial audiograms should be performed to monitor recovery. Patients with stable loss that shows no improvement after 3 to 6 months may benefit from amplification. Profoundly deafened ears may also use a CROS or Bi_CROS aid, depending on the degree of hearing in the opposite ear, to improve sound localization ability. Approximately 50% of patients have partial or total recovery; however, predicting which patients will recover can be difficult. Byl (1984) examined prognostic factors in hearing recovery and found that patients with profound hearing loss and delayed treatment, as well as those at the extremes of the age range had a much poorer prognosis for recovery. Unfortunately, sudden sensorineural hearing loss is a common disease and requires prompt evaluation and treatment, exclusion of retrocochlear pathology, and careful follow-up to detect contralateral disease. It is important that amplification not be provided too quickly as it may cause additional damage. Rather it is recommended that amplification be applied following confirmed stability of the patient's hearing thresholds.

Medical Management

Many patients who experience SSHL do not seek medical attention or they present long after the onset of symptoms. In many patients with SSHL, the hearing loss will resolve without intervention. However, it is difficult to predict which patients will have spontaneous recovery. Moderate to severe sloping hearing loss has the poorest prognosis and mild low-frequency hearing losses have the best prognosis (Mattox, 1980). For patients who do present for evaluation, treatment is directed at salvaging hearing through the use of steroids, which can be delivered systemically or through an intratympanic perfusion. Antivirals frequently are used in treatment as well; however, no clear therapeutic benefit of this approach has been shown consistently (Tucci, Farmer, Kitch, & Witsell, 2002). A host of other antioxidants and vasodilators have been used historically, but without proven efficacy.

Case 5–11: Sudden Sensorineural Hearing Loss

History

A 32-year-old male was seen for evaluation due to a sudden right-sided hearing loss. The patient reported a sudden onset of hearing loss approximately three weeks prior to his audiologic evaluation. He was initially treated by his primary care physician with antibiotics for otitis media with no improvement noted. He also reported constant tinnitus in the right ear coincident with the onset of his hearing loss, with no improvement in the tinnitus since its onset.

Audiology

An otoscopic check was unremarkable. Tympanograms were performed and revealed normal pressure, volume, and compliance, suggesting normal middle ear status bilaterally. A comprehensive audiologic evaluation demonstrated normal peripheral hearing sensitivity in the left ear and a moderately-severe mid-frequency sensorineural hearing loss in the right ear (Figure 5–11A). Word recognition was good in the left ear and poor in the right ear. Speech recognition thresholds were in good agreement with pure-tone averages bilaterally.

Medical Examination Result

The patient presented with an essentially normal otolaryngologic examination.

Impression

Sudden hearing loss with unknown etiology.

Audiologic Recommendations and Management

It was recommended that the patient undergo imaging to rule out retrocochlear involvement. Results from the MRI were negative.

DISORDER: Sudden Hearing Loss (Pretreatment)

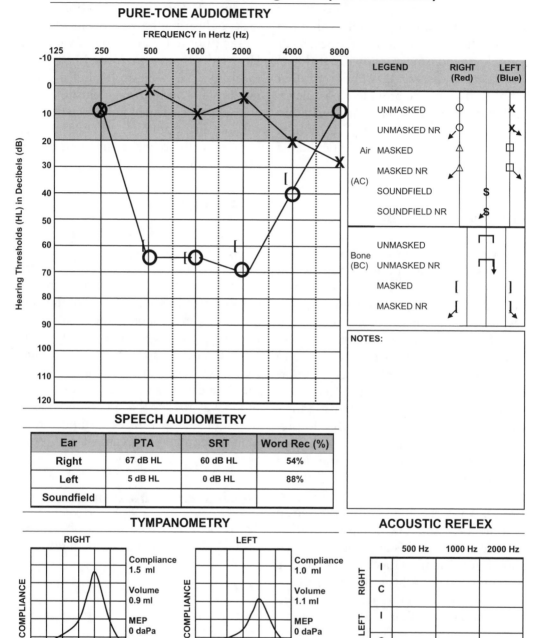

PURE-TONE AUDIOMETRY

SPEECH AUDIOMETRY

Ear	PTA	SRT	Word Rec (%)
Right	67 dB HL	60 dB HL	54%
Left	5 dB HL	0 dB HL	88%
Soundfield			

TYMPANOMETRY

RIGHT — Compliance 1.5 ml, Volume 0.9 ml, MEP 0 daPa

LEFT — Compliance 1.0 ml, Volume 1.1 ml, MEP 0 daPa

ACOUSTIC REFLEX

A

Figure 5–11. Pure-tone thresholds, speech audiometry, and tympanometry for a 32-year-old male (Case 5–11), who had experienced a sudden sensorineural hearing loss (**A**) and then improvement following treatment (**B**). continues

DISORDER: Sudden Hearing Loss (Posttreatment)

PURE-TONE AUDIOMETRY

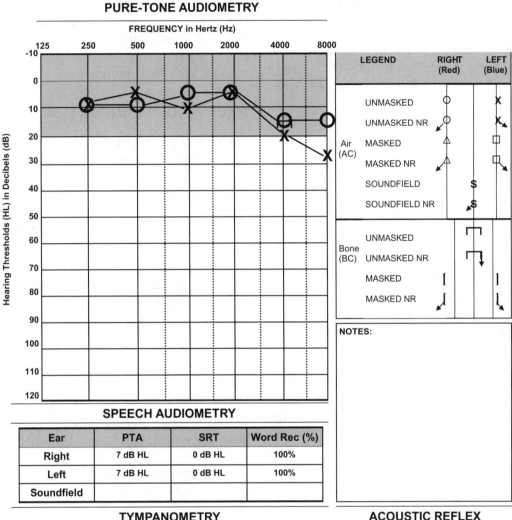

SPEECH AUDIOMETRY

Ear	PTA	SRT	Word Rec (%)
Right	7 dB HL	0 dB HL	100%
Left	7 dB HL	0 dB HL	100%
Soundfield			

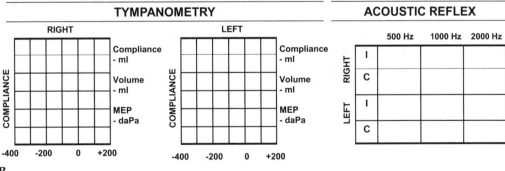

B

Figure 5–11. continued

Medical Recommendations and Management

The patient underwent a burst and taper prednisone treatment and an appropriate course of Famvir to treat for suspected viral pathology.

Additional Information

The patient responded well to treatment with complete recovery of auditory function and no subsequent hearing loss reported (Figure 5–11B).

Case 5–12: Sudden Sensorineural Hearing Loss

History

A 31-year-old female who was 29 weeks pregnant at the time of evaluation was seen for evaluation due to a sudden left-sided hearing loss without any known precipitating causes. She reported aural fullness, mild tinnitus, and episodic vertigo. No other significant history was reported.

Audiology

An otoscopic check was unremarkable. Tympanograms were performed and revealed normal pressure, volume, and compliance for both ears, suggesting normal middle ear status bilaterally. A comprehensive audiologic evaluation demonstrated normal peripheral hearing sensitivity in the right ear and a moderate low-frequency

sensorineural hearing loss in the left ear (Figure 5–12A). Word recognition was excellent bilaterally and speech recognition thresholds were in good agreement with the pure-tone averages.

Medical Examination Result

The patient presented with an essentially normal otolaryngologic examination.

Impression

Sudden hearing loss with unknown etiology.

Audiologic Recommendations and Management

It was medically recommended that the patient undergo a course of steroid treatment for the sudden sensorineural hearing loss.

Medical Recommendations and Management

After consultation with her OBGYN, the patient underwent a burst and taper prednisone treatment and an appropriate course of Famvir to treat for suspected viral pathology.

Additional Information

The patient responded well to treatment with complete recovery of auditory function and no subsequent hearing loss reported (Figure 5–12B).

DISORDER: Sudden Hearing Loss (Pretreatment)

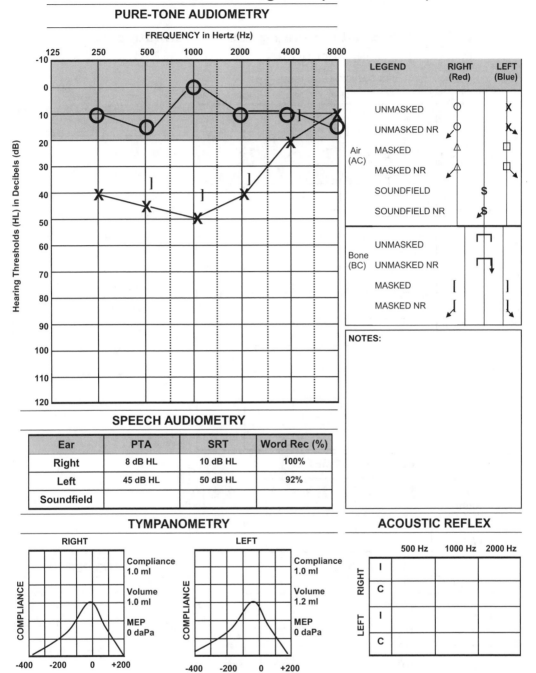

PURE-TONE AUDIOMETRY

SPEECH AUDIOMETRY

Ear	PTA	SRT	Word Rec (%)
Right	8 dB HL	10 dB HL	100%
Left	45 dB HL	50 dB HL	92%
Soundfield			

TYMPANOMETRY

RIGHT
Compliance 1.0 ml
Volume 1.0 ml
MEP 0 daPa

LEFT
Compliance 1.0 ml
Volume 1.2 ml
MEP 0 daPa

ACOUSTIC REFLEX

A

Figure 5–12. Pure-tone thresholds and speech audiometry for a 31-year-old female (Case 5–12) at the time of an initial audiologic evaluation for a sudden sensorineural hearing loss (**A**) and then following recovery (**B**). continues

DISORDER: Sudden Hearing Loss (Posttreatment)

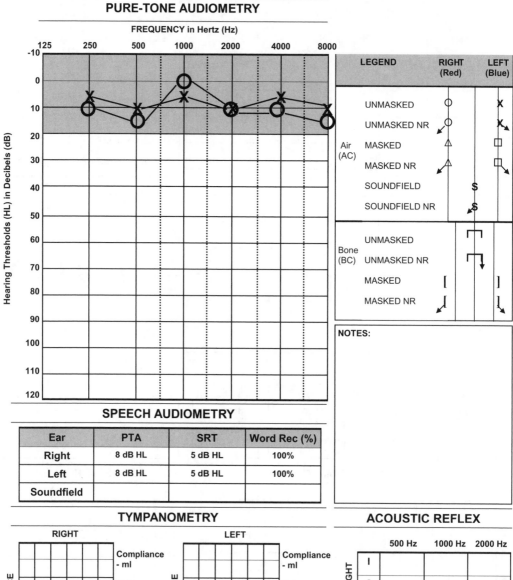

PURE-TONE AUDIOMETRY

FREQUENCY in Hertz (Hz)

LEGEND		RIGHT (Red)	LEFT (Blue)
Air (AC)	UNMASKED	○	X
	UNMASKED NR		
	MASKED	△	□
	MASKED NR		
	SOUNDFIELD	S	
	SOUNDFIELD NR	S	
Bone (BC)	UNMASKED		
	UNMASKED NR		
	MASKED	[	]
	MASKED NR		

NOTES:

SPEECH AUDIOMETRY

Ear	PTA	SRT	Word Rec (%)
Right	8 dB HL	5 dB HL	100%
Left	8 dB HL	5 dB HL	100%
Soundfield			

TYMPANOMETRY

RIGHT

Compliance - ml
Volume - ml
MEP - daPa

LEFT

Compliance - ml
Volume - ml
MEP - daPa

ACOUSTIC REFLEX

		500 Hz	1000 Hz	2000 Hz
RIGHT	I			
	C			
LEFT	I			
	C			

B

Figure 5–12. continued

OTHER DISORDERS AFFECTING THE COCHLEA

Diabetes Mellitus

The information on hearing loss and/or vestibular problems related to diabetes is rather limited. One would think that, because of the well known effects that diabetes has on vision, reports on the effects on auditory system would be as common, but this does not seem to be the case. Certainly, there are individuals with diabetes who likely have hearing loss related to the disease, but these associations are not easily documented.

The most common types of diabetes include type I and type II diabetes. Type I is an autoimmune disease where the cells that generate insulin are destroyed. This type of diabetes is sometimes known as juvenile onset diabetes, but it can occur at any age; however, the onset of type I diabetes is typically under 40 years of age. Individuals with type I diabetes usually must inject themselves with insulin daily. Type II diabetes is the more common type of diabetes with 85% of the individuals with this disease having this type, and it has a strong genetic factor. It is commonly treated with diet change, oral medication, and in advanced cases, insulin injections (Health*Insite*, 2010).

A third type of diabetes is referred to gestational diabetes mellitus, which is a carbohydrate intolerance condition that is first diagnosed during pregnancy through an oral glucose tolerance condition test. Although the carbohydrate intolerance often returns to normal after the birth, the mother has a significant risk of developing permanent diabetes later in life.

The etiology and pathology centers around elevated blood glucose levels and alterations of lipids and proteins. These conditions are likely related to microangiopathy or damage to small blood vessels and possible atherosclerosis. These vascular changes may affect the stria vascularis and other small vessels in the cochlea and central pathways (Lisowska, Namyslowski, Morawski, & Strojek, 2001).

The incidence of hearing loss directly related to diabetes is difficult to determine because it can be a challenge to distinguish this pathology from other etiologies that result in hearing loss (i.e., aging, noise exposure, etc.). Estimates of the incidence of hearing loss in individuals with diabetes range from 10 to 55% of the people diagnosed with the disease (see Jerger & Jerger, 1981).

The pathology is vascular in nature; hence, either the cochlea or the auditory nervous system can be involved. Typically, a bilateral sensorineural loss is noted in individuals with diabetes. The hearing loss tends to be slowly progressive and can range from mild to profound in degree. Dizziness may be present in approximately one-fifth of the patients with diabetes. Tympanograms usually are normal bilaterally and results of acoustic reflex testing vary depending on the site of maximum involvement and the degree of loss (i.e., they can align with either cochlear or retrocochlear findings) (Jerger & Jerger, 1981). Auditory brainstem response findings were found to be different for a diabetes group and a control group that included individuals less than 50 years of age (Konrad-Martin, Austin, Griest, McMillan, McDermott, & Fausti, 2010). In this study, the absolute latency of wave V was found to be delayed, as was the I–V interwave latency for the diabetes group. It also has been reported that the ABR reveals slower conduction times in individuals with diabetes, but without hearing loss (Lisowska et al., 2001). Specifically, delays of wave I and extensions of the I-V interwave intervals were reported in this study, indicating possible cochlear and/or retrocochlear involvement.

Perilymph Fistulas

Perilymph fistulas, also referred to as perilymphatic fistulas, are leaks of perilymph usually from either the oval or round window. (Superior canal dehiscence, which was discussed earlier in this chapter, is also considered a perilymph leak.) These leaks can be located at the ligament-type tissue around the oval window or as a result of a tear in the round window. Leaks in perilymph from either site often result in symptoms of hearing loss and/or of imbalance or dizziness. These symptoms may increase with activity and subside with rest (Hain, 2011). The diagnosis of perilymph fistula at times is difficult and controversial because the condition often cannot be confirmed—even at surgery.

Perilymph fistula is considered a rare disease, with a prevalence of less than 200,000 affected individuals at any given time in the United States (Wrong Diagnosis.com, 2011). The etiology of perilymphatic fistula is broad based. Chief among possible causes are head trauma, barotraumas (deep sea diving), severe straining (lifting), congenital conditions (malformations of the inner ear), surgical procedures (stapedectomy), and at times, even severe acoustic trauma (Hain, 2011). Pathophysiologically, secondary to the perilymph leak, the rupture of the oval or round window allows middle ear pressure changes to affect the inner ear (both auditory and vestibular portions) when ordinarily they do not. The drainage of

perilymph also may result in the changing of the relative pressure between the scala media and the scalae tympani and vestibuli. The decrease in perilymph that occurs as result of the fistula likely will create a greater relative pressure in the scala media vis a vis the other two scalae in the cochlea, a situation that is similar to that observed in endolymphatic hydrops. These pressure alterations can be variable as can be the related symptoms of sensorineural hearing loss, balance problems, and sometimes tinnitus (Hain, 2011; Møller, 2000). Because of the similarities in regard to pathology and symptoms, perilymph fistulas can easily be misdiagnosed as Ménière's disease.

The diagnosis of a perilymphatic fistula, as mentioned earlier, can be a challenge. A careful otologic exam and patient history is essential, as is the administration and interpretation of a CT scan. Audiology can also be of considerable help. An audiogram can reveal a sensorineural loss that is usually unilateral in nature. Also, the administration of a fistula test can provide valuable information that can lead to the diagnosis of a perilymph fistula. This test is done by varying the pressure in the ear canal (similar to tympanometry) and monitoring the movement of the eyes, usually under ENG, to see if nystagmus is created by the pressure changes or if the patient reports any vestibular symptoms. A regular ENG may also be useful as a hypofunction via caloric testing can show up on the involved side; however, how sensitive this diagnostic finding is remains to be determined. Although not routinely recommended for individuals at risk for this disorder, ABR testing, if done (perhaps for another reason or for differential diagnosis), should result in normal findings. The major challenge is to differentiate perilymph fistula from Ménière's disease and from the authors' perspective the history is key, especially if the reported symptoms are related to changes in activity rather than being truly episodic as would be noted in individuals with Ménière's disease.

The treatment for perilymph fistula can be nonsurgical or surgical (see Hain, 2011). The first approach is usually bed rest. It is felt that most of the time bed rest (a week or more) and the avoidance of any activity that will increase pressure in the middle or inner ear (e.g., heavy lifting, straining, coughing, etc.) can help resolve the fluid imbalance that occurs in the cochlea secondary to the perilymph leak. Placing a ventilation tube in the eardrum also may help by reducing the amount of pressure change in the middle ear (less eardrum movement). Finally, performing a tympanotomy to confirm if perilymph is leaking into the middle ear and then surgically patching the round window is currently viewed as a last resort to management of the fistula. Success rates of surgically covering the round widow with soft material are difficult to determine (Hain, 2011).

SUMMARY

This chapter provided information on some of the most significant disorders that can affect the cochlea. These include trauma, noise-induced hearing loss, ototoxicity, Ménière's disease, autoimmune inner ear disease, presbycusis, superior canal dehiscence syndrome, sudden idiopathic sensorineural hearing loss, diabetes, and perilymph fistula. The diagnostic protocols for most of these disorders (with the exception of autoimmune inner ear disease) have progressed to the point where they are essentially routine, but treatment approaches for these inner ear

disorders remain a challenge with progress slow to evolve. However, recent developments in our understanding of molecular biology, which has permitted an appreciation of free radicals and their effects on the inner ear, make the future seem promising.

Acknowledgments. The authors gratefully acknowledge the contributions of Matthew Bush, M.D., Assistant Professor, Department of Otolaryngology, University of Kentucky, and Michael E. Hoffer, MD, FACS, Department of Otolaryngology, Naval Medical Center, San Diego, to this chapter.

REFERENCES

American Academy of Otolaryngology. (1995). Committee on Hearing and Equilibrium guidelines for the evaluation of results of treatment of conductive hearing loss. *Otolaryngology-Head and Neck Surgery, 113*(3), 186–187.

Aetna. (2011). Clinical Policy Bulletin: Chronic Vertigo. Number 0238. Retrieved 6/15/11 from http://www.aetna.com/cpb/medical/data/200_299/0238.html.

Arenberg, I. K, Marovitz, W. F., & Shambaugh, G. E., Jr. (1970). The role of the endolymphatic sac in the pathogenesis of endolymphatic hydrops in man. *Acta Otolaryngologica, 275*(Suppl.), 1–49.

Arnold, W., Nadol, J. B., Jr., & Weidauer, H. (1981). Ultrastructural histopathology in a case of human ototoxicity due to loop diuretics. *Acta Otolaryngologica, 91*(5–6), 399–414.

Arnold, W., Pfaltz, R., & Altermatt, H. J. (1985). Evidence of serum antibodies against inner ear tissues in the blood of patients with certain sensorineural hearing disorders. *Acta Otolaryngologica, 99*(3–4), 437–444.

Baloh, R. W., Jacobson, K., & Winder, T. (1990). Drop attacks with Menière's syndrome. *Annals of Neurology, 28*(3), 384–387.

Beal, D. D., Hemenway, W. G., & Lindsay, J. R. (1967). Inner ear pathology of sudden deafness. Histopathology of acquired deafness in the adult coincident with viral infection. *Archives of Otolaryngology, 85*(6), 591–598.

Beaubien, A. R., Desjardins, S., Ormsby, E., Bayne, A., Carrier, K., Cauchy, M. J., . . . St Pierre, A. (1990). Delay in hearing loss following drug administration. A consistent feature of amikacin ototoxicity. *Acta Otolaryngologica, 109*(5–6), 345–352.

Beaubien, A. R., Ormsby, E., Bayne, A., Carrier, K., Crossfield, G., Downes, M., . . . Hodgen, M. (1991). Evidence that amikacin ototoxicity is related to total perilymph area under the concentration-time curve regardless of concentration. *Antimicrobial Agents and Chemotherapy, 35*(6), 1070–1074.

Berg, H. M., Cohen, N. L., Hammerschlag, P. E., & Waltzman, S. B. (1986). Acoustic neuroma presenting as sudden hearing loss with recovery. *Otolaryngology-Head and Neck Surgery, 94*(1), 15–22.

Berger, E. H. (1993). *EARlog #20–The naked truth about NRRs*. Southbridge, MA: Cabot Safety Corporation.

Black, F. O., & Nashner, L. M. (1985). Postural control in four classes of vestibular abnormalities. In M. Igarashi & F. O. Black (Eds.), *Vestibular and visual control of posture and locomotor equilibrium* (pp. 271–281). New York, NY: Krager.

Bohne, B. A., & Harding, G. W. (2000). Degeneration in the cochlea after noise damage: Primary versus secondary events. *American Journal of Otology, 21*(4), 505–509.

Bojrab, D. E., Bhansali, S. A., & Battista, R. A. (1994). Peripheral vestibular disorders. In R. K. Jackler & D. E. Brackmann (Eds.), *Neurotology* (pp. 629–650). St. Louis, MO: Mosby.

Brantberg, K., Bergenius, J., Mendel, L., Witt, H., Tribukait, A., & Ygge, J. (2001). Symptoms, findings and treatment in patients with dehiscence of the superior semicircular canal. *Acta Otolaryngologica, 121*(1), 68–75.

Brookhouser, P. E. (1994). Prevention of noise-induced hearing loss. *Preventative Medicine, 23*(5), 665–669.

Byl, F. M. (1977). Seventy-six cases of presumed sudden hearing loss occurring in 1973: Prognosis and incidence. *Laryngoscope, 87*(5, Pt. 1), 817–825.

Byl, F. M., Jr. (1984). Sudden hearing loss: Eight years' experience and suggested prognostic table. *Laryngoscope, 94*(5, Pt. 1), 647–661.

Carey, J. P., Minor, L. B., & Nager, G. T. (2000). Dehiscence or thinning of bone overlying the superior semicircular canal in a temporal bone survey. *Archives of Otolaryngology-Head and Neck Surgery, 126*(2), 137–147.

Chi, F. L., Ren, D. D., & Dai, C. F. (2010). Variety of audiologic manifestations in patients with superior semicircular canal dehiscence. *Otology and Neurotology, 31*(1), 2–10.

Claes, G. M., Wyndaele, M., De Valck, C. F., Claes, J., Govaerts, P., Wuyts, F. L., & Van de Heyning, P. H. (2008). Travelling wave velocity test and Ménière's disease revisited. *European Archives of Oto-Rhino-Laryngology, 265*(5), 517–523.

Cronberg, S. (1994). Simplified monitoring of aminoglycosides. *Journal of Antimicrobial Chemotherapy, 34*(5), 819–827.

da Silva, A. M., Latorre Mdo, R., Cristofani, L. M., & Odone Filho, V. (2007). The prevalence of hearing loss in children and adolescents with cancer. *Brazilian Journal of Otorhinolaryngology, 73*(5), 608–614.

Dahiya, R., Keller, J. D., Litofsky, N. S., Bankey, P. E., Bonassar, L. J., & Megerian, C. A. (1999). Temporal bone fractures: Otic capsule sparing versus otic capsule violating clinical and radiographic considerations. *Journal of Trauma, 47*(6), 1079–1083.

Daniel, E. (2007). Noise and hearing loss: A review. *Journal of School Health, 77*(5), 225–231.

Daniell, W. E., Fulton-Kehoe, D., Smith-Weller, T., & Franklin, G. M. (1998). Occupational hearing loss in Washington state, 1984–1991: I. Statewide and industry-specific incidence. *American Journal of Industrial Medicine, 33*(6), 519–528.

Davis, R. R., Kozel, P., & Erway, L. C. (2003). Genetic influences in individual susceptibility to noise: A review. *Noise Health, 5*(20), 19–28.

Di Girolamo, S., Picciotti, P., Sergi, B., D'Ecclesia, A., & Di Nardo, W. (2001). Postural control and glycerol test in Ménière's disease. *Acta Otolaryngologica, 121*(7), 813–817.

Don, M., Kwong, B., & Tanaka, C. (2005). A diagnostic test for Ménière's disease and cochlear hydrops: Impaired high-pass noise masking of auditory brainstem responses. *Otology and Neurotology, 26*(4), 711–722.

Donaldson, G. S., & Ruth, R. A. (1996). Derived-band auditory brain-stem response estimates of traveling wave velocity in humans. II. Subjects with noise-induced hearing loss and Ménière's disease. *Journal of Speech and Hearing Research, 39*(3), 534–545.

Edson, R. S., & Terrell, C. L. (1987). The aminoglycosides: Streptomycin, kanamycin, gentamicin, tobramycin, amikacin, netilmicin, and sisomicin. *Mayo Clinic Proceedings, 62*(10), 916–920.

Eggermont, J. J., & Roberts, L. E. (2004). The neuroscience of tinnitus. *Trends in Neurosciences, 27*(11), 676–682.

Fabiani, M., Mattioni, A., Saponara, M., & Cordier, A. (1998). Auditory evoked potentials for the assessment of noise induced hearing loss. *Scandinavian Audiology, 48*(Suppl.), 147–153.

Fausti, S. A., Wilmington, D. J., Gallun, F. J., Myers, P. J., & Henry, J. A. (2009). Auditory and vestibular dysfunction associated with blast-related traumatic brain injury. *Journal of Rehabilitation Research and Development, 46*(6), 797–810.

Fechter, L. D. (2004). Promotion of noise-induced hearing loss by chemical contaminants. *Journal of Toxicology and Environmental Health. Part A, 67*(8–10), 727–740.

Forge, A., & Schacht, J. (2000). Aminoglycoside antibiotics. *Audiology and Neurotology, 5*(1), 3–22.

Gaeth, J. (1945). *A study of phonemic regression associated with hearing loss* [Unpublished doctoral dissertation], Northwestern University, Evanston, IL.

Gates, G. A. (2006). Ménière's disease review 2005. *Journal of the American Academy of Audiology, 17*(1), 16–26.

Gelfand, S. A. (2001). *Essentials of audiology* (2nd ed.). New York, NY: Thieme.

Hain, T. C. (2011). *Perilymph fistula*. Retrieved 6/15/11 from http://www.dizziness-and-balance.com/disorders/unilat/fistula.html.

Hallpike, C. S., & Cairns, H. (1938). Observations on the pathology of Ménière's syndrome: (Section of Otology). *Proceedings of the Royal Society of Medicine, 31*(11), 1317–1336.

Harris, J. P., & Sharp, P. A. (1990). Inner ear autoantibodies in patients with rapidly progressive sensorineural hearing loss. *Laryngoscope, 100*(5), 516–524.

Harrison, R. V. (2001). The physiology of the cochlear nerve. In A. F. Jahn & J. Santos-Sacchi (Eds.), *Physiology of the ear* (pp. 549–573). San Diego, CA: Plural Publishing.

Hawkins, J. E., Jr. (1976). Drug ototoxicity. In W. D. Keidel & W. D. Neff (Eds.), *Handbook of sensory physiology* (Vol. 3, pp. 707–748). New York, NY: Springer.

Health*Insite* (2010). *Diabetes*. Retrieved 6/15/11 from http://www.healthinsite.gov.au/topics.

Helleman, H. W., Jansen, E. J., & Dreschler, W. A. (2010). Otoacoustic emissions in a hearing conservation program: General applicability in longitudinal monitoring and the relation to changes in pure-tone thresholds. *International Journal of Audiology, 49*(6), 410–419.

Hinshaw, H., & Feldman, W. (1945). Streptomycin in the treatment of clinical tuberculosis: A preliminary report. *Mayo Clinic Proceedings, 20*, 313.

Horner, K. C. (1995). Auditory and vestibular function in experimental hydrops. *Otolaryngology-Head and Neck Surgery, 112*(1), 84–89.

Huang, T., Cheng, A. G., Stupak, H., Liu, W., Kim, A., Staecker, H., . . . Van De Water, T. R. (2000). Oxidative stress-induced apoptosis of cochlear sensory cells: Otoprotective strategies. *International Journal of Developmental Neuroscience, 18*(2–3), 259–270.

Hughes, G. B., Barna, B. P., Calabrese, L. H., & Koo, A. (1993). Immunologic disorders of the inner ear. In B. J. Bailey (Ed.), *Head and Neck Surgery-Otolaryngology* (pp. 1883–1842). Philadelphia, PA: Lippincott.

Huizing, E. H., & de Groot, J. C. (1987). Human cochlear pathology in aminoglycoside ototoxicity—A review. *Acta Otolaryngologica, 436*(Suppl.), 117–125.

Huppert, D., Strupp, M., & Brandt, T. (2010). Long-term course of Menière's disease revisited. *Acta Otolaryngologica, 130*(6), 644–651.

Jacob, L. C., Aquiar, F. P., Tomiasi, A. A., Tschoeke, S. N., & Bitencourt, R. F. (2006). Auditory monitoring in ototoxicity. *Brazilian Journal of Otorhinolaryngology, 72*(6), 836–884.

Jaffe, B. F. (1973). Clinical studies in sudden deafness. *Advances in Oto-rhino-laryngology, 20,* 221–228.

Jerger, S., & Jerger, J. (1981). *Auditory disorders: A manual for clinical evaluation.* Boston, MA: Little, Brown.

Juhn, S. K., Ikeda, K., Morizono, T., & Murphy, M. (1991). Pathophysiology of inner ear fluid imbalance. *Acta Otolaryngologica, 485*(Suppl.), 9–14.

Kahlmeter, G., & Dahlager, J. I. (1984). Aminoglycoside toxicity—a review of clinical studies published between 1975 and 1982. *Journal of Antimicrobrial Chemotherapy, 13* (Suppl. A), 9–22.

Katzenell, U., & Segal, S. (2001). Hyperacusis: Review and clinical guidelines. *Otology and Neurotology, 22*(3), 321–326.

Kitahara, M., Takeda, T., Yazawa, Y., Matsubara, H., & Kitano, H. (1984). Pathophysiology of Meniere's disease and its subvarieties. *Acta Otolaryngologica, 406*(Suppl.), 52–55.

Konrad-Martin, D., Austin, D. F., Griest, S., McMillan, G. P., McDermott, D., & Fausti, S. (2010). Diabetes-related changes in auditory brainstem responses, *Laryngoscope, 120*(1), 150–158.

Kopke, R., Allen, K. A., Henderson, D., Hoffer, M., Frenz, D., & Van de Water, T. (1999). A radical demise. Toxins and trauma share common pathways in hair cell death. *Annals of the New York Academy of Sciences, 884,* 171–191.

Kopke, R. D., Coleman, J. K., Liu, J., Campbell, K. C., & Riffenburgh, R. H. (2002). Candidate's thesis: Enhancing intrinsic cochlear stress defenses to reduce noise-induced hearing loss. *Laryngoscope, 112*(9), 1515–1532.

Kopke, R. D., Jackson, R. L., Coleman, J. K., Liu, J., Bielefeld, E. C., & Balough, B. J. (2007). NAC for noise: From the bench top to the clinic. *Hearing Research, 226*(1–2), 114–125.

Korres, G. S., Balatsouras, D. G., Tzagaroulakis, A., Kandiloros, D., & Ferekidis, E. (2008). Extended high-frequency audiometry in subjects exposed to occupational noise. *British Journal of ENT, 4*(3), 147–155.

Kramer, S., Dreisbach, L., Lockwood, J., Baldwin, K., Kopke, R., Scranton, S., & O'Leary, M. (2006). Efficacy of the antioxidant N-acetylcysteine (NAC) in protecting ears exposed to loud music. *Journal of the American Academy of Audiology, 17*(4), 265–278.

Le Prell, C. G., Yamashita, D., Minami, S. B., Yamasoba, T., & Miller, J. M. (2007). Mechanisms of noise-induced hearing loss indicate multiple methods of prevention. *Hearing Research, 226*(1–2), 22–43.

Lee, F. S., Matthews, L. J., Dubno, J. R., & Mills, J. H. (2005). Longitudinal study of puretone thresholds in older persons. *Ear and Hearing, 26*(1), 1–11.

Lim, D. J., Dunn, D. E., Ferraro, J. A., & Lempert, B. L. (1982). Anatomical changes found in the cochleas of animals exposed to typical industrial noise. In R. P. Hamernick, D. Henderson & R. Salvi (Eds.), *New perspectives on noise-induced hearing loss* (pp. 23–48). New York, NY: Raven Press.

Lisowska, G., Namyslowski, G., Morawski, K., & Strojek, K. (2001). Early identification of hearing impairment in patients with type 1 diabetes mellitus. *Otology & Neurotology, 22*(3), 316–320.

Lynch, E. D., & Kil, J. (2005). Compounds for the prevention and treatment of noise-induced hearing loss. *Drug Discovery Today, 10*(19), 1291–1298.

Mancini, F., Catalani, M., Carru, M., & Monti, B. (2002). History of Meniere's disease and its clinical presentation. *Otolaryngologic Clinics of North America, 35*(3), 565–580.

Marangos, N. (1996). Hearing loss in multiple sclerosis: Localization of the auditory pathway lesion according to electrocochleographic findings. *Journal of Laryngology and Otology, 10*(3), 252–257.

Martin, J. S., & Jerger, J. F. (2005). Some effects of aging on central auditory processing. *Journal of Rehabilitation Research and Development, 42*(4, Suppl. 2), 25–44.

Mattox, D. (1980). Medical management of sudden hearing loss. *Otolaryngology-Head and Neck Surgery, 88*(2), 111–113.

McCabe, B. F., & McCormick, K. J. (1984). Tests for autoimmune disease in otology. *American Journal of Otology, 5*(6), 447–449.

McGee, T., & Olszewski, J. (1962). Streptomycin sulfate and dihydrostreptomycin toxicity. Behavioral and histopathologic studies. *Archives of Otolaryngology, 75*, 295.

Mendelsohn, M., & Katzenberg, I. (1972). The effect of kanamycin on the cation content of the endolymph. *Laryngoscope, 82*(3), 397–403.

Ménière, P. (1861a). Mémoiresur des lésions de l'oreille interne donnant lieu à des symptômes de congestion cérébraleapoplectiforme. *Gazette médicale (Paris, France), 16*, 597–601.

Ménière, P. (1861b). Sur uneforme de sourdité grave dépendantd'unelésion de l'oreille interne. *Gazette médicale (Paris, France), 16*, 29.

Minor, L. B. (2000). Superior canal dehiscence syndrome. *American Journal of Otology, 21*(1), 9–19.

Minor, L. B. (2005). Clinical manifestations of superior semicircular canal dehiscence. *Laryngoscope, 115*(10), 1717–1727.

Minor, L. B., Carey, J. P., Cremer, P. D., Lustig, L. R., Streubel, S. O., & Ruckenstein, M. J. (2003). Dehiscence of bone overlying the superior canal as a cause of apparent conductive hearing loss. *Otology and Neurotology, 24*(2), 270–278.

Minor, L. B., Cremer, P. D., Carey, J. P., Della Santina, C. C., Streubel, S. O., & Weg, N. (2001). Symptoms and signs in superior canal dehiscence syndrome. *Annals of the New York Academy of Sciences, 942*, 259–273.

Minor, L. B., Solomon, D., Zinreich, J. S., & Zee, D. S. (1998). Sound- and/or pressure-induced vertigo due to bone dehiscence of the superior semicircular canal. *Archives of Otolaryngology-Head and Neck Surgery, 124*(3), 249–258.

Moffat, D. A., & Ramsden, R. T. (1977). Profound bilateral sensorineural hearing loss during gentamicin therapy. *Journal of Laryngology and Otology, 91*(6), 511–516.

Møller, A. R. (2000). *Hearing: Its physiology and pathophysiology.* New York, NY: Academic Press.

Morata, T. C., Dunn, D. E., Kretschmer, L. W., Lemasters, G. K., & Keith, R. W. (1993). Effects of occupational exposure to organic solvents and noise on hearing. *Scandinavian Journal of Work Environment and Health, 19*(4), 245–254.

Morgan, W. E., Coker, N. J., & Jenkins, H. A. (1994). Histopathology of temporal bone fractures: Implications for cochlear implantation. *Laryngoscope, 104*(4), 426–432.

Morrison, A. W., Bailey, M. E., & Morrison, G. A. (2009). Familial Ménière's disease: Clinical and genetic aspects. *Journal of Laryngology and Otology, 123*(1), 29–37.

Mostafapour, S. P., Lahargoue, K., & Gates, G. A. (1998). Noise-induced hearing loss in young adults: The role of personal listening devices and other sources of leisure noise. *Laryngoscope, 108*(12), 1832–1839.

Murphy, K. W. (1970). Deafness after topical neomycin. *British Medical Journal, 2*(5701), 114.

National Institute on Deafness and Other Communication Disorders. (2010). *Presbycusis.* Retrieved 6/16/11 from http://www.nidcd.nih.gov/health/hearing/presbycusis.htm .

National Institutes for Occupational Safety and Health. (1998). *Criteria for a recommended standard: Occupational noise exposure.* Cincinnati, OH: U.S. Department of Health and Human Services, Public Health Service, Center for Disease Control, National Institutes for Occupational Safety and Health, DHHS (NIOSH) Publication No. 98–126.

Occupational Safety and Health Administration. (1983). Occupational noise exposure: Hearing conservation amendment. *Federal Register, 48*(46), 9738–9783.

Palmer, K. T., Griffin, M. J., Syddall, H. E., & Coggon, D. (2004). Cigarette smoking, occupational exposure to noise, and self reported hearing difficulties. *Occupational and Environmental Medicine, 61*(4), 340–344.

Pfammatter, A., Darrouzet, V., Gärtner, M., Somers, T., Van Dinther, J., Trabalzini, F., ... Linder T. (2010). A superior semicircular canal dehiscence syndrome multicenter study: Is there an association between size and symptoms? *Otology and Neurotology, 31*(3), 447–454.

Pichora-Fuller, M. K., & Souza, P. E. (2003). Effects of aging on auditory processing of speech. *International Journal of Audiology, 42*(Suppl. 2), 2S11–2S16.

Prasher, D. (1998). New strategies for prevention and treatment of noise-induced hearing loss. *Lancet, 352*(9136), 1240–1242.

Quick, C. A., & Duvall, A. J., 3rd. (1970). Early changes in the cochlear duct from ethacrynic acid: An electronmicroscopie evaluation. *Laryngoscope, 80*(6), 954–965.

Roosa, D., & John, S. (1875). Experiments concerning the effects of quinine upon the ear. *Transactions of the American Otological Society, 2,* 93.

Rosenhall, U., & Karlsson, A. K. (1991). Tinnitus in old age. *Scandinavian Audiology, 20*(3), 165–171.

Ruckenstein, M. J. (2004). Autoimmune inner ear disease. *Current Opinion in Otolaryngology & Head and Neck Surgery, 12*(5), 426–430.

Ruckenstein, M. J., Rutka, J. A., & Hawke, M. (1991). The treatment of Menière's disease: Torok revisited. *Laryngoscope, 101*(2), 211–218.

Rybak, L. P. (1993). Ototoxicity of loop diuretics. *Otolaryngologic Clinics of North America, 26*(5), 829–844.

Saraiya, P. V., & Aygun, N. (2009). Temporal bone fractures. *Emergency Radiology, 16*(4), 255–265.

Sataloff, J., Hawkshaw, M. J., & Sataloff, R. T. (2010). "Gun-shooting hearing loss": A pilot study. *Ear, Nose, and Throat Journal 89*(1), E15–E19.

Saumil, N., & Rosowski, J. J. (2008). Conductive hearing loss caused by third-window lesions of the inner ear. *Otology and Neurotology, 29*(3), 282–289.

Schuknecht, H. (1974). *Pathology of the ear.* Cambridge, MA: Harvard University Press.

Schuknecht, H. F., Kimura, R. S., & Naufal, P. M. (1973). The pathology of sudden deafness. *Acta Otolaryngologica, 76*(2), 75–97.

Schulman, J. B. (1979). Traumatic diseases of the ear and temporal bone. In V. Goodhill (Ed.), *Ear diseases, deafness and dizziness* (pp. 504–516). New York, NY: Harper & Row.

Schwabach, D. (1884). Uberbleiben de Storungenim Gehororgannach Chinin und Salicylgebrauch. *Deutsche Medizinische Wochenschrift, 10,* 163.

Schwaber, M. K. (2007). Vestibular disorders. In G. B. Hughes & M. L. Pensak (Eds.), *Clinical otology* (pp. 355–374). New York, NY: Thieme.

Schwaber, M. K., Hall, J. W., & Zealear, D. L. (1991). Intraoperative monitoring of the facial and cochleovestibular nerves in otologic surgery: Part II. *Insights in Otolaryngology, 6,* 108.

Schweitzer, V. G., Dolan, D. F., Abrams, G. E., Davidson, T., & Snyder, R. (1986). Amelioration of cisplatin-induced ototoxicity by fosfomycin. *Laryngoscope, 96*(9, Pt. 1), 948–958.

Sendowski, I. (2006). Magnesium therapy in acoustic trauma. *Magnesium Research, 19*(4), 244–254.

Silverstein, H., & Rosenberg, S. (1992). *Surgical techniques of the temporal bone and skull base.* Philadelphia, PA: Lea & Febiger.

Smullen, J. L., Andrist, E. C., & Gianoli, G. J. (1999). Superior semicircular canal dehiscence: A new cause of vertigo. *Journal of the Louisiana State Medical Society, 151*(8), 397–400.

Songer, J. E., & Rosowski, J. J. (2010). A superior semicircular canal dehiscence-induced air-bone gap in chinchilla. *Hearing Research, 269*(1–2), 70–80.

Sprinzl, G. M., & Riechelmann, H. (2010). Current trends in treating hearing loss in elderly people: A review of the technology and treatment options—a mini-review. *Gerontology, 56*(3), 351–358.

Stahle, J., Friberg, U., & Svedberg, A. (1991). Long-term progression of Menière's disease. *Acta Otolaryngologica, 485*(Suppl.), 78–83.

Strauss, M., Towfighi, J., Lord, S., Lipton, A., Harvey, H. A., & Brown, B. (1983). Cisplatinum ototoxicity: Clinical experience and temporal bone histopathology. *Laryngoscope, 93*(12), 1554–1559.

Suckfuell, M., Canis, M., Strieth, S., Scherer, H., & Haisch, A. (2007). Intratympanic treatment of acute acoustic trauma with a cell-permeable JNK ligand: A prospective randomized phase I/II study. *Acta Otolaryngologica, 127*(9), 938–942.

Suter, A. H., & von Gierke, H. E. (1987). Noise and public policy. *Ear and Hearing, 8*(4), 188–191.

Tsunoda, A., & Terasaki, O. (2002). Dehiscence of the bony roof of the superior semicircular canal in the middle cranial fossa. *Journal of Laryngology and Otology, 116*(7), 514–518.

Tucci, D. L., Farmer, J. C., Jr., Kitch, R. D., & Witsell, D. L. (2002). Treatment of sudden sensorineural hearing loss with systemic steroids and valacyclovir. *Otology and Neurotology, 23*(3), 301–308.

Tuzel, I. H. (1981). Comparison of adverse reactions to bumetanide and furosemide. *Journal of Clinical Pharmacology, 21*(11–12, Pt. 2), 615–619.

University of Texas Medical Branch Grand Rounds. (2001). Sudden sensorineural hearing loss. Retrieved 6/15/11 from http://www.utmb.edu/otoref/grnds/Sudden-HearingLoss-010613/SSNHL.htm.

Valente, M., Mispagel, K., Valente, L. M., & Hullar, T. (2006). Problems and solutions for fitting amplification for patients with Ménière's disease. *Journal of the American Academy of Audiology, 17*(1), 6–15.

Vasama, J. P., & Linthicum, F. H., Jr. (1999). Meniere's disease and endolymphatic hydrops without Meniere's symptoms: Temporal bone histopathology. *Acta Otolaryngologica, 119*(3), 297–301.

Vogel, I., Verschuure, H., van der Ploeg, C. P., Brug, J., & Raat, H. (2010). Estimating adolescent risk for hearing loss based on data from a large school-based survey. *American Journal of Public Health, 100*(6), 1095–1100.

Walker, E. M., Jr., Fazekas-May, M. A., & Bowen, W. R. (1990). Nephrotoxic and ototoxic agents. *Clinics in Laboratory Medicine, 10*(2), 323–354.

Watson, S. R., Halmagyi, G. M., & Colebatch, J. G. (2000). Vestibular hypersensitivity to sound (Tullio phenomenon): Structural and functional assessment. *Neurology, 54*(3), 722–728.

Whitaker, S. (1980). Idiopathic sudden hearing loss. *American Journal of Otology, 1*(3), 180–183.

Wiley, T. L., Cruickshanks, K. J., Nondahl, D. M., Tweed, T. S., Klein, R., & Klein, B. E. (1998). Aging and word recognition in competing message. *Journal of the American Academy of Audiology, 9*(3), 191–198.

Wilson, W. R., Byl, F. M., & Laird, N. (1980). The efficacy of steroids in the treatment of idiopathic sudden hearing loss. A double-blind clinical study. *Archives of Otolaryngology, 106*(12), 772–776.

Wladislavosky-Waserman, P., Facer, G. W., Mokri, B., & Kurland, L. T. (1984). Meniere's disease: A 30–year epidemiologic and clinical study in Rochester, MN, 1951–1980. *Laryngoscope, 94*(8), 1098–1102.

World Health Organization. (2005). Active ageing: A policy framework. *A contribution of the World Health Organization to the Second United Nations World Assembly on Ageing.* Madrid, Spain.

WrongDiagnosis.com. (2011). *Prevalence and Incidence of Perilymphatic fistula.* Retrieved 6/15/11 from http://www.wrongdiagnosis.com/p/perilymphatic_fistula/prevalence.htm.

Wynne, M. K. (2003). Sudden hearing loss. *The Hearing Journal, 56*, 10–15.

Xenellis, J. E., Linthicum, F. H., Jr., & Galey, F. R. (1990). Lermoyez's syndrome: Histopathologic report of a case. *Annals of Otology, Rhinology, and Laryngology, 99*(4, Pt. 1), 307–309.

Zenner, H. P., Reuter, G., Zimmermann, U., Gitter, A. H., Fermin, C., & LePage, E. L. (1994). Transitory endolymph leakage induced hearing loss and tinnitus: Depolarization, biphasic shortening and loss of electromotility of outer hair cells. *European Archives of Oto-Rhino-Laryngology, 251*(3), 143–153.

6

Auditory Nerve Disorders

INTRODUCTION

This chapter covers three main topics, including acoustic neuromas, auditory neuropathy, and vascular loops. These three topics are not the only disorders that can affect the auditory nerve, but they do represent relatively common occurrences and are well represented in the literature. These topics provide a snapshot of the spectrum of dysfunction of the auditory nerve and the great importance it plays in hearing. It was once commented on at a conference that the auditory nerve was a "bottleneck" for all auditory information coming from the cochlea. This was an astute comment as all auditory information processed in the cochlea is passed to the central auditory nervous system via the auditory nerve.

The auditory nerve is about 22 mm in length and is composed of 30,000 fibers in the adult human. It consists of type I fibers (90%) that connect to inner hair cells and type II fibers that connect to outer hair cells (10%). The more distal segment (fibers exiting the cochlea) is unmyelinated, with the more proximal portion (fibers projecting to the brain-

stem) myelinated in reference to type I fibers (i.e., the afferent fibers). The auditory nerve fibers project from the terminal buttons on the hair cells through the habenula perforata to Rosenthal's canal, which accommodates the spiral ganglion cells. These fibers form a trunk in the modiolus and then course through the internal auditory meatus before entering the cerebellopontine angle (CPA). The central projection of auditory nerve fibers is to the root entry zone in the brainstem between the anterior and posterior ventral cochlear nuclei. (For more information on the anatomy and physiology of the auditory nerve, see Musiek & Baran, 2007, and Chapter 2: Structure and Function of the Auditory and Vestibular Systems.)

ACOUSTIC NEUROMA

Introduction

Although historically referred to as acoustic neuromas, benign tumors of the eighth cranial nerve originating from Schwann cells are more accurately and currently referred to as vestibular schwannomas. These tumors occur, almost exclusively, on the vestibular branches of the vestibulocochlear nerve. Schwann cells produce myelin that insulates the nerve fibers subserving hearing and balance (Musiek & Baran, 2007). Although these tumors typically cause tinnitus, unilateral hearing loss, and disequilibrium, they may grow to considerable sizes and compress the brainstem leading to stroke, hydrocephalus, and even death. There has been a steady improvement in the early identification and surgical management of acoustic neuromas over the past several years as audiologists and otologists have worked in concert to improve the outcome for patients with acoustic neuromas and acoustic tumors from neurofibromatosis type 2 (NF2) (see the Etiology and Pathology section below and Chapter 9 for information on the genetic bases of NF2).

Symptoms

Tinnitus is the most common symptom in patients with vestibular schwannomas; however, hearing loss is often the presenting complaint in most patients. The hearing loss is classically a unilateral sensorineural hearing loss—the presence of which should signal the need for a workup for acoustic neuroma. The hearing loss in patients with acoustic tumors tends to be gradually progressive, with a decrease in word recognition performance that is out of proportion to the loss of pure-tone hearing sensitivity. Asymmetric sensorineural hearing loss reportedly occurs in 85% of confirmed tumor cases (see Tucci, 1997). However, others have reported that the presenting complaint for 75% of patients with acoustic tumors is hearing loss, but that when all patients with confirmed acoustic tumors are formally evaluated that 95% of the patients actually are found to have hearing loss (Angeli & Jackson, 1997). The high incidence of hearing loss in this population of patients is most likely the reason why the terms, acoustic neuroma and acoustic tumors, remain in common use.

Tucci (1997) reviewed the incidence of hearing loss in patients with vestibular schwannomas and found that 95% of patients with tumors larger than 3 cm had hearing loss, whereas patients with tumors 1 to 3 cm in size and those with tumors less than 1 cm in size had incidences of hearing loss of 88 and 77%, respectively.

Sudden hearing loss can occur in some patients with acoustic tumors, and some may even recover partially following treatment with steroids. However, less than 10% of patients with sudden sensorineural hearing loss will turn out to have acoustic neuromas on magnetic resonance imaging (MRI) (Ramos et al., 2005). On the other hand, up to 24% of patients with a diagnosis of acoustic neuroma present with sudden hearing loss as an initial complaint. For example, Pensak and colleagues reported that 15% of their patients with acoustic tumors had experienced a sudden loss of hearing (Pensak, Glasscock, Josey, Jackson, & Gulya, 1985). Sudden hearing loss, when it does occur, rarely improves even after treatment. In fact, the most common outcome is that the hearing loss progresses regardless of the chosen treatment.

Not every patient with an acoustic neuroma has hearing loss. Some patients maintain normal hearing sensitivity even when they are found to have surprisingly large tumors. Also, the degree and the rate of hearing loss do not correlate well with tumor size or growth rate. There are some patients (approximately 5%) with acoustic neuromas who have normal pure-tone findings for the ear on the side of the tumor (Musiek, Kibbe-Michal, Geurkink, Josey, & Glasscock, 1986; Welling, Glasscock, Woods, & Jackson, 1990). However, it is important to note that most of the patients with normal hearing sensitivity will have other complaints, such as vestibular problems and unilateral tinnitus that may signal the need to explore the possibility of retrocochlear pathology, such as a vestibular schwannoma. In some cases, unilateral tinnitus itself can be the initial symptom reported.

Disequilibrium is common in patients with acoustic tumors; however, true vertigo is rarely a presenting complaint. Because these tumors grow slowly, balance problems are usually subtle as ongoing central vestibular compensation occurs, and many patients will report disequilibrium only retrospectively. However, very large tumors can give rise to abnormal gait and ataxia due to compression of the cerebellum, which is the balance/coordination portion of the brain. The presence of ataxia or gross gait impairment usually signifies a large tumor and is a relatively serious neurological sign and should be addressed urgently (Pensak et al., 1985).

Facial nerve dysfuntion with involuntary spasms of the eyelids sometimes occurs. Paralysis of the facial nerve, however, is rare, and patients with facial paralysis along with an internal auditory canal lesion are likely to have a different type of tumor than a vestibular schwannoma. Facial nerve schwannomas commonly cause slow, progressive facial paresis along with the other auditory and vestibular symptoms. Patients with sudden and/or rapidly progressive facial paralysis may have malignant metastatic tumors and should undergo a thorough diagnostic evaluation.

Other symptoms of acoustic neuroma are caused by pressure against the adjacent cranial nerves, brainstem, and cerebellum (see House, 1997). These symptoms typically occur only when the tumors become quite large. Facial numbness or paresthesia (tingling sensation) is the result of pressure on the trigeminal or fifth cranial nerve. Headaches may also occur. In addition, very large tumors may cause drowsiness and even loss of consciousness from obstruction to the flow of cerebral spinal fluid. When this occurs, neurosurgical intervention is urgently required.

Incidence and Prevalence

Acoustic neuromas are the most common tumors of the CPA and they are also among the most common types of benign intracranial tumors, accounting for approximately 8% of all intracranial tumors (Gruskin, Carberry, & Chandrasekhar, 1997; Zulch, 1957). Nevertheless, their incidence is low, about 1–2 in 100,000 individuals. This equates to about 3,000 new cases of acoustic neuroma in the United States each year, of which only about 5% are bilateral (Pool, Palva, & Greenfield, 1970; Stangerup, Tos, Thomsen, & Caye-Thomasen, 2010).

Etiology and Pathology

A great deal has been learned about the etiology of acoustic neuromas in the last several years. As mentioned earlier, in most cases the "neuroma" is really a schwannoma—a proliferation of vestibular Schwann cells. The Schwann cells are the supporting cells that form a wrapping around the neurons and are important for conduction of neural signals. Schwann cell proliferation is regulated by a gene called

NF2, which encodes a tumor suppressor protein called merlin or schwannomin. This suppressor gene resides on chromosome 22q12. A variety of mutations may occur in this gene and the type of mutation present has been linked to the severity of disease. Loss of myelin function results in Schwann cell proliferation and tumor development. This may occur when both *NF2* gene copies contain mutations, which has been referred to as the "two-hit hypothesis" (see Scaravilli, 2003).

The vast majority of acoustic neuromas (>95%) occur sporadically, but 2 to 5% of tumors occur as part of a genetic hereditary syndrome, neurofibromatosis type 2 ("NF2"). Neurofibromatosis type 2 is believed to be inherited through an autosomal dominant pattern of inheritance with incomplete penetrance. (See Chapter 9, Hereditary and Congenital Hearing Loss, for additional information on genetics and inherited hearing loss). However, unlike the majority of other autosomal dominant conditions, where only a single copy of the affected gene is needed to result in the disorder, it appears that two copies of the *NF2* gene must be mutated for tumor formation in to occur (Genetics Home Reference, 2011). Most affected individuals inherit one defective copy of the tumor suppressor gene from one of their parents and a second copy is injured or mutated at some point during the individual's lifetime. Many NF2 patients may also develop spontaneous *NF2* mutations with no other affected family members. The presence of bilateral vestibular schwannomas is diagnostic of NF2; however, the Manchester criteria delineate the physical findings and family history necessary for a diagnosis of NF2 to be made (Baser et al., 2002). These individuals usually develop acoustic neu-

romas early in life and are prone to having multiple cranial nerve schwannomas, neuromas, spinal tumors, meningiomas, and other brain tumors as well. Additionally, they may present with clouding of the lens of the eye (juvenile posterior subcapsular lenticular opacities) and may develop early-onset cataracts (Baser et al., 2002). These unfortunate individuals usually require multiple surgical procedures and often end up with bilateral deafness, which usually cannot be corrected by cochlear implantation. Genetic counseling is of paramount importance in these patients because the gene can be passed on by the parent to his/her offspring in an autosomal dominant fashion (see Pensak et al., 1985, and Scaravilli, 2003).

Site of Lesion

Acoustic neuroma is the most common "retrocochlear" lesion. As such, site-of-lesion tests that differentiate retrocochlear from cochlear conditions are used in the audiologic diagnosis of acoustic neuroma. Acoustic tumors arise from the vestibular portion of the eighth cranial nerve about 90% of the time. These tumors typically originate in the internal auditory canal and as they grow they extend medially into the CPA and/or erode the bone of the internal canal (Gruskin et al., 1997). However, as mentioned earlier, the vast majority of acoustic neuromas reside in the CPA.

It is important to note that tumors greater than 2 cm in maximum diameter are likely to eventually contact and compress the brainstem and cerebellum (Musiek & Kibbe, 1986). In this situation, the central auditory nervous system becomes involved and additional auditory and/or vestibular symptoms may appear.

Audiology

Although the auditory brainstem response (ABR) is typically recognized as the standard test protocol for use in the assessment of auditory nerve function, the audiology of acoustic neuromas includes more than just the ABR. There is valuable information to be gained from the pure-tone audiogram and word recognition test scores. In addition, acoustic reflexes and otoacoustic emissions (OAEs) can be of help. Therefore, each of these tests are discussed along with the various permutations of the ABR that may be observed in patients with acoustic neuromas.

Pure-Tone Threshold and Speech Recognition Tests

It has been reported that over 90% of patients with acoustic tumors present with unilateral sensorineural loss (Lustig & Jackler, 1997). However, only a very small percentage of individuals with unilateral sensorineural loss actually will have an acoustic neuroma (estimates range from less than 1% to slightly more than 1%) (National Institutes of Health Consensus Conference, 1991). Therefore, to use unilateral sensorineural loss as a key criterion for referral can be problematic. The most common audiometric configuration for acoustic neuromas is a sloping high-frequency loss, which occurs almost two-thirds of the time (Johnson, 1977). Speech recognition scores vary widely, but interestingly in one large study, 35% of the patients studied had scores of 0% (Johnson, 1977). The classic audiologic signs of unilateral sensorineural hearing loss and reduced speech recognition scores remain important warning signs of acoustic neuroma; however, the sensitivity and specificity of these measures do not permit them to be highly diagnostic.

An important issue regarding pure-tone thresholds is what criteria should be used to determine if further workup is indicated. This issue here centers around the degree of asymmetry that should exist between the two ears before a referral for further testing is made. There are a variety of criteria that have been proposed for this purpose. Obholzer, Rea, and Harcourt (2004) reviewed six different criteria that have been used and offered yet another set of criteria. Their criteria require that the thresholds for two adjacent frequencies to be more than 15 dB poorer in one ear than the other when the better ear pure-tone average is equal to or greater than 30 dB HL for the audiometric frequencies between 250 and 8000 Hz. If the pure-tone average across these frequencies is greater than 30 dB HL, then the criterion changes to a 20 dB difference between the two ears for two neighboring frequencies. Application of these criteria revealed a high sensitivity (>90%), but a moderately poor specificity, which is typical of all such criteria. However, in spite of the moderately poor specificity, the Obholzer et al. criteria seem to be of some value when determining the need for follow-up in patients presenting with asymmetrical sensorineural hearing losses.

Otoacosutic Emissions and Acoustic Reflexes

Otoacoustic emissions, including transient otoacoustic emissions (TEOAEs) and distortion product otoacoustic emissions (DPOAEs), are generated by the outer hair cells in the cochlea. This being the case, it would seem logical to assume that OAEs would be normal in acoustic neuromas; however, it is not always that straightforward. The likely reason is that in many cases of acoustic neuroma there is coexisting cochlear hearing loss. This could be from the tumor pressing on the vertebrobasilar blood supply in the internal auditory meatus and reducing the blood supply to the inner ear, or, alternatively, to the comorbid presence of a cochlear hearing loss from another cause such as noise exposure. Therefore, what is observed in large studies of patients with acoustic neuromas are findings that are consistent with both cochlear hearing loss (where the OAEs are usually absent) and/or eighth nerve involvement (where the OAE responses are better than the audiometric thresholds) (Telischi, Roth, Stagner, Lonsbury-Martin, & Balkany, 1995).

Acoustic reflexes (AR) are typically elevated or absent in patients with acoustic neuromas when the stimulus is presented to the affected ear. Also, acoustic reflex decay, which can only be assessed if acoustic reflexes are present, can be excessive, indicating retrocochlear involvement (again the decay, if present, would be observed when the stimulus is presented to the affected ear). The sensitivity and specificity of the AR threshold and decay measures hovers around 80% in terms of detecting acoustic neuromas (Johnson, 1977; Wilson & Margolis, 1999). However, the sensitivity and specificity of these measures is influenced by the degree of hearing loss. In general, as hearing loss becomes greater, the number of false positives increases—especially when the hearing loss is greater than 60 dB HL. The most reliable frequencies in testing for acoustic neuromas are 500, 1000, and 2000 Hz, and abnormalities should be observed for both ipsilateral and contralateral in patients with acoustic neuromas

when the test stimulus is presented to the ear that has the acoustic neuroma (see Wilson & Margolis, 1999).

Auditory Brainstem Response (ABR)

Clearly the best audiologic test for acoustic neuromas is the ABR. In fact, it has been shown that for acoustic neuromas the best procedure is the ABR alone. When it is combined with other tests overall test efficiency suffers (Turner, Frazer, & Shepard, 1984). The ABR indices that are most telling in acoustic neuroma patients are the I–III and the I–V interwave intervals and the interaural latency difference (ILD). These indices individually or in combination will yield hit rates of approximately 90% or better and false positive rates of usually less than 20% (Musiek, Shinn, & Jirsa, 2007). In many cases of acoustic neuromas the ABR is totally absent even when the audiogram reveals reasonably good hearing sensitivity. Another diagnostic protocol that has started to emerge in the audiologic assessment of the patient considered to be at risk for an acoustic neuroma is the comparison of the puretone thresholds with the ABR thresholds. If there is a large discrepancy between these measures (that is, if behavioral thresholds are considerably better than ABR thresholds), then retrocochlear involvement should be considered (Bush, Jones, & Shinn, 2008).

There has been concern about missing very small tumors with ABR for some time (Wilson, Hodgson, Gustafson, Hogue, & Mills, 1992). To this end, Don and colleagues developed the stacked ABR, which better accounts for low-frequency contributions (or lack of thereof) to the electrophysiologic response than does the conventional ABR, thus permitting a better sensitivity for diagnosing small lesions (Don, Kwong, Tanaka, Brackmann, & Nelson, 2005). The difficulty surrounding the stacked ABR procedure is that it does require considerable time to complete the procedure. In an attempt to address this difficulty, a new "chirp" stimulus has been introduced in research circles and we await the studies using this stimulus (see Bell, Allen, & Lutman, 2002).

It is important to consider utilization of the ABR, with its impressive record of high sensitivity for acoustic tumors, in the assessment of patients who may be considered to be at risk for acoustic tumors. Its use may help to reduce the number of overreferrals for MRIs that are made based on findings of asymmetrical hearing loss alone. The ABR test can also be used in cross checking radiologic results in that it has now been shown that MRIs are not without flaws. A recent report highlights a false positive result for acoustic neuroma based on MRI where ABR results were normal (House, Bassim, & Schwartz, 2008). This report adds to a growing number of reports revealing false positive MRI results in patients with asymmetrical sensorineural hearing losses. These false positive MRI cases involve very small lesions (1–2 mm) that mimic vestibular schwannomas and may even have unilateral auditory symptoms; however, they lack a discrete tumor during surgery. Also there are many individuals who cannot undergo MRIs or CTs for a number of reasons, and in these cases, the application of ABR test procedures would be essential. In addition, the ABR is a physiologic measure, whereas the MRI is not, and there are many cases of auditory nerve dysfunction that show nothing significant on MRI as this diagnostic procedure does not assess physiologic function. Auditory brainstem response testing is

therefore considered to be important adjunct to imaging procedures because to effectively manage the patient with eighth nerve involvement, physiologic dysfunction must be confirmed and quantified.

There are various disorders that can affect the auditory nerve that are not acoustic neuromas. These could possibly be categorized under the well-known term, auditory neuropathy. However, auditory neuropathy is defined by a constellation of audiologic test findings, which include pure-tone threshold test results that can range from normal hearing to profound hearing loss, speech recognition scores that are typically significantly reduced, and normal OAEs (unless there is some comorbid cochlear involvement), as well as totally absent ABRs (at least in most cases) with no obvious anatomic or pathologic indicators. Certainly, vascular problems, infections, neural degeneration, and trauma can damage the auditory nerve and will likely yield abnormal ABRs. However, within the present classification system, these disorders would not provide the audiologic profile that would deem them an auditory neuropathy. The main point here, however, is that a variety of disorders can cause auditory nerve dysfunction; and although they might not be found via imaging, they can be identified by utilizing ABR. This is a critical point too often ignored in today's diagnostic world (see Musiek et al., 2007). One of these disorders that deserves mention here is vascular loop syndrome. In this situation, a blood vessel may be positioned so that it places pressure on the auditory nerve. This in turn can result in associated tinnitus, hearing loss, and in some cases hemifacial spasm (see later discussion).

The ABR is also a highly useful tool in intraoperative monitoring during acoustic neuroma surgery. This is especially the case when there is an attempt to preserve hearing; however, some controversy surrounds this issue. The maintenance of an ABR waveform, specifically the preservation of wave V, during acoustic neuroma surgery usually indicates that the auditory nerve has not been compromised and hearing likely has been preserved. It should be noted, however, that the loss of wave V does not necessarily mean there has been a loss of hearing. In addition, timely feedback to the surgeon during surgery is valuable in the process of preserving hearing. Utilizing ABR for intraoperative monitoring during the surgery for acoustic tumors has become commonplace in many major medical centers (see Martin & Yong-bin Shi, 2007; Phillips, Kobylarz, De Peralta, Stieg, & Selesnick, 2010).

Vestibular Evaluation

Videonystagmography (VNG) can be of value in quantifying vestibular function in cases of acoustic neuroma. One of the important findings is that of unilateral paresis on the involved side. This is especially noteworthy if the patient has minimal vestibular symptoms, which may be the case with acoustic neuromas. The status of the function of the vestibular system is helpful to know in acoustic neuroma cases in regard to predicting how stable the patient may be after surgery. To elaborate, individuals with good preoperative vestibular function who undergo sectioning of the vestibular nerve may have a longer adjustment period postoperatively than those who have poor vestibular function before surgery. This is likely due to the fact that those with intact vestibular function preoperatively are likely to require more time for central vestibular compensation to occur following surgery; however, the extent and rate of this cen-

tral compensation also may be influenced by patient age and other factors. Sharing this information with the patient prior to surgery can help the patient establish realistic expectations for postsurgical adjustment and recovery and result in a better outcome for the patient. Finally, central vestibular findings (eye tracking abnormalities) may be also observed on eye tracking tests is some patients with acoustic neuromas if there is secondary brainstem involvement due to the locus or size of the lesion.

Vestibular evoked myogenic potentials (VEMPs) are considered in the evaluation of acoustic neuromas because the inferior vestibular nerve is critical to the generation of this potential. Amplitudes of the VEMPs are decreased on the side of involvement, but latencies seem not to be affected in most cases. At best, the hit rate for acoustic tumors using VEMP is around 80%, but overall test efficiency suffers due to the high variability of amplitude measures. The most commonly used, and likely the best, VEMP indice is the interaural amplitude comparison (see Aiken & Murnane, 2008, for more information).

Medical Examination

The physical examination should include examination of the ears, nose, throat, and cranial nerves, as well as the patient's balance and gait. The ENT exam is usually normal. The cranial nerve exam, however, will generally indicate a hearing loss on the side of the tumor, which should be confirmed audiometrically. Extraocular movements are generally normal and double vision or impairment of extraocular movement should signify another type of tumor, such as a meningioma. The fifth nerve (or trigeminal nerve) is examined by light touch and pinprick over the three divisions of the face. Loss of sensation over part of the face is sign of a large tumor pressing on the trigeminal nerve. The corneal reflex may be absent on the affected side as well. Facial nerve function is usually intact. The presence of facial nerve weakness usually signifies facial nerve tumor rather than acoustic neuroma. A careful search for muscle fasciculations, especially around the upper and lower eyelids, should also be made. The facial nerve has sensory fibers as well as motor fibers. Loss of sensation to light touch around the posterior edge of the external auditory meatus ("Hitselberger's sign") is a sensitive early sign of acoustic neuroma (Hitselberger & House, 1966). Eighth nerve function involves balance as well as hearing. Nystagmus, a beating eye movement, is the cardinal sign of a balance system impairment. However, because balance deficits are usually well compensated, nystagmus is a rare finding. Brun's nystagmus, which can occur in patients with cerebellar involvement, is an asymmetrical nystagmus in which there is little or no spontaneous nystagmus in the primary position, but an asymmetry exists at the extremes of lateral gaze (Robinson, Zee, Hain, Holmes, & Rosenberg, 1984). This could be a sign of a very large tumor that is exerting pressure on the cerebellum. Gait ataxia or inability to walk arises from pressure on the cerebellum and brainstem. The lower cranial nerves, which are responsible for swallowing, the gag reflex, vocal fold function, and tongue function, are rarely involved.

Once a retrocochlear lesion is indicated by audiometric testing, the most appropriate diagnostic test is an MRI scan of the internal auditory canals with gadolinium enhancement. Magnetic resonance imaging will typically detect even the smallest tumors (approximately 1 mm in size). Gadolinium is important as a contrast agent because it is concentrated by the tumor and shows up as a very bright spot on the image. Techniques of MRI using high resolution and avoiding gadolinium have been used, but the diagnosis is then contingent on the quality of the scan and the experience of the radiologist. At the present time, gadolinium-enhanced scanning remains the diagnostic gold standard.

An acoustic neuroma will typically manifest as a bright lesion in the internal auditory canal that extends out into the CPA. The tumor has a pear-shaped appearance. The canalicular component is narrower and somewhat triangular and the extracanalicular component extends like a mushroom cap to fill the space between the temporal bone and the brain (see case studies for this chapter). Most tumors arise in the internal auditory canal and so the canalicular component is an important diagnostic finding. The absence of this raises a suggestion of meningioma or some other type of tumor of the CPA.

Audiologic Management

Audiologic management of patients with acoustic neuromas depends to a great extent on the symptoms of the patient after surgery. This could include auditory and/or vestibular management. If hearing has been partially or totally lost after surgery, then appropriate audiologic steps should be pursued. This may include a hearing aid fitting and counseling. Also, auditory training may be useful and appropriate in some cases.

If the patient has balance difficulties after surgery, then vestibular rehabilitation approaches may be initiated. Vestibular exercises can be of value in helping stabilize the patient. It is also useful to help the patient connect with others who have had this surgery for support. Patient groups across the country have been formed and provide valuable assistance in this regard.

Medical Management

The treatment options for acoustic neuroma include surgical removal, stereotactic radiation therapy, or serial observation (see Luxford, 1997). The choice of treatment depends on the size of the tumor, the age and general health of the patient, the patient's hearing status, and (increasingly) the patient's preference.

Surgical removal of an acoustic neuroma is usually performed as a team approach between a neurotologist and a neurosurgeon. The surgery can be done by one of three approaches; translabyrinthine, retrosigmoid (or suboccipital), or middle cranial fossa. The choice of approach depends on the size of the tumor, the desire to preserve hearing, and the surgeon's preference.

The translabyrinthine approach is done through a postauricular incision. Following a complete mastoidectomy, the drilling is extended through the semicircular canals and the posterior petrous bone to access the CPA and the internal auditory canal. Hearing is always lost during this approach. The main virtue of this approach is that the facial nerve is identified early as it exits the internal auditory canal and the tumor can be separated easily from the facial nerve in this location, ensuring safety to the nerve. Tumors of almost any size and location can be removed through this approach.

The retrosigmoid or suboccipital approach is through a craniotomy or bony opening posterior to the sigmoid sinus and inferior to the lateral sinus behind the ear. After bone removal, the dura is incised and cerebral spinal fluid is allowed to egress. This allows the cerebellum to relax posteriorly and provides a good view of the tumor in the CPA, but not in the internal auditory canal. A drill has to be used to remove part of the temporal bone to obtain access to the canalicular portion of the tumor. The tumor is then incised and its internal contents removed. Once the tumor is reduced in size, the facial nerve and the auditory nerve can be identified and dealt with. Tumors that extend laterally into the internal auditory canal cannot be fully accessed through this approach and place the patient at risk for tumor recurrence. This approach allows for preservation of hearing in cases where the tumor can be successfully separated from the cochlear division of the eighth nerve; however, in general, the hearing preservation rate is reported to be in the 30% range (see Glasscock, Bohrer, & Steenerson, 1997; Kaylie, Gilbert, Horgan, Delashaw, & McMenomey, 2001).

The middle cranial fossa approach is appropriate for accessing tumors that are small and limited to the internal auditory canal when hearing preservation is a goal. A 4×4 cm bony opening is made in the skull above the ear and the dura of the temporal lobe of the brain is gently lifted and retracted. A drill is used on the roof of the temporal bone to outline the internal auditory canal. Once the canal is open, the facial nerve is separated from the tumor and the tumor is removed. The goal of surgery is to remove the tumor completely and to preserve the facial nerve and the auditory branch of the eighth nerve. Additionally, this approach can be utilized to decompress the internal auditory canal for patients with tumors in an only hearing ear in which tumor growth has been demonstrated and hearing is declining. Hearing preservation of this approach ranges from 80 to 90% when careful patient selection is employed (Arts, Telian, El-Kashlan, & Thompson, 2006), Preservation of auditory function in these patients depends on having good hearing and good ABR waveform morphology preoperatively, and being able to anatomically separate the tumor from the cochlear division of the auditory nerve without entering the inner ear. This can only be accomplished in selected cases. Facial nerve preservation occurs in the majority of cases of small to median size tumors—better than 90% in experienced hands. Total tumor removal is usually achieved except in the case of very large tumors, where adherent tumor may be left on the facial nerve so as to not sacrifice facial function. The regrowth rate after successful tumor removal is in the 3 to 4% range (Dew, Shelton, & Hitselberger, 1997).

Surgery carries certain risks in addition to facial paralysis and hearing loss. Patients will routinely experience unilateral loss of vestibular function, which results in vertigo and nausea with head movement in the first 3 to 7 days postoperatively, and imbalance lasting for several weeks following surgery. Some patients, especially elderly patients, will require more time to recover, and may need vestibular rehabilitation therapy. Most will regain their balance function to near-normal levels with time, and can generally return to work in about a six-week timeframe. However, some patients will continue to experience transient loss of balance with rapid head movement, but these patients tend to learn to compensate for this deficit without much modification of daily activities of life.

Other complications of surgery include cerebral spinal fluid leak in about 10% of cases, prolonged headaches, meningitis, loss of other cranial nerve function (fifth and sixth cranial nerves are most common), stroke, and serious neurological problems. The mortality rate in experienced hands is less than 1%, and is much improved over the early days of acoustic neuroma surgery (see Charpiot, Tringali, Zaouche, Ferber-Viart, & Dubreuil, 2010).

Stereotactic radiotherapy, also known as gamma knife, CyberKnife, Linac, and "radiosurgery," is a nonsurgical method that has gained increasing popularity (Luxford, 1997). Originally introduced in Denmark in the 1970s, stereotatic radiotherapy has become increasingly prevalent in this country in the last 10 to 15 years. The goal is to deliver a highly focused beam of radiation to the carefully delineated treatment area that conforms to the tumor while avoiding the surrounding bone and brain. Acoustic neuromas are benign tumors and are not radiosensitive *per se*; however, radiation may induce fibrosis and destruction of tumor vasculature, and thus have a direct effect on the tumor cells. The tumor, therefore, typically does not disappear, but its growth is arrested. Radiation therapy has been reported successful in a high percentage (approximately >90%) of cases (University of Pittsburgh, 2009), and Authurs and colleagues (2011) in a systematic review of papers published between 2004 and 2009 found that hearing preservation was accomplished in 44 to 66% of cases undergoing radiosurgery and that only 2 to 4% of the patients studied required additional treatment. When fractionated radiotherapy was performed, these authors found hearing preservation rates of 59 to 94%, with 3 to 7% of the patients requiring additional treatment.

Additional Information

Acoustic neuromas constitute about 80 to 85% of tumors occurring in the CPA, and about 90% of tumors involving the internal auditory canal (see Hain, 2011, for review). The differential diagnosis of lesions occurring in these locations includes meningiomas, epidermoid tumors, lipomas, schwannomas of other cranial nerves (facial, trigeminal), and arachnoid cysts. Other rare lesions may occur, including malignancies (primary or metastatic), chordomas, vascular tumors, or inflammatory conditions. Menigiomas and other benign tumors are treated in a similar fashion to acoustic neuromas (i.e., surgical excision with attempted preservation of adjacent neural structures). Smaller lesions can sometimes be simply observed if they are asymptomatic. Arachnoid cysts are generally treated conservatively unless they become very large and cause compressive symptoms. Malignant lesions are usually managed with the assistance of an oncologist and involve multiple modes of treatment, such as surgery, radiation, and/or chemotherapy. The selection of treatment is individualized according to tumor type, grade, stage, and patient status (Luxford, 1997).

Case 6–1: Acoustic Neuroma

History

A 44-year-old female presented with problems of imbalance, lightheadedness, and vertigo. These symptoms reportedly were first experienced following a sailing trip 2 months prior to the current evaluation. The patient's husband reported concerns regarding a decrease in his wife's hearing sensitivity and the patient reported some hypersensitivity to sound. She additionally reported severe headaches and unilateral left-sided tinnitus.

Audiology

An otoscopic check was unremarkable bilaterally. A comprehensive audiologic evaluation indicated essentially normal peripheral hearing sensitivity bilaterally with normal word recognition scores and tympanometry results for both ears (Figure 6–1A). Speech recognition thresholds were in good agreement with pure-tone averages bilaterally. A routine ABR test was completed with test results revealing normal absolute and interwave latencies bilaterally. However, when a threshold ABR was obtained (Figure 6–1B) and compared to behavioral thresholds for the click stimulus, the right ear demonstrated good agreement between the behavioral and electrophysiologic thresholds. However, the electrophysiologic threshold for the left ear was significantly elevated (30 dB) above the behavioral threshold for the same ear suggesting retrocochlear involvement. A VNG was also performed and was unremarkable.

Medical Examination Result

The otolaryngologic exam revealed an abnormal Romberg examination with the patient leaning significantly to the left. Given the patient's reported symptoms and her audiologic test results, an MRI with contrast was performed to rule out retrocochlear involvement. However, test results revealed a small left-sided acoustic tumor (Figure 6–1C).

Impression

Small left-sided acoustic neuroma.

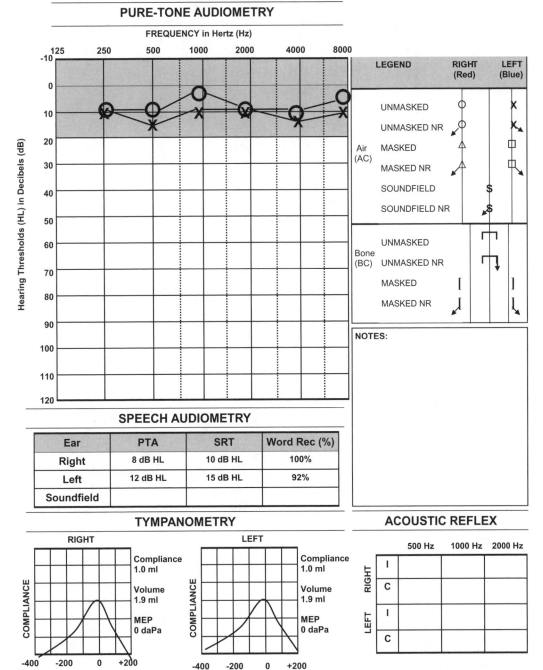

Figure 6–1. *Pure-tone thresholds, speech recognition scores, and tympanometry results (A), an ABR showing better approximation of threshold for the right ear than for the left ear (B), MRI results showing a small acoustic neuroma on the left side (see arrow) (C) for a 44-year-old female with a small left-sided acoustic neuroma (Case 6–1).* continues

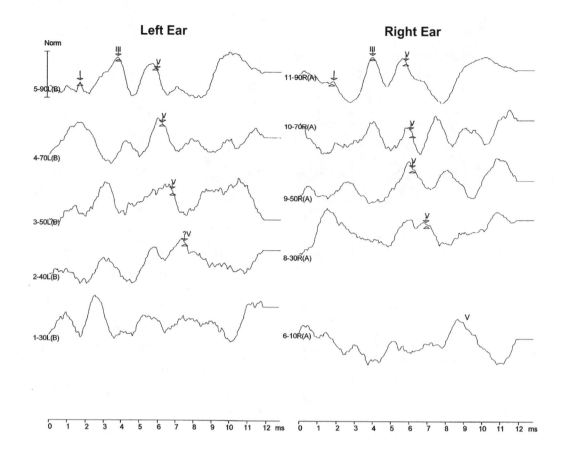

		Left Ear	Right Ear
Absolute Latencies (msec)			
	I	1.7	1.8
	III	3.93	3.9
	V	6.0	5.75
Interwave (msec)			
	I-III	2.22	2.1
	III-V	2.08	1.85
	I-V	4.3	3.95
	V ILD	.25 msec	
Threshold Comparisons (Behavioral— Electrophysiological)		30 dB	10 dB

B

Figure 6–1. continues

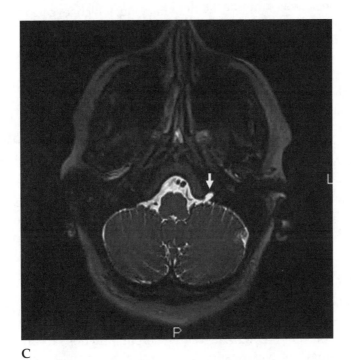

C

Figure 6–1. continued

Audiologic Recommendations and Management

Continue to monitor hearing sensitivity.

Medical Recommendations and Management

Given the small size of the acoustic neuroma, the decision was made in consultation with the patient to continue to monitor for any progression of the tumor. The patient was to be seen for annual audiologic evaluations and MRIs to monitor for any changes in the tumor.

Case 6–2: Acoustic Neuroma

History

This 41-year-old female was seen for an audiologic evaluation as part of her work requirements as a flight nurse. She had no previous evaluations on record. She indicated no concerns regarding hearing sensitivity on the right side, but reduced hearing and aural fullness on the left side. These symptoms were reported as having been experienced for the past 2 years. She denied any other significant audiologic or otologic history.

Audiology

An otoscopic check was unremarkable bilaterally. Tympanometry was performed and revealed normal pressure, volume, and compliance bilaterally (Figure 6–2A). A comprehensive audiologic evaluation revealed a mild low-frequency sensorineural hearing loss for the right ear, and a mild to moderate high-frequency sensorineural hearing loss for the left ear (see Figure 6–2A). Word recognition was excellent for the right ear and poor for the left ear. A significant asymmetry was noted for both pure-tone thresholds and word recognition scores.

Medical Examination Result

The otolaryngologic exam was essentially normal. Tympanic membranes were normal, extraocular muscle movement was full, and no nystagmus was observed. The patient's Romberg, Gait, and Tandem walk were all within normal limits. Facial nerve function was normal and symmetric. Given the degree of asymmetry in the hearing thresholds for the two ears and the age of the patient, no ABR was done. Rather the patient was sent directly for imaging, which revealed a left-sided acoustic neuroma (Figures 6–2C and 6–2D).

Impression

Left-sided acoustic neuroma.

Audiologic and Medical Recommendations and Management

The patient was presented with management options, which included observation, traditional surgery, or Gamma Knife radiosurgery, and possible audiologic follow-up, if and when warranted.

Additional Information

The patient chose to undergo traditional surgical removal of the acoustic neuroma. The surgery was successful with respect to the surgery and the patient did well postoperatively. However, no hearing could be preserved in the left ear as is reflected in Figure 6–2B.

DISORDER: Acoustic Neuroma Pre-Op

PURE-TONE AUDIOMETRY

SPEECH AUDIOMETRY

Ear	PTA	SRT	Word Rec (%)
Right	25 dB HL	15 dB HL	92%
Left	43 dB HL	45 dB HL	24%
Soundfield			

TYMPANOMETRY

RIGHT
Compliance 1.0 ml
Volume 1.3 ml
MEP 0 daPa

LEFT
Compliance 1.0 ml
Volume 1.4 ml
MEP 0 daPa

ACOUSTIC REFLEX

		500 Hz	1000 Hz	2000 Hz
RIGHT	I			
	C			
LEFT	I			
	C			

A

Figure 6–2. Preoperative (A) and postoperative (B) audiograms for a 41-year-old patient who had an acoustic neuroma removed (Case 6–2). Also shown are T1-weighted gadolinium-contrasted coronal (C) and axial (D) MRI images documenting the presence and location of the acoustic neuroma. continues

DISORDER: Acoustic Neuroma Post-Op

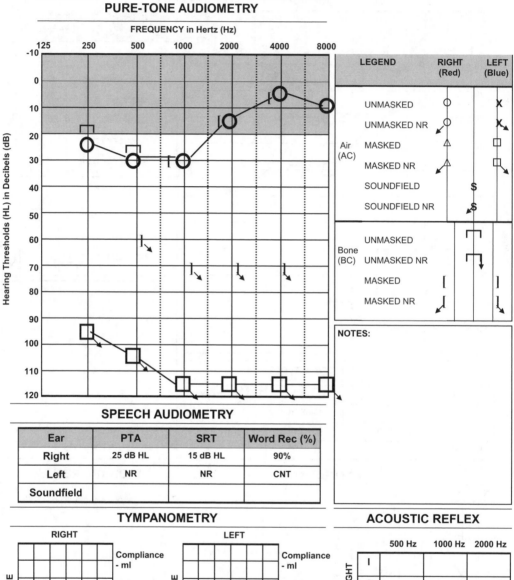

PURE-TONE AUDIOMETRY

SPEECH AUDIOMETRY

Ear	PTA	SRT	Word Rec (%)
Right	25 dB HL	15 dB HL	90%
Left	NR	NR	CNT
Soundfield			

TYMPANOMETRY

ACOUSTIC REFLEX

B

Figure 6–2. continues

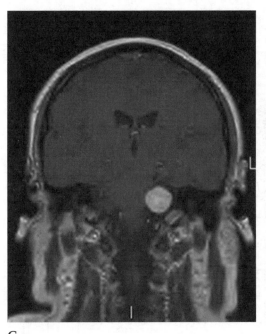

C

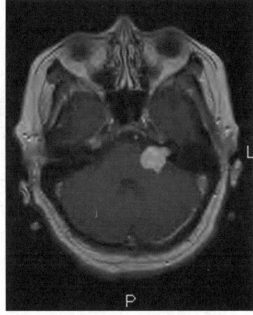

D

Figure 6–2. continued

Case 6–3: Acoustic Neuroma

History

This case is one of a 52-year-old woman who had a history of tinnitus and progressive hearing loss on the left side for several years. She also suffered for some time with imbalance. No other significant audiologic or otologic history was reported.

Audiology

An otoscopic check was unremarkable bilaterally. Pure-tone thresholds showed a mild to moderate sensorineural loss with no measurable speech recognition at suprathreshold levels on the left side. A speech recognition threshold was obtained in this ear, but only at a high intensity level, which was inconsistent with the pure-tone findings (Figure 6–3A). The right ear pure-tone and speech audiometry test results were normal. Radiology revealed a large acoustic neuroma in the left cerebellopontine angle (Figure 6–3B). The right ear ABR was normal except for poor morphology of the IV–V complex (Figure 6–3C). In the left ear no response was observed after wave I. Note: inserts were used in this case; hence, there will be a delay of 0.9 msec in the latencies on these waveforms. Distortion product otoacoustic emissions were essentially normal bilaterally (Figure 6–3D).

Medical Examination Result

The otolaryngologic exam revealed balance difficulties and tinnitus. Tympanic membranes were normal. Facial nerve function was questionable. Radiologic follow-up was recommended.

DISORDER: Acoustic Neuroma

PURE-TONE AUDIOMETRY

FREQUENCY in Hertz (Hz)

Hearing Thresholds (HL) in Decibels (dB)

LEGEND		RIGHT (Red)	LEFT (Blue)
Air (AC)	UNMASKED	◯	X
	UNMASKED NR	◯	X
	MASKED	△	☐
	MASKED NR	△	☐
	SOUNDFIELD		S
	SOUNDFIELD NR		S
Bone (BC)	UNMASKED		
	UNMASKED NR		
	MASKED	[	]
	MASKED NR		

NOTES:

SPEECH AUDIOMETRY

Ear	PTA	SRT	Word Rec (%)
Right	12 dB HL	10 dB HL	100%
Left	40 dB HL	75 dB HL	0%
Soundfield			

TYMPANOMETRY

RIGHT

COMPLIANCE

Compliance - ml
Volume - ml
MEP - daPa

-400   -200   0   +200

LEFT

COMPLIANCE

Compliance - ml
Volume - ml
MEP - daPa

-400   -200   0   +200

ACOUSTIC REFLEX

		500 Hz	1000 Hz	2000 Hz
RIGHT	I			
	C			
LEFT	I			
	C			

A

Figure 6–3. Pure-tone audiogram and speech recognition scores (**A**), MRI (**B**), ABR tracings (**C**), and DPOAEs (**D**) for a 52-year-old female with a left-sided acoustic neuroma (Case 6–3). continues

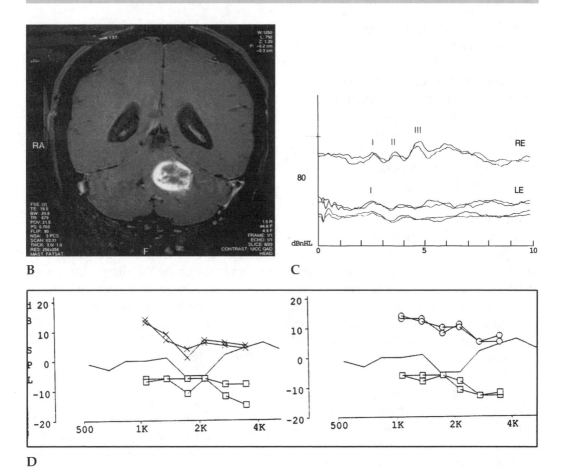

B   **C**

D

Figure 6–3. continued

Impression

Left-sided acoustic neuroma.

Audiologic and Medical Recommendations and Management

The patient was presented with management options, which included traditional surgery or Gamma Knife radiosurgery, and possible audiologic follow-up, if and when warranted.

AUDITORY NEUROPATHY/ DYS-SYNCHRONY (AUDITORY NEUROPATHY SPECTRUM DISORDER)

Introduction

Auditory neuropathy/auditory dys-synchrony (AN/AD), also referred to in recent publications as auditory neuropathy spectrum disorder, is perhaps one of the most difficult disorders to discuss as there is considerable controversy that surrounds this particular auditory nerve disorder. Therefore, it is a challenge to present a fair and balanced picture of this disorder. There is no question that the present authors have a perspective on this disorder and this perspective is likely biased toward certain notions about AN/AD. One of the difficulties with AN/AD is the way that it is defined. The neurological definition of neuropathy is impaired function of the peripheral nerves and the only peripheral nerve in the auditory system is the auditory nerve. Therefore, in a strict sense AN/AD means dysfunction of the auditory nerve. If that is the case, then all of the disorders mentioned earlier, including acoustic neuromas, could be interpreted as AN/AD. It is difficult to determine if those investigating AN/AD would agree or disagree with this interpretation. This, therefore, presents a problem in terms of classification and discussion of auditory nerve disorders. Should all these disorders be bundled and discussed under AN/AD or should they be treated separately? From a common usage or popular interpretation only discussing AN/AD might be best, but from a pathophysiology standpoint perhaps each disorder or type of disorder should be individually presented. This is a dilemma in regard to presentation for which it is difficult to determine the best answer. The present authors doubt if most people would say that the acoustic neuroma or vascular loop is an auditory neuropathy, yet both could meet the audiologic criteria mentioned earlier. The same could be said for the rare case of multiple sclerosis that attacks the myelinated portion of the auditory nerve (for discussion of additional sites of lesions for multiple sclerosis, please refer to Chapter 7: Disorders Affecting the Central Auditory

Nervous System). Another disorder that presents a challenge is hyperbilirubinemia, or in its severe pathologic state, kernicterus, which is often considered an AN/AD (see Dublin, 1986, and Rapin & Gravel, 2003). Although this disorder can affect the auditory nerve, the primary site of lesion (in the auditory system) is the cochlear nuclei located in the lower brainstem (Dublin, 1986; Møller, 2000). This is why this disorder is discussed in the central auditory chapter and not in this chapter. These questions re: the definition and classification of this disorder obviously influence much of the discussion about AN/AD, such as its incidence and prevalence, etiology, site of lesion, and so forth.

Symptoms

Hearing loss is the main symptom of AN/AD. However, depending on the etiology, the hearing loss may take on various characteristics and degrees of involvement. Some individuals will offer complaints of severe distortion of speech and extreme difficulty hearing in noise, and yet will demonstrate fairly good hearing sensitivity. Others will have complete or near complete loss of hearing sensitivity. Again, depending on the etiology, there may be other associated symptoms, such as vestibular problems, tinnitus, and other sensory or motor difficulties. Auditory neuropathy/auditory dys-synchrony is frequently diagnosed in newborns. Therefore, there is often limited information regarding the associated symptoms as these patients are not able to describe their experiences.

Incidence and Prevalence

As alluded to earlier, the incidence or prevalence of AN/AD is difficult to determine because it depends on the breadth of the inclusion criteria. For example, if one includes hyperbilirubinemia, then the incidence/prevalence would be higher. Cone-Wesson and Rance (2000) in a review article, related the incidence of AN/AD to be slightly over 2% for infants with risk factors for hearing loss. However, this figure includes those infants with hyperbilirubinemia. Others would argue that true AN/AD is much rarer than 2% (Rapin & Gravel, 2003).

Etiology and Pathology

As mentioned earlier, if one entertains the neurological definition of neuropathy, then the etiology of AN/AD could essentially be any disorder that damages the auditory nerve. It has been proposed that specific dysfunction of the auditory nerve is the likely basis for AN/AD. This dysfunction can include: (1) injury to the synaptic junctions between inner hair cells and the dendrites of the spiral ganglion, (2) damage to spiral ganglion dendrites directly, (3) direct injury to spiral ganglion neurons, and/or (4) axonal damage to the auditory nerve (which in turn cascades damage to more rostral (brainstem) nuclei (Shaia, Bojrab, & May, 2009). These types of auditory nerve damage are often related to various disorders or conditions, such as anoxia, hypoxia, low birth weight, prematurity, family history of AN/AD, viral disease, seizure, high fever, Friedrich's ataxia, Stevens-Johnson syndrome, Ehlers-Danlos syndrome, and Charcot-Marie-Tooth syndrome (Shaia et al., 2009). Hyperbilirubinemia is commonly included in this group, but the present authors would maintain that this disorder is primarily one of the central nervous system, and if involved at all, the auditory nerve is involved only secondarily.

Site of Lesion

By definition, AN/AD implicates the auditory nerve as its site of lesion. However, it has been shown that damage to the inner hair cells, but not the outer hair cells, can yield audiologic results consistent with those noted in AN/AD (Salvi, Wang, Ding, Stecker, & Arnold, 1999).

It also is well known that some researchers and clinicians advocate for diagnosing dysfunction of the auditory neurons in the lower brainstem as AN/AD (see Rapin & Gravel, 2003). The problem simply stated is: Why wouldn't these disorders be classified as a central as opposed to a peripheral auditory disorder? It is the opinion of the authors that disorders affecting the auditory neurons of the brainstem should be classified among the central auditory disorders.

There are several possible sites of lesion in the auditory nerve as reported by Rapin and Gravel (2003). These include the following:

➤ myelin sheath
➤ axon
➤ axon and myelin sheath
➤ neuronal cell body

Audiology

Auditory neuropathy/auditory dyssynchrony is most often defined by a constellation of audiologic test findings, including variable degrees of hearing loss (most often reduced), poor speech recognition ability in relation to the degree of hearing loss, and normal otoacoustic emissions (at least in the vast majority of cases), as well as totally absent ABRs (although in some cases, the later waves may be present, but abnormalities of the earlier waves are evident). This disorder is not currently defined by anatomical or pathologic indicators. Certainly, vascular problems, infections, neural degeneration, and trauma can damage the auditory nerve and will likely yield abnormal ABRs, implicating auditory nerve involvement. However, within the present classification system, these disorders may not provide the audiologic findings that would classify them as AN/AD disorders. The main point here, however, is that a variety of disorders may cause auditory nerve dysfunction that can, and should, be detected by utilizing ABR and not by imaging. This is a critical point too often ignored in today's diagnostic world (see Musiek et al., 2007).

Pure-tone thresholds can be highly variable in AN/AD, ranging from normal to a profound loss of hearing sensitivity. When hearing loss is greater than 30 to 40 dB HL and OAEs are normal, the interpretation is that of retrocochlear involvement, such as in AN/AD. A recent study reported that about 3% of AN/AD cases had normal pure-tone hearing and 15% had profound hearing loss (Berlin et al., 2010). These results demonstrate the wide range of hearing losses that can be found in patients with AN/AD.

Speech recognition performance, like pure-tone thresholds, has been reported as highly variable; however, the majority of patients for whom speech testing can be completed generally show reduced scores and/or scores that are poorer than expected based on the audiogram (Hood, 2007).

Acoustic reflexes are often absent in AN/AD cases (nearly 90% of the time), but there are also exceptions to this. Otoacoustic emissions are generally present in AN/AD (approximately 75% of the time), but there also have been reports showing them to be absent and/or changing over time (Berlin et al., 2010).

As mentioned earlier, AN/AD is currently defined by patient performance on a constellation of audiologic tests. Perhaps the most important of these tests is

the ABR. The strictest interpretation for ABR in AN/AD is no response, but with a recordable cochlear microphonic (CM), and most reports on AN/AD show totally absent ABRs (Hood, 2007). It is our view, that when ABR waves are present, but delayed or of poor morphology, the diagnosis of AN/AD may not be as definitive as if there was no response. Often, imaging procedures will not show anything abnormal in cases of AN/AD; hence, there is an emphasis on the ABR results in these cases. At times there can be confusion between the CM and a wave I of the ABR. Changing polarity will "flip or reverse" the CM, but not wave I. Also, the CM does not change in latency as one decreases stimulus intensity, but wave I does (see Hood, 2007). Therefore, if there is any question whether one is observing the CM or wave I, one or both of these strategies should be employed.

Recent reviews have promoted the use of transtympanic electrocochleography for helping to determine if the AN/AD is related to presynaptic versus true neural (auditory nerve) dysfunction. This technique is not used routinely in many clinics, but it use may prove useful in better determining the underlying mechanisms for AN/AD (Berlin et al., 2010).

There appears to be a high incidence of bilateral involvement in cases of AN/AD. A recent study revealed that 92% of 260 cases of AN/AD had both ears involved. Interestingly, in the small number of cases that were unilaterally involved, there were twice as many left ears involved (Berlin et al., 2010).

Medical Examination

Because AN/AD can have many causes, otologic consultation/examination is recommended. A careful review of the patient's medical records and a medical examination can help determine the cause and whether there is any medical treatment for the particular etiology of AN/AD that has been identified. Genetic testing, as well as various blood tests, may be performed to help determine the basis of the problem. In many cases, however, the actual cause of the problem will remain undetermined.

Medical and Audiologic Management

If there is an ongoing underlying medical problem that is linked to AN/AD, then otologic management is key. Once this is attended to, or if there is no known medical factor, then management will typically involve a hearing aid fitting or a cochlear implant. One of the main considerations in the management of AN/AD is the realization that some patients with this disorder will present with an overall auditory performance that is often much poorer than would be predicted by their pure-tone thresholds. In some patients with AN/AD, speech recognition ability can be very poor even when hearing sensitivity is good (Berlin et al., 2010; Rance & Barker, 2008). In these cases, the benefits received from traditional amplification may be limited.

A number of children with AN/AD have been managed with cochlear implants. Although the overall results have certainly been worthwhile, there is great variability in outcomes. This is related to the highly heterogeneous nature of the AN/AD population. Some of the reasons for the variability in patient outcomes include various sites of lesion for the disorder; the duration, degree, and type of hearing loss (especially the hearing status of the nonimplanted ear); the duration of implant use; and the age and linguistic and cognitive abilities of the patient.

A key factor in predicting cochlear implant success is the result of various preimplant electrical stimulation procedures, such as electrical ABRs and/or electrical promontory stimulation. Clearly, those individuals that demonstrate robust responses to electrical stimulation do better than those who yield meager or no responses. A recent study shows better speech understanding for those with robust electrically evoked action potentials (EEAPs) compared to those with absent or poor EEAPs (Teagle et al., 2010).

Most children with AN/AD demonstrate improved speech recognition after implantation, but not all do so. The heterogeneous factors mentioned earlier make it difficult to grasp general and consistent trends for hearing improvement. Generally, the longer the patient wears the implant, the better the speech recognition; however, again this is not always a consistent finding with many notable exceptions (Teagle et al., 2010).

Those who do poorly after implantation are of the most interest in terms of predictive and habilitative techniques. Research aimed at determining the reasons why some individuals do not experience positive outcomes following implantation can help professionals establish better candidacy criteria. The findings from these types of research efforts will advance the success rate of cochlear implantation as a rehabilitative intervention for individuals diagnosed with AN/AD.

Auditory training and counseling can prove most helpful in the habilitation of the patient with AN/AD who has been implanted (Chute & Nevins, 2000). Key factors are the age and the linguistic level of the child or adult. Auditory training approaches need to start at levels that are consistent with the age and language status of the individual and then progress to more advanced levels. Training should start at the level of detection. This can include presenting a wide variety of sounds in varying contexts. This then can be followed by auditory discrimination tasks with the focus on same versus different decisions. Both various environmental sounds and speech segments can be utilized. Next, the identification of sounds/speech can be targeted, again using a wide variety of stimuli in varying contexts. The comprehension of language is the final step and requires appropriate thinking about the speech stimulus and responding verbally. There are a number of auditory training techniques presently used in intervention for children with central auditory processing disorders that would be excellent procedures for use with children with cochlear implants (see Musiek, Shinn, & Hare, 2002).

Hearing aids can be of help for at least a subset of the children and adults who present with AN/AD. Because of the wide range of abilities of those with AN/AD, individual monitoring and frequent follow-up is critical. Berlin et al. (2010) reported that 61% of the patients diagnosed with AN/AD in their study received no benefit from hearing aids. Therefore, monitoring for the achievement of the appropriate language milestones with hearing aid use is essential when working with young children. If the child's performance lags or does not reach expected milestones, then a cochlear implant becomes a consideration. Hearing aids can be fitted on a trial basis when the audiologist is attempting to decide on a hearing aid(s) versus a cochlear implant (Teagle et al., 2010). When hearing aids are fitted, they should provide access to and understanding of speech. If this is not accomplished, then consideration for cochlear implants becomes more viable. Because in AN/AD the audiogram may be misleading, one must be careful in fitting

"power hearing aids" as they may damage peripheral hearing. This is where the applications of OAEs and ABRs become valuable as the finding of normal or near normal test results should serve as a contraindication for the fitting of "power hearing aids."

Case 6–4: Auditory Neuropathy/Dys-synchrony

History

A 31-year-old female presented with problems of bilateral facial nerve palsy, severe balance disturbance, and auditory symptoms of severe distortion of speech and some loss of hearing sensitivity, all with simultaneous onset approximately 10 years prior to her current audiologic evaluation. The patient reported recovery of the facial nerve palsy, but not the auditory symptoms, which reportedly became progressively more severe following the onset of symptoms.

Audiology

An otoscopic check was unremarkable bilaterally. Results of a comprehensive audiologic evaluation indicated a moderate to mild low-frequency sensorineural hearing loss with normal tympanometric findings bilaterally (Figure 6–4A). Speech recognition thresholds were in agreement with the pure-tone averages for the two ears, whereas speech recognition scores at suprathreshold levels were fair in the right ear and very poor in the left ear. In addition, both ipsilateral and contralateral acoustic reflexes were absent in both ears at all frequencies tested (500, 1000, and 2000 Hz). Severe deficits were also observed on the Dichotic Digits Test (8% left, 78% right) and the Dichotic Rhyme Test (13% left, 20% right), and

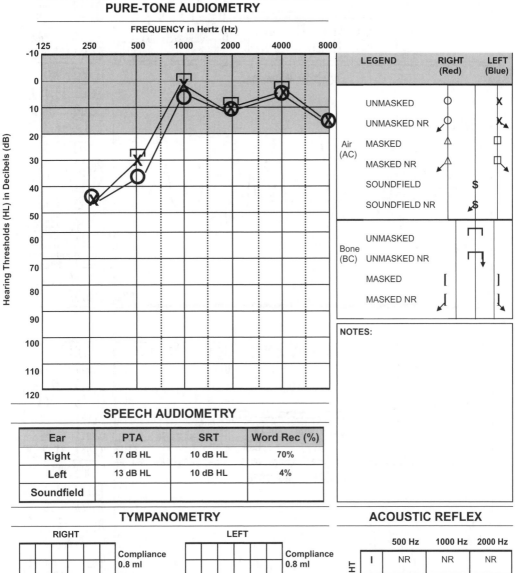

DISORDER: Auditory Neuropathy/Dys-synchrony

PURE-TONE AUDIOMETRY

SPEECH AUDIOMETRY

Ear	PTA	SRT	Word Rec (%)
Right	17 dB HL	10 dB HL	70%
Left	13 dB HL	10 dB HL	4%
Soundfield			

TYMPANOMETRY

RIGHT
Compliance 0.8 ml
Volume 1.1 ml
MEP 0 daPa

LEFT
Compliance 0.8 ml
Volume 1.1 ml
MEP 0 daPa

ACOUSTIC REFLEX

		500 Hz	1000 Hz	2000 Hz
RIGHT	I	NR	NR	NR
	C	NR	NR	NR
LEFT	I	NR	NR	NR
	C	NR	NR	NR

A

Figure 6–4. Pure-tone audiogram and speech recognition scores (**A**), TEOAEs (**B**), and ABR tracings (**C**) for a 31-year-old female with auditory neuropathy/auditory dys-synchrony (Case 6–4). continues

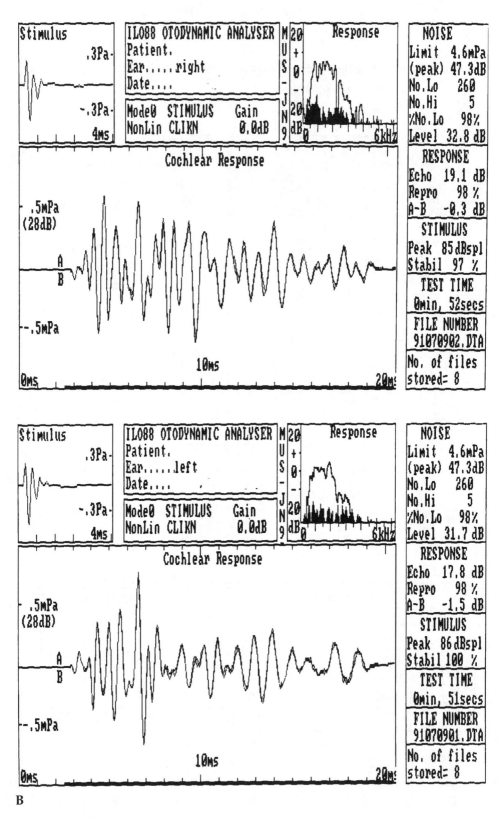

Figure 6–4. continues

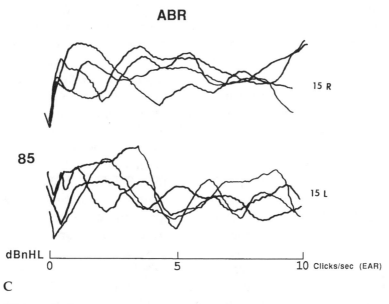

ABR

85

15 R

15 L

dBnHL

0   5   10   Clicks/sec (EAR)

C

Figure 6–4. continued

the patient was not able to complete the Frequency Pattern Test in either the verbal or hummed conditions for either ear. Middle latency response testing was completed and responses were essentially absent bilaterally for three electrode sites (C_z, C_3, C_4). Both TEOAEs and ABRs also were administered. The TEOAE results were normal for both ears (Figure 6–4B) and the ABRs were totally absent bilaterally (Figure 6–4C).

Medical Examination Result

An otolaryngologic examination was unremarkable, as were the results of CT, MRI, and EEG testing.

Impression

Auditory neuropathy/auditory dyssynchrony secondary to a likely viral insult of the seventh and eighth cranial nerves based on exclusion.

Audiologic Recommendations and Management

An assistive listening device was suggested along with a wide variety of listening strategies and auditory training.

Medical Recommendations and Management

None.

VASCULAR LOOP SYNDROME

Introduction

Vascular loops or vascular loop syndrome can affect the auditory nerve. The vascular loop syndrome was popularized by the work of Peter Jannetta, a neurosurgeon, in the mid to late 1960s (Jannetta, 1967). In this vascular condition, the auditory and adjacent cranial nerves may be compressed by a vessel in the CPA and this compression is believed to result in auditory, vestibular, and/or facial symptoms. The audiologic findings in patients with vascular loops can be variable and will depend on the degree of involvement. After surgical decompression, audiologic results often improve (Møller, 2000). However, more research with audiologic testing needs to be done to gain better insight into the audiologic profile associated with this particular disorder. It has been argued that this disorder can mimic symptoms of Ménière's disease and other auditory disorders. This makes the diagnosis difficult and renders this disorder controversial (see Hain, 1999).

Symptoms

Vascular loops can result in auditory symptoms of loss of hearing sensitivity, speech perceptual distortions, tinnitus, and hyperacusis. In addition, hemifacial spasm, and in some cases, facial pain on the side of lesion can be experienced. These latter two symptoms are usually related to the involvement of the trigeminal nerve. Patients with vascular loop compression can also present with vestibular symptoms that can be severe in degree in some patients. Compression effects secondary to vascular loops can result in many or all of the symptoms just mentioned or they may result in any one of them; however, facial spasm and/or pain are the symptoms that are considered most indicative of the disorder (Bergsneider & Becker, 1995; Møller, 2000).

Incidence and Prevalence

It is important to understand that not all vascular loops that come into contact with the auditory nerve in the CPA will result in auditory symptoms. That is, some vascular loops that are apparently in a position to affect the auditory nerve do not. Therefore, it is difficult to determine the incidence of auditory compromise associated with vascular loops. Makins, Nikolopoulos, Ludman, and O'Donoghue (1998) reported that, "In the general population, evidence of contact between vascular loops and CN VIII has been shown in 7% by computer tomographic cisternography, 12% by post-mortem dissections and 14% by MRI—this suggests that contact is normal." (p. 1740). Although these data provide information as to the incidence of "contact" between vascular loops and the auditory nerve, they do not address the percentage of patients with auditory symptoms. It is also difficult to determine the incidence of vascular loops that result in any of the symptoms mentioned above; however, it has been estimated that trigeminal neuralgia and hemifacial spasm associated with vascular loops occur at rates of 0.5 and 0.8 per 100,000 (see Møller, 2000). Lingawi (2003), who examined at the incidence of vascular loop contact with the auditory/vestibular, facial, and trigeminal nerves, noted that: "Forty-two of 540 nerves (8%) showed evidence of impingement, 108 of 540 nerves (20%) showed evidence of abutment, and 390 of 540 nerves (72%) were normal. Among the 42 impinged nerves, 38 (90.5%) were facial/vestibulocochlear complex; 4 (9.5%) were trigeminal, and 1 (2.0%) had all 3 nerves impinged. No bilateral impingements were detected. Of the 108 volunteers with vascular abutment of the nerves, 101 nerves (93.5%) were facial/

vestibulocochlear complex; 7 (6.5%) were trigeminal, and 3 (2.7%) had abutment of all 3 vessels." (p. 21).

Etiology and Pathology

It appears that in most cases the vascular loop originates from the anterior inferior cerebellar artery (AICA). It is the compression on the eighth nerve and adjacent nerves, as well as the irritation of these nerves that may eventually result in demyelination of the nerve fibers and the auditory, vestibular, and facial symptoms (Makins et al., 1998). As mentioned earlier, many people with vessel contact with cranial nerves in the CPA do not have symptoms of any sort. For example, Hardy and Rhoton (1978) found vessel contact with the trigeminal nerve in 60% of 50 cadavers examined, none of which had trigeminal complaints before their deaths. This suggests that there must be a constellation of factors present for symptoms to be manifested, and currently it is not known what factors are necessary to yield symptoms (Møller, 2000).

Site of Lesion

In vascular loop compression the site of involvement is the CPA—more specifically the porus acousticus or opening of the internal auditory canal. At this site, the vascular loop can affect the nerves exiting the internal auditory canal, which include the vestibular, auditory, and facial nerves. The trigeminal nerve can also be affected by vascular loops; however, this nerve is generally more rostral than the seventh (facial) and eighth (auditory and vestibular) nerves. Hence, the likelihood of a slightly different locus for trigeminal

neuralgia associated with vascular loop compression exists (Møller, 2000). McDermott and colleagues reported results on vascular loops that were classified based upon their sites of lesion (McDermott, Dutt, Irving, Pahor, & Chavda, 2003). Using an anatomic classification to type the loops, these authors reported that there were 412 type I loops within the CPA, 202 type II loops at the porus acousticus that extended up to 50% of IAC, and 50 type III loops that extended to greater than 50% of IAC.

Audiology

There has been some evidence pointing to a mid-frequency pure-tone hearing loss in patients with vascular loop compression. However, many individuals with this syndrome will demonstrate normal pure-tone thresholds. So, the hearing thresholds of patients with vascular loops can be variable. Given the potential effect of a vascular loop on the auditory nerve the ABR is a valuable procedure in helping to establish a diagnosis of vascular compression. The ABR is often abnormal in patients with vascular loops that impinge on the auditory nerve. When abnormalities are noted, the abnormalities typically involve an extension of the interwave intervals between waves I and II and/or waves I and III for the involved side. These findings implicate auditory nerve involvement, a situation that is likely to resolve following surgical intervention. After surgery, it is common for both the auditory symptoms and the ABR to improve (Møller, 2000).

Møller (2000) also advocates performing acoustic reflex testing in patients who may have this disorder. Interestingly, Shinn, Bush, and Jones (2009) reported a case of vascular loop that yielded decreased performance on a central auditory test battery, which helped in the localization of the abnormality. The audiologic testing of these patients garners some emphasis because radiology (MRI) does not always prove helpful in documenting vascular compression in the CPA. If vestibular complaints are reported, VNG examination should also be performed.

Medical Examination

As alluded to earlier, vascular loops can present with symptoms similar to acoustic neuromas or Ménière's disease as well as other neurologic or otologic problems. Hence, otologic/neurologic consults are essential. An extensive case history and an otologic and neurologic exam should be done. Ruling in or out a retrocochlear disorder is done in the usual manner with appropriate audiologic and radiologic (usually MRI) procedures.

Medical Treatment

Although treatment with anticonvulsant drugs, such as carbamazepine and baclofen can prove helpful (Hain, 1999), surgery has been the most documented treatment based on the original approach by Jannetta (1967). However, the surgery is risky as there is the need to expose the brainstem, which is usually done by a retrosigmoid craniotomy, and should only be considered in extreme cases. The surgery results in moving the vessel away from the nerve or in some way buffering the nerve from the vessel (usually by inserting small pieces of Teflon) to prevent the

vessel from migrating back to its original position (Jannetta, 1967). This is a "decompression" of the nerve and the result is diminished symptoms. For example, Bergsneider and Becker (1995) reported that 22 out of 41 patients with severe vertigo had excellent improvement of symptoms after surgical decompression of the eighth cranial nerve and Brackmann, Kesser, and Day (2001) reported marked improvement for 16 out of 20 patients with disabling vertigo and tinnitus following surgical intervention. Part of the hesitancy in recommending surgery for vascular loops is believed to be related to the uncertainty surrounding the diagnosis of this disorder that was discussed earlier. Perhaps the strongest support for this syndrome is the relatively impressive results from surgery. As mentioned earlier, other disorders can result in the symptoms similar to vascular loop syndrome and more research is needed to differentiate these other disorders from vascular loop problems.

Case 6–5: Vascular Loop Syndrome

History

A 49-year-old female was seen for a central auditory processing evaluation due to persistent concerns regarding hearing in her right ear in spite of normal peripheral hearing sensitivity as measured by routine audiologic tests. This patient reported that this has been a long-standing concern. Additional audiologic history included constant bilateral tinnitus, occasional vertigo, and imbalance. She also reported the need for constant repetition of auditory information, difficulty hearing in background noise, and poor localization abilities. Other medical history included migraines with associated facial weakness and a poor sense of smell.

Audiology

An otoscopic check was unremarkable bilaterally and results of a comprehensive audiologic evaluation indicated essentially normal peripheral hearing sensitivity bilaterally (Figure 6–5A). Of note, however, was an asymmetry on the order of 10 dB HL across the frequency range. Word recognition in quiet was excellent bilaterally.

Five tests of central auditory function were performed on the patient (Figure 6–5B). They included the Dichotic Rhyme Test, the Dichotic Digits Test, the Competing Sentences Test, the Duration Patterns Test, and the Low-Pass Filtered Speech Test. Results from the auditory processing evaluation demonstrated a right ear deficit on the Dichotic Digits Test, the Competing Sentences Test, and the Low-Pass Filtered Speech Test. In addition, an unexplained left ear deficit was also obtained for the Competing Sentences Test.

An ABR test was also performed in ipsilateral and contralateral recording conditions with insert receivers (Figure 6–5C). Results for the left ear were within normal limits with respect to absolute and interwave latencies. The right ear response was abnormal with the absence of a wave I cautiously interpreted. Waves II through V were present at normal latencies and a normal III–V interwave interval was noted for the right ear.

Medical Examination Result

The patient presented with an essentially normal otolaryngologic examination. Imaging revealed a very prominent anterior inferior paracerebellar artery on the right side (Figure 6–5D).

Impression

Vascular loop syndrome.

Audiologic Recommendations and Management

It was recommended that the patient undergo aural rehabilitation to include intense training exercises to build skills in binaural integration and the processing of degraded speech. This was particularly important for this patient as she is employed as an operating room nurse. In addition, a mild gain hearing aid was recommended in order to assist with the auditory processing deficit. Although the patient considered both recommendations, she opted not to proceed with any intervention at the time of her evaluation. However, she continues to be monitored annually.

Medical Recommendations and Management

The option of microvascular decompression of the vascular loop away from the facial nerve and vestibulocochlear nerve complex along with the risks and benefits of surgery were discussed with the patient. The patient continues to be seen for otologic evaluations annually as she elected to forego surgery.

DISORDER: Vascular Loop

PURE-TONE AUDIOMETRY

FREQUENCY in Hertz (Hz)

Hearing Thresholds (HL) in Decibels (dB)

LEGEND		RIGHT (Red)	LEFT (Blue)
Air (AC)	UNMASKED	○	X
	UNMASKED NR	○	X
	MASKED	△	□
	MASKED NR	△	□
	SOUNDFIELD		S
	SOUNDFIELD NR		S
Bone (BC)	UNMASKED		Γ
	UNMASKED NR		Γ
	MASKED	[	]
	MASKED NR	[	]

NOTES:

SPEECH AUDIOMETRY

Ear	PTA	SRT	Word Rec (%)
Right	15 dB HL	0 dB HL	100%
Left	3 dB HL	5 dB HL	100%
Soundfield			

TYMPANOMETRY

RIGHT

Compliance - ml
Volume - ml
MEP - daPa

-400   -200   0   +200

LEFT

Compliance - ml
Volume - ml
MEP - daPa

-400   -200   0   +200

ACOUSTIC REFLEX

		500 Hz	1000 Hz	2000 Hz
RIGHT	I			
	C			
LEFT	I			
	C			

A

Figure 6–5. Pure-tone audiogram and speech recognition scores (**A**), central auditory behavioral test results (**B**), the ABR with ipsilateral recordings in the upper tracings and contralateral recordings in the lower tracings for each ear (**C**), and the MRI (**D**) for a 49-year-old female with a right-sided vascular loop syndrome (Case 6–5). Reproduced with permission from J. B. Shinn, M. L. Bush, & R. O. Jones. Correlation of central auditory processing deficits and vascular loop syndrome. Ear, Nose, & Throat Journal, 88(10), E34-E37. Copyright 2009 Ear, Nose, and Throat Journal. continues

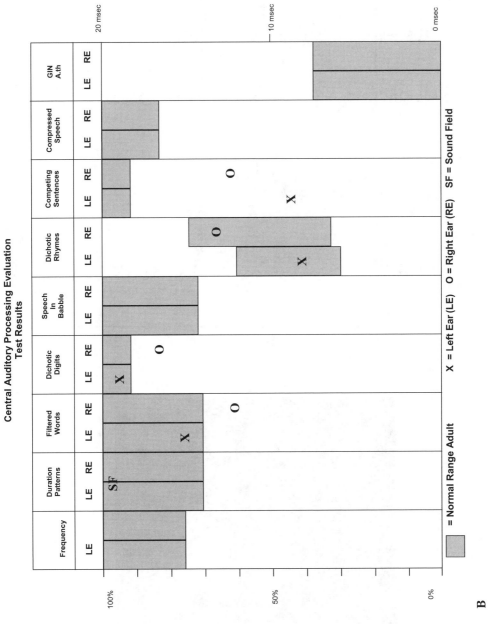

Figure 6–5. continues

273

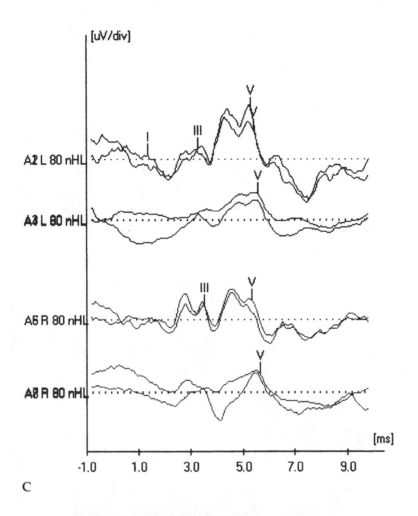

C

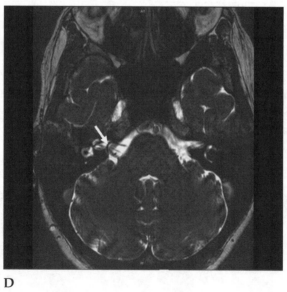

D

Figure 6–5. continued

SUMMARY

Acoustic neuromas (vestibular schwannomas), auditory neuropathy/auditory dys-synchrony, and vascular loops (compression) are all disorders that can compromise auditory nerve function. Acoustic neuromas require early detection so they can be managed optimally. Early detection is dependent on interaction between audiologists and otologists. Audiologists also can be involved in monitoring and managing these patients after surgery. The main treatments, however, are surgery, radiation, and monitored observation. Auditory neuropathy/auditory dys-synchrony remains, at least from some perspectives, somewhat controversial. It affects newborns as well some older children and adults. It is defined by behavioral, electroacoustic, and electrophysiologic audiologic test results. Cochlear implants have provided significant help to many of the patients with this disorder. Vascular loops or vascular compression syndrome results from pressure on the eighth and/or adjacent cranial nerves resulting from a misplaced blood vessel in the CPA. Hearing loss, hemifacial spasm, tinnitus, vestibular problems, and even facial pain can be symptoms. Although commonly diagnosed and treated, the nature and characterization of this disorder remain controversial.

Acknowledgment. The authors gratefully acknowledge Eric Smouha, MD, Associate Professor, Department of Otolaryngology, Director of Otology-Neurotology, Mount Sinai School of Medicine for his contributions to this chapter.

REFERENCES

Akin, F. W., & Murnane, O. D. (2008). Vestibular evoked myogenic potentials. In G. P. Jacobson & N. T. Shepard (Eds.), *Balance function: Assessment and management* (pp. 405–434). San Diego, CA: Plural Publishing.

Angeli, S. I., & Jackson, C.A. (1997). Neurotological evaluation. In W. F. House, C. M. Luetje, & K. J. Doyle (Eds.), *Acoustic tumors: Diagnosis and management* (2nd ed., pp. 85–93). San Diego, CA: Singular Publishing.

Arthurs, B. J., Fairbanks, R. K., Demakas, J. J., Lamoreaux, W. T., Giddings, N. A., Mackay, A. R., . . . Lee, C. M. (2011). A review of treatment modalities for vestibular schwannoma. *Neurosurgical Review, 34*(3), 265–279.

Arts, H. A., Telian, S. A., El-Kashlan, H., & Thompson, B. G. (2006). Hearing preservation and facial nerve outcomes in vestibular schwannoma surgery: Results using the middle cranial fossa approach. *Otology and Neurotology, 27*(2), 234–241.

Baser, M. E., Friedman, J. M., Wallace, A. J., Ramsden, R. T., Joe, H., & Evans, D. G. (2002). Evaluation of diagnostic criteria for neurofibromatosis 2. *Neurology, 59*(11), 1759–1765.

Bell, S. L., Allen, R., & Lutman, M. E. (2002). An investigation of the use of band-limited chirp stimuli to obtain the auditory brainstem response. *International Journal of Audiology, 41*(5), 271–278.

Bergsneider, M., & Becker, D. P. (1995). Vascular compression syndrome of the vestibular nerve: A critical analysis. *Otolaryngology-Head and Neck Surgery, 112*(1), 118–124.

Berlin, C. I., Hood, L. J., Morlet, T., Wilensky, D., Li, L., Mattingly, K. R., . . . Frisch, S. A. (2010). Multi-site diagnosis and management of 260 patients with auditory neuropathy/dys-synchrony (auditory spectrum disorder). *International Journal of Audiology, 49*(1), 30–43.

Brackmann, D. E., Kesser, B. W., & Day, J. D. (2001). Microvascular decompression of the vestibulocochlear nerve for disabling positional vertigo: The House Ear Clinic experience. *Otology and Neurotology, 22*(6), 882–887.

Bush, M. L., Jones, R. O., & Shinn, J. B. (2008). Auditory brainstem response threshold differences in patients with vestibular schwannoma: A new diagnostic index. *Ear, Nose, and Throat Journal, 87*(8), 458–462.

Charpiot, A., Tringali, S., Zaouche, S., Ferber-Viart, C., & Dubreuil, C. (2010). Perioperative complications after translabyrinthine removal of large or giant vestibular schwannoma: Outcomes for 123 patients. *Acta Otolaryngologica, 130*(11), 1249–1255.

Chute, P. M., & Nevins, M. E. (2000). Cochlear implants in children. In M. Valente, H. Hosford-Dunn, & R. J. Roeser (Eds.), *Audiology: Treatment* (pp. 511–536), New York, NY: Thieme.

Cone-Wesson, B., & Rance, G. (2000). Auditory neuropathy: A brief review. *Current Opinion in Otolaryngology and Head and Neck Surgery, 8*(5), 421–425.

Dew, L. A., Shelton, C., & Hitselberger, W. E. (1997). Partial versus total removal of acoustic tumors. In W. F. House, C. M. Luetje, & K. J. Doyle (Eds.), *Acoustic tumors: Diagnosis and management* (2nd ed., pp. 205–214). San Diego, CA: Singular Publishing Group.

Don, M., Kwong, B., Tanaka, C., Brackmann, D., & Nelson, R. (2005). The stacked ABR: Sensitive and specific screening tool for detecting small acoustic tumors. *Audiology and Neurotology, 10*(5), 274–290.

Dublin, W. B. (1986). Central auditory pathology. *Otolaryngology-Head Neck Surgery, 95* (3, Pt. 2), 363–424.

Genetic Home Reference. (2011). *Your guide to understanding genetic conditions.* Retrieved 6/15/11 from http://ghr.nlm.nih.gov/.

Glasscock, M. F., Bohrer, P. S., & Steenerson, R. L. (1997). A history of acoustic tumor surgery: 1961–present. In W. F. House, C. M. Luetje, & K. J. Doyle (Eds.), *Acoustic tumors: Diagnosis and management* (2nd ed., pp. 21–26). San Diego, CA: Singular Publishing.

Gruskin, P., Carberry, J. N., & Chandrasekhar, S. S. (1997). Pathology of acoustic tumors. In W. F. House, C. M. Luetje, & K. J. Doyle (Eds.), *Acoustic tumors: Diagnosis and management* (2nd ed., pp. 27–85). San Diego, CA: Singular Publishing.

Hain, T. C. (1999). Microvascular compression syndrome, *Otoneurology Index.* Retrieved 6/15/11 from http://www.tchain.com/otoneurology/disorders/unilat/microvascular.htm/.

Hain, T. C. (2011). Acoustic neuroma. *Dizziness Tumor Index.* Retrieved 6/15/11 from http://www.dizziness-and-balance.com/disorders/tumors/acoustic_neuroma.htm/.

Hardy, D. G., & Rhoton, A. L., Jr. (1978). Microsurgical relationship of the superior cerebellar artery and the trigeminal nerve. *Journal of Neurosurgery, 49*(5), 669–678.

Hitselberger, W. E., & House, W. F. (1966). Acoustic neuroma diagnosis: External ear canal hypethesia as an early sign. *Archives of Otolaryngology, 83*(3), 50–53.

Hood, L. J. (2007). Auditory neuropathy and dys-synchrony. In R. F. Burkard, M. Don, & J. J. Eggermont (Eds.), *Auditory evoked potentials: Basic principles and clinical application* (pp. 275–290). Philadelphia, PA: Lippincott Williams & Wilkins.

House, W. F. (1997). A history of acoustic tumor surgery: 1800–1961. In W. F. House, C. M. Luetje, & K. J. Doyle (Eds.), *Acoustic tumors: Diagnosis and management* (2nd ed., pp. 1–20). San Diego, CA: Singular Publishing.

House, J. W., Bassim, M. K., & Schwartz, M. (2008). False positive magnetic resonance imaging in the diagnosis of vestibular schwannoma. *Otology and Neurotology, 29*(8), 1176–1178.

Jannetta, P. J. (1967). Arterial compression of the trigeminal nerve at the pons in patients with trigeminal neuralgia, *Journal of Neurosurgery, 26*(1 Suppl.), 159–162.

Johnson, E. W. (1977). Auditory test results in 500 cases of acoustic neuroma. *Archives of Otolaryngology, 103*(3), 152–158.

Kaylie, D. M., Gilbert, E., Horgan, M. A., Delashaw, J. B., & McMenomey, S. O. (2001).

Acoustic neuroma surgery outcomes. *Otology & Neurotology, 22*(5), 686–689.

Lingawi, S. (2003). The presence of vascular impingement of the trigeminal, facial and vestibulo-cochlear nerves in healthy volunteers. *Journal of the Hong Kong College of Radiology, 6,* 20–24.

Lustig, L., & Jackler, R. (1997). Benign tumors of the temporal bone. In G. B. Hughes & M. L. Pensak (Eds.), *Clinical otology* (2nd ed., pp. 313–334). New York, NY: Thieme.

Luxford, W. (1997). Surgical decision making in acoustic tumor surgery. In W. F. House, C. M. Luetje, & K. J. Doyle (Eds.), *Acoustic tumors: Diagnosis and management* (2nd ed., pp. 135–142). San Diego, CA: Singular Publishing.

Makins, A. E., Nikolopoulos, T. P., Ludman, C., & O'Donoghue, G. M. (1998). Is there a correlation between vascular loops and unilateral auditory symptoms? *Laryngoscope, 108*(11, Pt. 1), 1739–1742.

Martin, W., & Yong-bin Shi, B. (2007). Intraoperative monitoring. In R. F. Burkard, M. Don, & J. J. Eggermont (Eds.), *Auditory evoked potentials: Basic principles and clinical application* (pp. 355–384). Philadelphia, PA: Lippincott Williams & Wilkins.

McDermott, A. L., Dutt, S. N., Irving, R. M., Pahor, A. L., & Chavda, S. V. (2003). Anterior inferior cerebellar artery syndrome: Fact or fiction. *Clinical Otolaryngology and Allied Sciences, 28*(2), 75–80.

Møller, A. R. (2000). *Hearing: Its physiology and pathophysiology.* New York, NY: Academic Press.

Musiek, F. E., & Baran, J. A. (2007). *The auditory system: Anatomy, physiology, and clinical correlates.* Boston, MA: Allyn & Bacon.

Musiek, F. E., & Kibbe, K. (1986). Auditory brain stem response wave IV–V abnormalities from the ear opposite large cerebellopontine lesions. *American Journal of Otology, 7*(4), 253–257.

Musiek, F. E., Kibbe-Michal, K., Geurkink, N. A., Josey, A. F., & Glasscock, M., 3rd. (1986). ABR results in patients with posterior fossa tumors and normal pure-tone hearing. *Otolaryngology-Head and Neck Surgery, 94*(5), 568–573.

Musiek, F. E., Shinn, J., & Hare, C. (2002). Plasticity, auditory training, and auditory processing disorders. *Seminars in Hearing, 23*(4), 263–275.

Musiek, F. E., Shinn, J. B., & Jirsa, R. E. (2007). The auditory brainstem response in auditory nerve and brainstem dysfunction. In R. F. Burkard, M. Don, & J. J. Eggermont (Eds.), *Auditory evoked potentials: Basic principles and clinical application* (pp. 291–312). Philadelphia, PA: Lippincott Williams & Wilkins.

National Institutes of Health. (1991). *Acoustic Neuroma.* Consensus Statement Online, 9(4), 1–24. Retrieved 6/15/11 from http://consensus.nih.gov/1991/1991Acoustic Neuroma087html.htm/.

Obholzer, R. J., Rea, P. A., & Harcourt, J. P. (2004). Magnetic resonance imaging screening for vestibular schwannoma: Analysis of published protocols. *Journal of Laryngology and Otology, 118*(5), 329 –332.

Pensak, M. L., Glasscock, M. E., 3rd, Josey, A. F., Jackson, C. G., & Gulya, A. J. (1985). Sudden hearing loss and cerebellopontine angle tumors. *Laryngoscope, 95*(10), 1188–1193.

Phillips, D. J., Kobylarz, E. J., De Peralta, E. T., Stieg, P. E., & Selesnick, S. H. (2010). Predictive factors of hearing preservation after surgical resection of small vestibular schwannomas. *Otology and Neurotology, 31*(9), 1463–1468.

Pool, L. J., Palva, A. A., & Greenfield, E. C. (1970). Acoustic nerve tumors: Early diagnosis and treatment (2nd ed.). Springfield, IL: Charles C. Thomas.

Ramos, H. V., Barros, F. A., Yamashita, H., Penido Nde, O., Souza, A. C., & Yamaoka, W.Y. (2005). Magnetic imaging in sudden deafness. *Brazilian Journal of Otorhinolaryngology, 71*(4), 422–426.

Rance, G., & Barker, E. J. (2008). Speech perception in children with auditory neuropathy/dyssynchrony managed with either hearing aids or cochlear implants. *Otology and Neurotology, 29*(2), 179–182.

Rapin, I., & Gravel, J. (2003). "Auditory neuropathy": Physiologic and pathologic evidence calls for more diagnostic specificity.

International Journal of Pediatric Otorhinolar-yngology, 67(7), 707–728.

Robinson, D. A., Zee, D. S., Hain, T. C., Holmes, A., & Rosenberg, L. F. (1984). Alexander's law: Its behavior and origin in the human vestibulo-ocular reflex. *Annals of Neurology, 16*(6), 714–722.

Salvi, R. J., Wang, J., Ding, D., Stecker, N., & Arnold, S. (1999). Auditory deprivation of the central auditory system resulting from selective inner hair cell loss: Animal model of auditory neuropathy. *Scandinavian Audiology, 51*(Suppl.), 1–12.

Scarivilli, F. (2003).The pathology of the vestibular system In L. Luxon, J. M. Furman, A. Martini, & D. Stephens (Eds.) *Audiological medicine* (pp. 641–654). London, UK: Martin Dunitz.

Shaia, W. T., Bojrab, D. I., & May, J. G. (2009). Auditory neuropathy. *Medscape reference: Drugs, diseases and procedures*. Retrieved 6/15/11 from http://emedicine.medscape.com/article/836769-overview/.

Shinn, J. B., Bush, M. L., & Jones, R. O. (2009). Correlation of central auditory processing deficits and vascular loop syndrome. *Ear, Nose, and Throat Journal, 88*(10), E34–E37.

Stangerup, S., Tos, M., Thomsen, J., & Caye-Thomasen, P. (2010). True incidence of vestibular schwannoma? *Neurosurgery, 67,* 1335–1340.

Teagle, H. F., Roush, P. A., Woodard, J. S., Hatch, D. R., Zdanski, C. J., Buss, E., & Buchman, C. A. (2010). Cochlear implanta-tion in children with auditory neuropathy spectrum disorder. *Ear and Hearing, 31*(3), 325–335.

Telischi, F. F., Roth, J., Stagner, B. B., Lons-bury-Martin, B. L., & Balkany, T. J. (1995). Patterns of evoked otoacoustic emissions associated with acoustic neuromas. *Laryngoscope, 105*(7, Pt. 1), 675–682.

Tucci, D. L. (1997). Audiologic testing. In W. F. House, C. M. Luetje, & K. J. Doyle (Eds.), *Acoustic tumors: Diagnosis and management* (2nd ed., pp. 93–105). San Diego, CA: Singular Publishing.

Turner, R. G., Frazer, G. J., & Shepard, N. T. (1984). Formulating and evaluating audiological protocols. *Ear and Hearing, 5*(6), 321–330.

Welling, D. B., Glasscock, M. E., 3rd, Woods, C. I., & Jackson, C. G. (1990). Acoustic neuroma: A cost-effective approach. *Archives of Otolaryngology-Head and Neck Surgery, 103*(3), 583–585.

Wilson, D. F., Hodgson, R. S., Gustafson, M. F., Hogue, S., & Mills, L. (1992). The sensitivity of the auditory brainstem response testing in small acoustic neuromas. *Laryngoscope, 102*(9), 961–964.

Wilson, R. H., & Margolis, R. H. (1999). Acoustic-reflex measurements. In F. E. Musiek & W. F. Rintelmann (Eds.), *Contemporary perspectives in hearing assessment* (pp. 131–166), Boston, MA: Allyn & Bacon.

Zulch, K. (1957). *Brain tumors: Their biology and pathology.* New York, NY: Springer.

7

Disorders Affecting the Central Auditory Nervous System

INTRODUCTION

In considering disorders of the central auditory nervous system (CANS), it must be understood that it is not necessarily the type of disorder but rather the location of the lesion and the specific effects of the disorder on the CANS (i.e., disease mechanisms) that are the crucial issues. Anatomically, the central auditory nervous system begins at the level of caudal pons, specifically at the cochlear nucleus. At a similar level, but located deep in the pons, is the next major group of nuclei, the superior olivary complex, which projects fibers along the lateral lemniscus, a major brainstem pathway that also has a group of nuclei in the upper half of the pons. The next major nucleus is the inferior colliculus, which is located in the midbrain and receives input from practically all the more caudally located nuclei and projects to the underside of the thalamus to the medial geniculate body (MGB). The MGB sends fibers to the cortex, specifically Heschl's gyrus and secondary auditory areas such as the insula. The corpus callosum connects the two hemispheres and has a specific auditory region where impulses are exchanged between the two hemispheres.

Many disorders can result in audiologic deficits if they damage the auditory neural substrate within the CANS. However, the effects of CANS damage often result in audiologic findings that are not unique to a particular disorder, but rather to the site of the CANS lesion. Some of the more significant disorders that can result in central auditory deficits are discussed in this chapter. Many of these disorders are often overlooked by health care professionals as resulting in auditory deficits. In some cases, these disorders may not result in hearing deficits, but in others they certainly can and do. When they do, it is important to determine the nature and degree of the deficit so that optimal medical and/or audiologic treatment can be realized.

Audiology

The audiology sections in this chapter are organized in a slightly different manner than in previous chapters. This was done for efficiency. We discuss the audiologic profiles associated with various types of CANS disorders as has been done in other chapters; however, due to the similarity of the audiologic findings in mass and vascular lesions, rather than dedicating a separate section to the audiologic findings for each lesion site, the discussion is combined. Audiologic findings are provided separately for the following lesion types: degenerative disorders, neurotoxicity, traumatic brain injury, temporal lobe epilepsy, surgical compromise of the CANS, and learning problems.

Anatomic Factors

In the assessment of various disorders of the CANS, it is useful to understand that various tests have anatomic limitations. Some tests are efficient for the assessment of brainstem involvement, whereas others may be better suited for use with cortical or interhemispheric involvement. Also, some disorders may manifest their dysfunction primarily in one of these three anatomic regions, whereas others may affect two or all three regions. This, of course, influences the types of tests selected for administration during evaluation of the patient. For example, a small tumor of the low brainstem would have a focal effect in the pons. On the other hand, heavy metal neurotoxicity could involve the entire auditory system. Therefore, the selection of the tests to be administered to a particular patient will depend on the patient's case history and present-

ing symptomatology, as well as the results of any tests that are administered during the patient's evaluation as these may indicate that additional testing is needed to explore different auditory processes and/or sites of lesion.

Types of Tests

Two main categories of central tests are discussed in this chapter. These are psychophysical (i.e., behavioral) tests and electrophysiologic tests. The psychophysical test category includes dichotic listening, temporal processing, low redundancy speech, and binaural interaction tests, whereas the electrophysiologic procedures to be discussed include the auditory brainstem response (ABR), the middle latency response (MLR), the N1 and P2 late potentials, and the P300 (also referred to as the P3 potential). On occasion, a brief discussion of other auditory evoked potentials also is included.

In cases of CANS involvement, the goals of testing generally are not to make the diagnosis, as in many instances the disorder is already known and many medical procedures are better at defining the lesion than are the central auditory tests. However, there are three major goals of using audiologic tests when CANS involvement is either suspected or confirmed. The first is as a screener. The audiologist may be the first professional to see a patient with a CANS disorder and therefore has the responsibility to make the appropriate referral. This, of course, cannot be done unless central dysfunction is determined. Although not a common occurrence, this situation does happen and when it does appropriate follow-up and management of the patient is essential. The second major goal in utilizing central tests in CANS disease is to determine if the auditory (central) system is involved. For example, a patient with a long-standing diagnosis of multiple sclerosis might seek audiologic assessment because of a new symptom of hearing difficulty. The key here is to determine if this new symptom is really auditory in nature or not, and if it is, whether it is due to peripheral or central system compromise. The third goal of central auditory assessment is to corroborate the medical and communicative symptoms and/or complaints of the patient with test measures. All three of these goals lead to another important aspect of audiology, that is, the proper management of the patient. Without the appropriate diagnostic information, proper management of the patient with confirmed or suspected CANS involvement is difficult.

Brain Plasticity

Plasticity of the CANS is a factor in all brain lesions. Natural compensation by the brain for central dysfunction often occurs over time. Therefore, some lesion effects may not be as severe if the patient is assessed at some time after the initial occurrence of the CANS disorder as they would have been had the patient been assessed closer in time to the original disease process or CANS compromise. On the other hand, some CANS lesions may progress, creating greater problems over time, as potentially would be the case in progressive CANS disorders such as multiple sclerosis. Given these considerations, central auditory testing can be used not only to initially document the auditory deficits associated with CANS

involvement, but also to monitor subsequent changes in the patient's audiologic profile that may result as a function of brain plasticity, audiologic intervention, or disease progression.

MASS LESIONS

Introduction

Essentially, mass lesions are space-occupying lesions within the brain. Lesions that are located within or close to the auditory areas of the brain, of course, are at risk for influencing central auditory function. Sometimes, vascular lesions such as aneurysms and hematomas could be viewed as mass lesions in that they can be space occupying as they often are quite large. However, these types of lesions are classified as vascular disorders. In the brainstem, mass lesions are divided into intra-axial and extra-axial categories depending on whether the tumor resides primarily within or outside the brain tissue. The first reports on central auditory disorders by Bocca, Calearo, and Cassinari (1954) were on patients with temporal lobe tumors. In many cases, these patients reported varying auditory symptoms depending on the characteristics of their tumors.

Symptoms

The symptoms related to mass lesions of the central nervous system depend on the size, location, type, and consistency of the tumor (Young, 1983). In terms of general symptoms, headaches, nausea and vomiting, seizures (usually at later stages), dizziness, and altered mentation can occur (Perkins, 2002). Tumors that specifically affect the CANS can result in the same symptoms, but they also may create subtle complaints of difficulty hearing in noise, tinnitus, auditory hallucinations, difficulty understanding speech, decreased appreciation of music, sound distortions, and so forth. In some cases, however, patients with CANS compromise may experience no auditory symptoms. The specific auditory symptoms experienced depend on such factors as the location of the lesion, its size and duration, the presence and amount of brain plasticity, and the age of the patient. Often, auditory symptoms are overshadowed by more overt symptoms and the patient may have to be asked specifically about hearing abilities before any auditory difficulties are acknowledged (Bamiou et al., 2006; Musiek, Baran, & Pinheiro, 1994; Perkins, 2002).

Incidence and Prevalence

The incidence of benign brain tumors is about 7.9 per 100,000 with females being slightly more commonly affected than males (i.e., 9.7 and 5.8 per 100,000 for females and males, respectively) (Ries et al., 2007). Malignant brain tumor incidence in adults is approximately 6.4 per 100,000 (National Cancer Institute, 2000). When all tumor types are combined, there is definitely an age influence on the incidence of tumor occurrence with greater occurrence reported for the elderly population than for children. However, certain tumor types are more prevalent in children. There is a monotonic function for age ranging from those under 20 years

to those 85 years and older (Ries et al., 2007). There also is an anatomic factor in the occurrence of cerebral tumors. Most tumors occur in the frontal lobe, followed by the temporal, parietal, and occipital lobes (Larjavaara et al., 2007).

In the brainstem, intra-axial tumors arise from within the brainstem structures themselves, often near the midline. Gliomas are the most common type of intra-axial brainstem tumor and include many subtypes such as astrocytomas, ependymomas, and medulloblastomas (McLeod & Lance, 1989). These mass lesions vary in prognosis, often are difficult to manage, and, because of their location, usually result in compromise of brainstem auditory function (Jerger & Jerger, 1981).

Extra-axial tumors often are meningiomas, astrocytomas, or schwannomas. These tumors occur outside the brainstem and encroach on the brainstem and cranial nerves. Probably the most common schwannoma that often affects auditory function is the vestibular schwannoma. A vestibular schwannoma larger than 2 cm will compress the brainstem and can be considered an extra-axial tumor.

Etiology and Pathology

Reeves (1981) outlines the pathophysiology of mass lesions. Initially, mechanical displacement of the particular brain structure is involved. This can result in stretching of the nerve fibers' myelin and potentially demyelination of the nerve fibers, which in turn causes impaired or altered impulse propagation and velocity. Mechanical pressure evolves and results in impeded axon function and blood flow and over time can lead to the development of hydrocephalus. Swelling also evolves, thus creating increased mechanical pressure. At times, there can be bleeding into the tumor itself. Obviously, with increases in the involvement of a particular brain structure, there comes the likelihood that more of these pathologic actions will occur, which in turn would increase the likelihood of compromised auditory function.

Site of Lesion

Mass lesions and vascular disorders can take place anywhere in the CANS and can directly affect auditory function. Mass lesions also can result in indirect effects on CANS structures from compression or shifting of the brain. For example, due to its size and location, a large frontal lobe tumor could also compress the temporal and parietal lobes. Vascular lesions such as strokes tend to be more anatomically precise than mass lesions, but these also can have indirect influences. An example of this would be what is known as "vascular steal" effects. However, most of the time mass and vascular lesions will result in the greatest amount of dysfunction in the anatomic area where the lesion is located.

Medical Diagnosis

Medical diagnosis is first concerned with determining whether the tumor is malignant or not. Approaches include a detailed general medical and neurologic history. This generally is followed by a neurologic exam. Radiologic investigation relies primarily on magnetic resonance imaging (MRI) with contrast enhancement, but occasionally computerized tomography (CT) is used (see Chapter 3, Audiological, Vestibular, and Radiologic Procedures). MRI can provide considerable information about tumor size, type, and location, which can inform the need for surgical intervention. Several tumors have such typical findings on MRI that a diagnosis can be made without a formal biopsy. This is particularly true for extra-axial tumors, such as vestibular schwannomas. However, on occasion, a biopsy in the operating room may be needed. Surgical approaches for biopsy can take a variety of forms, a discussion of which is beyond the scope of this book. However, it is important to note that surgical biopsy often is necessary for differentiating malignant from benign mass lesions.

Medical Management

As related by Perkins (2002) management of the patient with a mass lesion often depends on whether the lesion is benign or malignant. In the case of benign lesions, surgical excision is typically the most direct course of treatment. However, this approach is dependent on the age and overall health of the patient, as well as the location, type, and size of the tumor and its neurologic effects. Sometimes, careful observation is the most appropriate course of action, particularly in patients who are elderly or poor surgical candidates, as well as in cases where the tumor is slow growing and causing minimal neurologic disturbance.

For malignant tumors that are amenable to surgery, surgical resection is usually combined with radiation treatments and/or chemotherapy. Gamma knife surgery, a relatively new treatment, involves the targeted radiologic destruction of the tumor. As this does not involve traditional surgical procedures (i.e., surgical incisions are not required), the patient is not exposed to the side effects or risks of invasive surgery. However, radiation damage to tissue around the lesion often yields side effects. Gamma knife surgery can also be used to treat benign tumors as an alternative to surgery for small- or medium-sized tumors and the patient prefers a nonsurgical approach. It may also have applications for large tumors in some cases.

Audiology

With the advances in radiology, diagnostic audiology is not the best approach to diagnose mass lesions. However, the audiologist may be the first person to see a patient with a mass lesion, especially if auditory symptoms are the patient's major complaint. If this is the case, assessment of the patient's central auditory function is key to the diagnosis of central auditory dysfunction, and ultimately to the appropriate referral for medical follow-up.

A role more commonly played by the audiologist when working with patients with diagnosed brain tumors is to determine if the tumor has compromised the auditory system. If surgery is being recommended for a given patient, the audiologist also may be involved in the pre- and postsurgical assessment of auditory function to determine the status of the patient's auditory function following surgery. This determination is important for the overall welfare of the patient. In addition to patients who have undergone traditional surgical procedures, those who have

undergone Gamma knife surgery, chemotherapy, and radiologic treatments for tumors that are located in or in close proximity to the auditory areas of the brain should be evaluated for potential postsurgical compromise of central auditory function and then managed appropriately.

VASCULAR DISORDERS

Introduction

Vascular disorders are among the most common disorders that affect the CANS. These disease processes typically result in a reduction of the blood supply to the neural substrate served by the vascular system affected. Because blood supply provides oxygen and glucose to the cells, removes waste matter, and is essential to overall cell metabolism, normal or unrestricted blood supply to the brain structures is critical for the normal function of these structures. Pathologic conditions of blood vessels in the brain are referred to collectively as cerebrovascular disorders.

The major types of cerebrovascular brain disease have been reviewed by Kaufman (1990) and Perkins (2002). Vascular disorders can be broadly grouped into two major categories: ischemic and hemorrhagic. Ischemic disorders occur when blood flow to an area of brain tissue is diminished. If diminished blood flow is prolonged, the condition can result in tissue infarction (referred to as an ischemic stroke). Ischemic stroke typically occurs when cerebral arteries are occluded as a result of vessel narrowing due to atherosclerosis, or due to the lodging of a blood clot in a vessel. However, compromise of arterial supply due to tumor, infection, vessel spasm, or inflammation (vasculitis) also can cause ischemic stroke. Hemorrhagic vascular lesions occur when a blood vessel ruptures and bleeds into the brain. Intracerebral hemorrhage (hemorrhagic stroke) results from damage to blood vessels, often due to high blood pressure, and results in loss of blood flow to associated brain tissue, as well as a mass effect in the brain. Hemorrhagic vascular lesions also can occur as a result of an aneurysm, which is the "ballooning" of a vessel usually because of a weakness or damage along the vessel wall. These aneurysms can bleed, resulting in intracerebral or subarachnoid hemorrhage. All types of stroke result in loss of blood supply to neural substrate, and can lead to either reversible or irreversible neural damage depending on their duration.

Symptoms

Symptoms of vascular disease are dependent on the locus of the problem, the number and types of vessels involved, the degree of involvement, and patient factors such as age, general health, and activity level. One of the key symptoms of vascular disease is transient ischemic attacks (TIAs), which are caused by a temporary decrease in blood supply to an area of the brain that results in temporary or transient symptoms. These TIAs can be a warning of impending stroke in 10 to 30% of the cases in which they occur (McLeod & Lance, 1989). Other symptoms related to stroke can be headache, confusion, drowsiness, parasthesias, hemiplegia, sensory deficits, aphasia, vomiting, and dizziness (McLeod & Lance, 1989). Specific auditory symptoms will result when

the blood supply is decreased to areas of the CANS. Symptoms that may occur when the auditory areas of the brain are compromised include tinnitus (central), hallucinations, loss of hearing sensitivity, poor hearing in noise, confusion following directions and understanding speech, localization difficulties, and changes in music appreciation. In extreme cases, total central deafness can occur when major vascular deficits affect both sides of the central auditory tracts in the brainstem or cerebral hemispheres (see Musiek et al., 1994; Musiek & Lee, 1998).

Incidence and Prevalence

Prevalence of vascular disease varies with age, occurring in only 1 in 100,000 for those under 35 years of age and 840 in 100,000 for those over 35 years. About 80% of vascular accidents occur in individuals 65 years of age or older. Vascular problems in younger age groups are more common in men, but in older age groups the incidence of vascular problems is essentially equal between genders. Transient ischemic attacks are more common in men than women (Jerger & Jerger, 1981).

Etiology and Pathology

Occlusive disease often manifests as atherosclerosis, which narrows or occludes arteries. This evolves over time due to the increasing amounts of fatty materials and fibrous tissue that progressively build up within the blood system, especially at the branching points of the arteries. Atherosclerosis can damage artery walls, which triggers thrombus formation from platelets and collagen. It often is seen in the internal carotid and vertebral basilar systems, but is not as common in the middle cerebral artery (MCA). Another occlusive problem can be a cardiac embolism, a type of clot that can travel from the heart to the brain where it becomes a brain embolism that arrests the blood supply to the brain structures supplied by the particular artery affected. Vasoconstriction also can affect small vessels by reducing the lumen of the vessel and restricting blood flow through the vessel. Medications, drugs, and even natural physiologic responses such as fear can cause this action (Chaves & Jones, 2005).

When blood supply is disrupted, time becomes a key factor. In 30 seconds ischemia develops and brain metabolism is altered. After 1 minute of no blood supply, neural tissue ceases normal activity, and after 5 minutes of arrested circulation, neural substrate becomes anoxic leading to infarction (Toole, 1979). Smoking, poor diet, drugs, drinking, hereditary factors, and lack of exercise all can contribute to occlusive disease by accelerating atherosclerosis (Chaves & Jones, 2005).

Intracerebral hemorrhage can result in hematomas and edema, which can compress brain tissue (see Chaves & Jones, 2005; Perkins, 2002). This condition evolves quickly (usually in hours) and is related to degeneration of the blood vessel walls, a condition that can be acquired or congenital. General weakness of the vessel walls is worsened by conditions such as high blood pressure, which can further weaken the vessels. In addition, emboli fragments can cause ischemia of artery walls, which would result in a weakening of these walls. Other conditions, such as tumors and trauma, may result in intracerebral hemorrhage. Use of anticoagulants and antiplatelet agents can worsen this

condition; hence, it must be differentiated from other disorders, such as occlusive disease (for which antiplatelet therapy is usually recommended) (Perkins, 2002).

There are five subtypes of aneurysms: saccular (sac-shaped; most common), fusiform (spindle-like outpouching), dissecting (longitudinal splitting of the artery), traumatic (secondary to trauma), and infectious (related to infection). These weakened blood vessels, commonly form at branching sites, are space occupying, and can result in improper blood supply to certain areas of the brain. Importantly, they also can rupture resulting in subarachnoid bleeding, which can be fatal, and they also can be a site of emboli, which can result in occlusion of various vessels (Steel, Thomas, & Strollo, 1982).

Site of Lesion

Vascular disorders that are located near auditory regions of the central nervous system are of concern to hearing function. Sometimes a "vascular steal" takes place, which can affect regions far from the actual vascular site of damage. The vertebral-basilar vascular system supplies the auditory brainstem pathways via branches primarily from the basilar artery. These branches are circumferential proceeding to the posterior brainstem where the auditory structures are located. Branches of the middle cerebral artery (MCA) supply the auditory cortex and the fronto-opercular artery supplies the insula.

Medical Management

Chaves and Jones (2005) outline the medical management of occlusive disease. This includes a neurologically oriented history and examination, as well as determination of the anatomic site of involvement, usually with CT and/or MRI. Commonly, cardiac function assessment and ultrasound of carotid arteries or MR or CT-angiography to look for vascular occlusion are performed. On occasion, CT perfusion studies also are indicated. Treatment can be prophylactic, primarily with antiplatelet therapy (aspirin, Plavix) and aggressive management of cholesterol and blood pressure, or surgical, such as carotid endarterectomy, angioplasty, or the use of stents to keep arteries open. In patients with atrial fibrillation (which can cause clots to form in the heart that can embolize to the brain) or disorders of normal clotting function (which also may result in clot formation), anticoagulation medication often is recommended. In unusual cases, neurologists may consider cerebral vasculitis as the cause of the vascular disorder. If this condition is suspected, it is evaluated with blood tests and angiography and it can be treated with immunosuppressive drugs.

In cases of potential hemorrhage or aneurysm, history and medical examination focusing on such factors as hypertension, smoking, and alcohol use should be considered. It also is important to watch for use of anticoagulants (i.e., warfarin, heparin), as urgent reversal of anticoagulation may be required to stop bleeding. Treatment for intracerebral hemorrhage is usually to lower blood pressure and watch for signs of increased intracranial pressure or increased hematoma size. Surgical decompression and evacuation of hematoma sometimes is required. Treatment of ruptured aneurysm involves surgical repair of the aneurysm, followed by close clinical observation for signs of

cerebral vasospasms/arterial occlusion, which can occur after many aneurysmal bleeds (Hreib & Jones, 2005; Sung, 2006).

AUDIOLOGY: MASS AND VASCULAR LESIONS

Behavioral Test Procedures

Dichotic Listening Tests

There are several commonly used tests of dichotic listening such as dichotic digits (Musiek, 1983a), the dichotic word listening test (DWLT) (Meyers et al., 2002), the staggered spondaic word test (Katz et al. 1963), and many others (see Baran & Musiek, 1999).

Dichotic speech tests can be sensitive to brainstem involvement, but are most noted for their sensitivity in detecting hemispheric and corpus callosum dysfunction (see Baran & Musiek, 1999). Typical findings are ipsilateral or bilateral deficits for low brainstem lesions and contralateral effects for cortical lesions. Perhaps most importantly, the paradoxical left ear deficit is known to implicate the corpus callosum (i.e., a left ear dichotic deficit with a left hemisphere lesion that involves the corpus callosum). Although tests vary in terms of their sensitivity, dichotic listening tests are considered to have moderately good diagnostic power.

A large number of studies support the value of dichotic speech tests in the evaluation of mass and vascular lesions of the cortex and subcortex. Findings show a definite contralateral deficit in adults (i.e., unless the corpus callosum is involved where left ear deficits are commonly noted) (Cohen, Hynd, & Hugdahl,

1992; Kimura, 1961; Lynn & Gilroy, 1975; Musiek, 1983b; Musiek et al., 1994; Raeder, Helland, Hugdahl, & Wester, 2005; Speaks, Gray, & Miller, 1975; and others). Cohen et al. (1992) also showed contralateral effects from hemispheric involvement in children similar to those noted in adults. Investigations of mass and vascular lesions of the brainstem have yielded somewhat mixed results as to the type of deficits typically detected, but predominately ipsilateral and bilateral deficits have been noted on these dichotic tests (Musiek, 1983b; Musiek & Baran, 2004; Musiek & Geurkink, 1982). However, the sensitivity of dichotic listening tests to brainstem involvement is less than the sensitivity of these tests to cortical and interhemispheric dysfunction (see Baran & Musiek, 1999, and Chermak & Musiek, 2011, for reviews).

Temporal Processing Tests

Temporal processing tests include tests that assess temporal sequencing, temporal resolution, temporal integration, and temporal masking. This chapter focuses on examples of the first three test categories, that is, pattern perception, gap detection, and integration of tonal stimuli. Frequency and duration patterns are commonly used tests that are highly dependent on temporal sequencing as well as other functions such as auditory discrimination and linguistic labeling (see Baran & Musiek, 1999). These tests require processing of the acoustic stimuli in both hemispheres if a verbal response to the test stimuli is required even though the tests commonly are administered monaurally (in some cases they can be administered in a sound field). When a verbal response to the test stimuli is required, the right hemisphere is involved in contour

recognition and sequencing of the stimuli and the left hemisphere is involved in the linguistic labeling of the processed stimuli. In order for accurate processing and a response to occur, information processed in the right hemisphere needs to be transferred to the left hemisphere via the corpus callosum. Related to these concepts and observations is that dysfunction or compromise in either hemisphere or the corpus callosum typically yields bilateral deficits when a verbal response is required (Musiek, Pinheiro, & Wilson, 1980). If an alternative type of response is used, such as humming the pattern, then the test procedure taps primarily right hemisphere function as there is no need to transfer across the corpus callosum to the left hemisphere. If a patient is unable to accurately hum the patterns being presented, then a right hemisphere compromise would be implicated.

A number of studies have shown frequency and duration pattern perception tests to be sensitive and specific tests for mass and vascular lesions of the auditory regions of each hemisphere. These studies demonstrate primarily, but not exclusively, bilateral deficits (Baran, Bothfeldt, & Musiek, 2004; Fallis-Cunningham, Keith, & Warnick, 1998; Musiek et al., 1990; Musiek & Pinheiro, 1987). Poor performance on pattern perception also has been observed in patients with vascular lesions of the insula (Bamiou et al., 2006). As would be expected, patients with corpus callosum damage typically show extremely low scores for verbal report, but they can often hum the patterns without difficulty (Musiek et al., 1980). Although auditory pattern perception is affected by hemispheric and interhemispheric mass and vascular lesions, it appears that these tests are not highly sensitive to brainstem involvement (Musiek & Geurkink, 1982; Musiek & Pinheiro, 1987).

The Gaps-in-Noise test (GIN) (Musiek et al., 2005) is an example of a temporal resolution test. The ability to detect extremely brief interruptions of an ongoing broadband signal (gaps) requires integrity of the CANS. It has been shown that individuals with vascular lesions of the CANS (including the insula and brainstem) do not perform well on gap detection procedures, requiring longer silent gaps than controls for accurate perception (Bamiou et al., 2006; Efron, Yund, Nichols, & Crandall, 1985; Musiek et al., 2005).

Temporal integration is not a commonly used test procedure for mass and vascular involvement of the CANS, but it probably should be. This procedure requires the measurement of threshold for long (500 ms) and short (20 ms) tones and the determination of the difference between these thresholds. This test procedure has been shown to be sensitive to CANS involvement secondary to vascular/mass lesions (Baru & Karaseva, 1972). However, Cranford, Stream, Rye, and Slade (1982) modified the test to include a frequency difference limen for short and long tones, which made the procedure more sensitive to CANS problems. It is difficult to understand why this simple, straightforward procedure is not utilized more in clinical settings. To date, the available evidence suggests that the procedure is sensitive to cortical damage, but to our knowledge, no data are available on brainstem involvement.

Monaural Low Redundancy Speech Tests

Monaural low redundancy speech tests (often referred to as distorted speech tests) include such procedures as filtered, compressed, or interrupted speech signals as well as speech signals presented in the presence of noise or other speech signals. Filtered (usually low-pass filtered) and compressed speech tests have been shown to yield contralateral ear deficits for individuals with mass and vascular auditory cortex lesions. However, as a group, these procedures are not as sensitive to cortical lesions as the tests discussed above (Bocca et al., 1954; Karlsson & Rosenhall, 1995; Lynn & Gilroy, 1972, 1975; see Baran and Musiek, 1999, for review).

Monaural low redundancy speech procedures are not highly dependent on interhemispheric transfer; therefore, even individuals with split brains typically do well on these tests (Musiek, Kibbe, & Baran, 1984). However, for brainstem involvement, speech in noise and the synthetic sentence identification with ipsilateral competing message (SSI-ICM) have been shown to be sensitive to a variety of central lesions, including mass and vascular disorders (Jerger & Jerger, 1974; Morales-Garcia & Poole, 1972; Rintelmann, 1985). In addition, filtered speech, interrupted speech, and compressed speech tests have been shown to statistically separate control groups from patients with confirmed vascular lesions of the brainstem (Karlsson & Rosenhall, 1995).

Binaural Interaction Tests

Auditory tasks that require functional interrelationships between the two ears that are not the classically defined dichotic speech tests fit into the category of binaural interaction tests. Masking level differences (MLDs), interaural timing tests, and localization and lateralization tasks are the primary test procedures in this test category. These tests require fine acoustic comparisons by the two ears usually for time, intensity, and/or phase cues. The use of these tests has been directed primarily toward assessment of brainstem functions through the use of localization and lateralization tasks that are sensitive to both brainstem and cerebral dysfunctions.

The classic localization study on cortical lesions with primarily, but not exclusively, vascular etiology was conducted Sanchez-Longo, Forster, and Auth (1957). These investigators used a simple bedside localization task and found deficits in the auditory field opposite the involved hemisphere. This finding also has been documented in a subsequent localization study (Cranford, Diamond, Ravizza, & Whitfield, 1971). In addition, Pinheiro and Tobin (1969) reported asymmetric lateralization findings in stroke patients for a clinically oriented task utilizing interaural intensity differences.

The MLD procedure has a long clinical history. In a mixed clinical population of both mass and vascular lesions of the brainstem, Lynn, Gilroy, Taylor, and Leiser (1981) showed high sensitivity and specificity for the MLD using CVs as stimuli. This classic study also demonstrated that individuals with midbrain and cortical lesions revealed MLDs similar to those demonstrated by their control group.

Electrophysiologic Tests

Auditory Brainstem Response

Early on in its history the auditory brainstem response (ABR) was shown to be sensitive to mass or vascular lesions of the brainstem (Starr & Achor, 1975). Subsequent reports have supported this early finding with larger numbers of patients. Sensitivity and specificity have been in the 80% range with some variability noted in the reports (Chiappa, 1988; Karlsson & Rosenhall, 1995; Musiek & Lee, 1995). The standard one channel electrode array is sufficient to obtain these kinds of sensitivity and specificity rates. Waves III through V are generated by pontine auditory structures; hence, latency delays or absence of these waves (especially with wave I normal) or the presence of an extended III–V interwave latency likely indicate brainstem involvement, although a III–V extension also could indicate auditory nerve dysfunction, but this is unlikely. Amplitude measures have not been used widely with ABR to identify abnormal brainstem function as amplitude measures tend to be quite variable. On the other hand, absolute and interwave latency measures have been shown to be more sensitive and specific and tend to be used more commonly for diagnostic purposes. Mass or vascular lesions that are intra-axial often result in very high hit rates for ABR (Musiek, 1991).

Mass and vascular lesions of the thalamocortical tracts and auditory cortices are best assessed by the middle latency response (MLR) and the late potentials (N1, P2, P3), respectively. In considering brainstem involvement, the auditory brainstem response (ABR) is the evoked potential of choice, but it is of little value for assessing lesions rostral to the pons.

Middle Latency Response

The middle latency response (MLR) has been shown to be relatively sensitive to lesions of the auditory cortex and thalamo-cortical connections. Hit rates in the mid-70% range or better have been reported (Musiek, Charette, Kelly, Lee, & Musiek, 1999; Scherg & von Cramon, 1986). When assessing the MLR, it is most useful to use electrodes positioned in midline (Cz) and lateral positions relative to the auditory cortex (e.g., C3, C4, or T3, T4) as this allows electrode comparisons from each side of the head (i.e., intrasubject comparisons). Usually, the electrode positioned closest to the lesion site will show a compromised response (i.e., an electrode effect) when the MLR is assessed, hence the importance of using this type of electrode placement when assessing patients at risk for auditory cortex or thalamo-cortical pathway compromise. It is clear that amplitude measures are better diagnostically than latency measures for the MLR and that this potential benefits from the type of intrasubject comparison described above (Kileny, Paccioretti, & Wilson, 1987; Musiek et al., 1999). Significant amplitude differences for hemispheric comparisons is a common finding with unilateral cerebral lesions and investigators have demonstrated that the MLR results in the best sensitivity measures when measures such as the electrode effect with amplitudes are applied (Musiek et al., 1999; Scherg & von Cramon, 1986).

The MLR can be recorded simultaneously with the ABR, which can be a major advantage in diagnostic utility. Under these testing conditions, the ABR can readily serve as a benchmark for the MLR waves indicating integrity of the more caudal auditory nervous system.

Late Responses (N1, P2)

The N1 and P2 auditory evoked potentials are generated mostly from the auditory cortex. In vascular and mass lesions, these potentials can be compromised by changes in their amplitude as well as latency. Electrodes should be placed laterally as was described above for the MLR. A study on left hemisphere stroke patients interestingly demonstrated reduced N1 amplitudes over both hemispheres for right, but not for left ear stimulation (Ilvonen et al., 2001). The N1 also has been shown to have good differential capability. Studies have shown the N1 to be reduced in temporal lobe strokes significantly more often than when the parietal or frontal lobes are similarly affected (Knight, Hillyard, Woods, & Neville, 1980; Knight, Scabini, Woods, & Clayworth, 1988). As with the MLR, N1, P2 responses generally are smaller in amplitude for the electrode that is near the lesion site. In addition, the latency of the response for the electrode nearer the site of lesion is likely to be delayed compared to that observed for the other hemispheric electrode (see Musiek & Lee, 1999, for review).

P300 Response

The P300 generators are not well known, but it seems logical that there are many throughout the brain. Auditory regions of the temporal cortex play a role, as probably do the frontal lobe and hippocampus (see Musiek & Lee, 1999). The P300 does not appear to provide distinct laterality information like the MLR and N1, P2. This may be because of the multiple generator sites for the P300 response (Musiek, Baran, & Pinheiro, 1992). The P300 is highly sensitive to aging and dementia. It also is sensitive to lesions of the auditory cortical areas of the brain. Both amplitude and latency effects are noted for P300s in individuals with mass and/or vascular lesions (Musiek et al., 1992; Obert & Cranford, 1990). The P300 has been shown to differentiate parietal from temporo-parietal lesions with the latter severely compromising latency and amplitude measures (Knight, Scabini, Woods, & Clayworth, 1989). The oddball paradigm that is used to acquire the P300 is a powerful approach and allows the simultaneous recording of the N1, P2 and P300 evoked potentials. The electrode arrangement for the P300 classically is midline anterior to posterior (Fz, Cz, Pz). However, because the N1 and P2 can be recorded with the P300 electrodes in lateral positions (C3, C4, and/or T3, T4), the use of these types of electrode arrays could prove useful.

Case 7–1: Temporal Lobe Tumor

History

This patient was a young adult who developed seizures secondary to a temporal lobe tumor. She reported left arm numbness for years and difficulty with motor movements on the left side. In addition, she complained of light-headedness and often feeling as if she was about to pass out. She stated that the hearing in her left ear was worse than in her right, yet hearing sensitivity was better in her left ear on the audiogram.

Audiology

The patient had normal hearing sensitivity for pure tones in the left ear and a very mild conductive loss for the right ear with excellent speech recognition bilaterally. Central auditory behavioral tests showed rather marked left ear deficits for dichotic listening tests (digits and rhyme tests)

and a bilateral deficit for duration patterns (Figure 7–1A).

Medical Examination

Neurologically, there was documentation of a seizure disorder. Radiologically, a CT scan showed a right posterior temporal lobe tumor that can readily be seen in Figure 7–1B. This tumor was approximately 2 × 2 × 4 cm in size. Note how the tumor has affected the right lateral ventricle by compressing it (see Figure 7–1B).

Impression

This patient has central auditory involvement secondary to a right temporal lobe tumor and the patient's related subjective complaints of hearing difficulty for the left ear. A very mild conductive loss is present in the right ear. Interestingly, the left ear (i.e., contralateral to the involved hemisphere) was reported by the patient as being poorer than the right ear (i.e., the ear with the mild conductive loss). These central test findings are consistent with expectations for a right posterior temporal lobe lesion in that they revealed a classic contralateral ear effect.

Case 7–2: Temporoparietal Stroke

History

At the time of evaluation, this middle-aged woman was several months post a right temporoparietal stroke. She was bothered by dizziness episodes, difficulty hearing soft voices, and hearing in the presence of background noise to the point that audiologic consultation was sought.

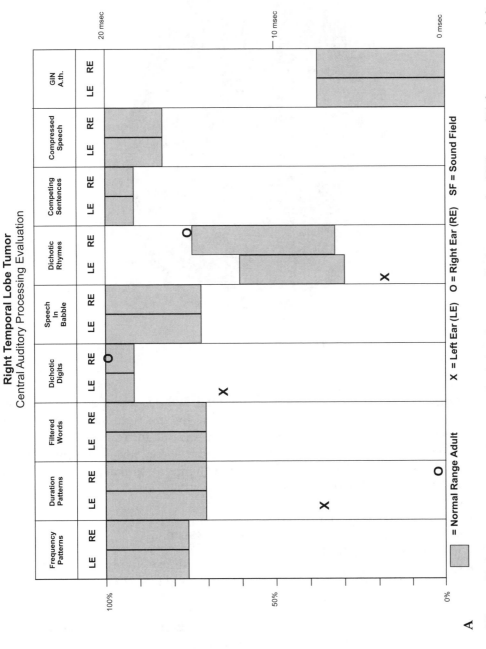

Figure 7–1. *Central behavioral tests results (A) and computerized tomography (CT) scan (B) for a young adult with a right temporal lobe tumor (Case 7–1) (note the temporal lobe tumor at 8 o'clock).* continues

293

Right Temporal Lobe Tumor

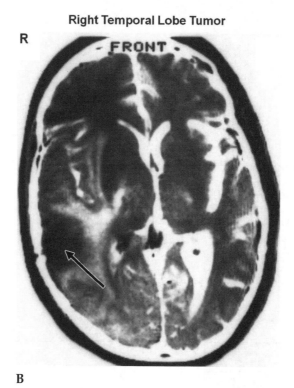

B

Figure 7–1. continued

Audiology

This patient's pure-tone thresholds were normal and her speech recognition ability was excellent bilaterally. Behavioral central auditory test results showed the classic contralateral effect on dichotic speech tests and a bilateral deficit on frequency patterns (Figure 7–2A). Central auditory electrophysiologic tests included ABR-MLR testing performed simultaneously using a click stimulus (Figure 7–2B). The ABR was normal bilaterally, whereas the MLR showed an ear effect with the right ear Pa responses essentially present at all electrode sites and the left ear showing an absent Pa response with a meager Na that if present, would be delayed at all recording sites.

The ENG test results for this patient showed some mild smooth pursuit tracking abnormalities and a stronger caloric response for the right side that did not reach clinical significance. The CT scan revealed a lesion site in the right hemisphere (temporoparietal area) (see arrows in Figures 7–2C and 7–2D).

Impression

Central auditory involvement consistent with temporal lobe stroke.

Medical Examination and Management

This patient was being followed and managed neurologically poststroke. She also had weakness for the left extremities, but was ambulatory.

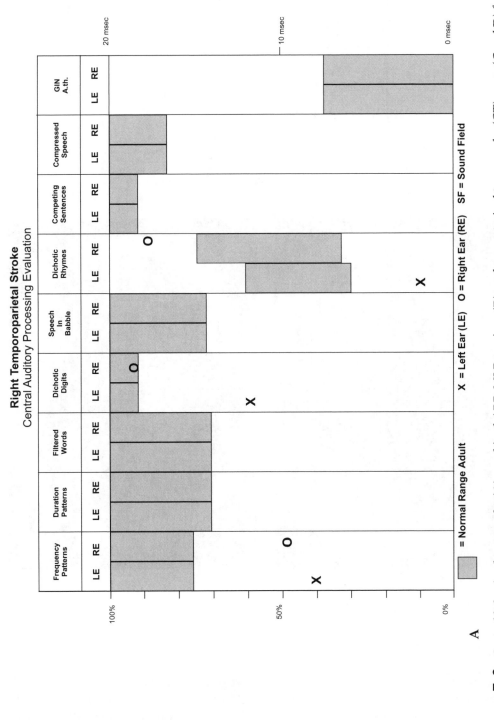

Figure 7–2. *Central behavioral test results (A), combined ABR-MLR tracings (B), and computerized tomography (CT) scans (C and D) for a middle-aged woman with a right-sided temporoparietal stroke (Case 7–2). Key: V = ABR wave V, Pa = MLR wave V, Pa = MLR wave, Cz, C3, C4 = electrode sites.* continues

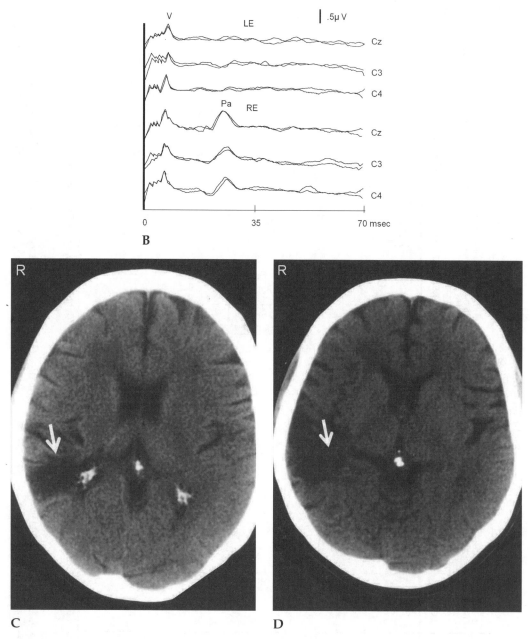

Figure 7–2. continued

Audiologic Management

At the time of her evaluation, the patient was counseled on the use of assistive listening devices, enhancing the listening environment, and home auditory training techniques, and arrangements were made for follow-up and consultations closer to her home.

DEGENERATIVE DISORDERS

Introduction

A variety of degenerative disorders can compromise the CANS. However, in this chapter, the focus is on two relatively common degenerative disorders that can affect the CANS: multiple sclerosis (MS) and Alzheimer's disease (AD). Multiple sclerosis is a chronic, progressive autoimmune disease that results in myelin destruction, which primarily affects young adults. The severity is highly variable, and some patients have prolonged periods of total remission. MS patients can have flares (i.e., transient episodes of focal demyelination) that can last days to weeks. Thus, the symptoms can be relapsing and remitting over time, but generally present with an overall progressive decline. Because it is a disease affecting the myelin sheathing of nerve fibers, MS can affect any system or region of the nervous system that has myelinated nerves. Of note is the fact that only a portion (medial) of the auditory nerve is myelinated. Therefore, this disease more commonly involves the CANS rather than the peripheral auditory system.

Alzheimer's disease (AD) is the most common cause of dementia and is classified as a degenerative cognitive disorder, but it also affects other systems in the central nervous system. Generally, older adults are affected by the disease, but it can attack middle-aged individuals as well. There is tendency for the disease to run in families (see Zabar, 2005).

Symptoms

In MS, the symptoms are related to the locus of the disease. That is, wherever the myelin is attacked and plaques (a type of scarring of myelin) form, symptoms related to that area of the brain can emerge. As mentioned above, the motor and sensory symptoms associated with MS can come and go. When the symptoms become worse, it is called an exacerbation. This situation is accompanied by swelling around the plaque and a related increase in dysfunction. All neural systems can be affected. Auditory symptoms often are overlooked by both the patient and the clinician because they tend to be more subtle than other motor or sensory symptoms. Initial onset is usually in the 20- to 40-year-old age bracket and common symptoms include paresthesias, motor weakness, diplopia, blurred vision, ataxia, vertigo (or balance disturbance), and hearing difficulties (Jerger & Jerger, 1981; Merritt & Antunes, 1979).

In patients with AD, different symptoms emerge, and in the early stages of this neurodegenerative disease process, it is quite likely that the symptoms may not be noticed. However, in time, short-term memory loss, loss of organizational skills, decreased language function, the need for frequent repetition of conversational statements and verbal requests, impaired visual spatial skills, and hearing difficulties will become obvious and progress to the point where the patient becomes dependent (see Zabar, 2005).

Incidence and Prevalence

It is interesting to note that MS is more common in cold as opposed to warm geographic regions. For example, in Southern states the incidence is 6 to 14 per 100,000, whereas in Northern states it is 40 to 60 per 100,000. MS is not found in native born Africans and is rare in the populations of Japan, Taiwan, and India. It is more common in women than men and the mean age of onset is usually between 20 to 30 years of age (Poser, 1979).

Alzheimer's disease is present in about 50% of the population over 85 years of age. There are about 4 million cases in the United States and the risk of developing the disease doubles every 5 years after age 65 (Zabar, 2005).

Etiology and Pathology

The etiology for MS is unknown but results in the demyelination of nerves (with secondary axonal degeneration occurring as a result). MS is classified as an autoimmune disease, and it appears that lymphocytes and macrophages play a role in the disease process by attacking myelin (Calabresi, 2006). Demyelination due to inflammatory plaques results in reduced and/or delayed neural impulses. In turn, this affects the specific system that is involved. The brain is capable of repairing areas of demyelination, which is why periods of exacerbation and remission (i.e., a period of time when the symptoms are not manifested) are noted in many patients with MS, especially those in the earlier stages of this disease. However, if the inflammation is severe, recurrent, or prolonged, it can cause axonal damage that becomes permanent.

The exact etiology of AD is not known. However, a common finding with this disease is an excess of beta-amyloid protein, which can impair synaptic function. It appears that the excess of beta-amyloid proteins is a factor in the development of amyloid plaques, which are commonly seen in AD brains. However, it is unclear if beta-amyloid alone is enough to trigger AD. Inflammation and free radical damage also appear to play a role. One hall-mark of AD is the presence of neuronal inclusions called neurofibrillary tangles that contain tau, a protein that can cause cell damage. Another factor in AD is the reduction in acetylcholine, which is observed in patients with AD and may be related to some of the conditions mentioned above (Zabar, 2005).

There are risk factors that are associated with AD. These include age, family history, hypertension, stroke, diabetes, and head injury (Zabar, 2005). In addition, patients with Down syndrome also commonly develop AD, with the onset of the degenerative processes frequently occurring in these individuals when they are in their 40s (Zabar, 2005).

Site of Lesion

In MS there is not a relationship between the disease and any particular nerve tract. Because MS is a disease of myelin, it will often be found where there is an abundance of white matter, such as in the corpus callosum, the medial longitudinal fasiculus, and a periventricular region of the brain referred to as the trigone (Muriello, Jones, & Chaves, 2005; Rubens, Froehling, Slater, & Anderson, 1985).

In AD, the frontal, temporal, and parietal lobes often are the first structures to become involved. However, with time the entire cerebrum eventually undergoes degenerative processes. When this degeneration occurs, the gyri become thin and the sulci become large and the subcortical areas also degenerate (Zabar, 2005).

Medical Diagnosis

In MS, a neurologic history will check for intermittent and relapsing symptoms, such as ocular, vestibular and/or auditory problems, "electric shock" sensations, numbness, tingling, weakness, motor problems, and fatigue. Several tests are used to make the diagnosis including MRI (to visualize plaques), lumbar puncture, and evoked potentials. Usually, evidence of lesions in at least two areas of the central nervous system and a minimum of two separate neurologic episodes must have occurred for the diagnosis to be made (Muriello et al., 2005).

There are no definitive tests for AD. However, careful evaluation of mental status is critical. Trends of cognitive impairment and decline are important to document. Neuropsychological studies in regard to cognitive (reasoning) and memory functions are central in the evaluation of AD. In advanced AD, CT or MRI can show cortical atrophy. In addition, other studies, such as positron emission tomography (PET), cerebrospinal fluid analysis for beta-amyloid and tau, single photon emission computed tomography (SPECT), functional MRI (fMRI), electroencephalography (EEG), and P300 evoked potentials occasionally are used for diagnosis (Musiek et al., 1994; Zabar, 2005).

Medical Management

In the treatment of MS, pharmaceutical management is the main course. The mainstay of MS therapy is treatment with injectable interferon-beta or glitaramer acetate, which has been shown to be effective in reducing exacerbations. Several new drugs that modulate the immune system are becoming available. In severe cases, azathioprine, cyclosporine, cyclophosphamide, and methotrexate have been recommended (Muriello et al., 2005).

Alzheimer's disease is treated by initiating good all around health habits such as exercise, good nutrition, and social activities. Current medications such as Aricept, Exelon, and Razadyne seem to focus on arresting the breakdown of acetylcholine. These medications are not a cure for AD, but there are some indications of improved mental function for patients taking these drugs (Web MD, Alzheimer's Disease Guide, 2009).

Audiology

A wide variety of degenerative disorders can affect the CANS. However, in this section of this chapter we focus on multiple sclerosis (MS) and Alzheimer's disease (AD). It is important to realize that hearing difficulties occur much more often in patients with MS than was originally believed (Jerger, Oliver, Chmiel, & Rivera, 1986). Musiek, Gollegly, Kibbe, and Reeves (1989) reported that approximately 40% of the patients with MS in their study had some type of hearing complaint, but only 18% had abnormal pure-tone audiograms. In another study, Luxon (1980) showed abnormal audiograms in over 50% of the MS patients she studied.

Although not a common occurrence, sometimes hearing difficulties can be the first sign of MS. Usually, the hearing problems are subtle and become more obvious in noisy listening situations (Luxon, 1980; Musiek et al., 1989). Tinnitus and vestibular symptoms can also be experienced by patients with MS.

Alzheimer's disease (AD) has come to the forefront of audiology recently due to the interesting findings that have been reported by George Gates. Gates and his colleagues have demonstrated that central auditory test results are often abnormal in patients with AD compared to matched controls (Gates, Anderson, Feeney, McCurry, & Larson, 2008). In addition, it appears that poor performance on central auditory tests may precede the onset of AD or at least the diagnosis of AD. This in turn has raised the question that perhaps central auditory testing may have some predictive value in regard to AD. Based on their findings, Gates and colleagues (2008) have argued strongly for including central auditory tests in the hearing evaluation of the elderly.

Behavioral Test Procedures in MS

Dichotic Listening Tests. There is a generous amount of literature pertaining to MS and dichotic listening. It is well known that dichotic listening requires action in the corpus callosum, a structure that is highly myelinated. As myelin is the target of MS, this is a likely locus for the manifestation of the disease. Both recent as well as early reports support the claim that the corpus callosum is a common lesion site in MS, as do studies that document the classic finding of left ear deficits on dichotic listening in patients with MS (Gadea et al., 2009; Rubens et al., 1985). The left ear deficit can be variable and depends on the amount and locus of interhemispheric disruption caused by the MS plaques. Dichotic listening to speech stimuli is one of the best procedures for detecting auditory dysfunction in MS (Gadea et al., 2009; Musiek et al., 1989).

Temporal Processing Tests. Temporal processing tests have not been utilized as much as dichotic speech tests in MS. At best, auditory pattern perception and gap

detection procedures have revealed only moderate sensitivity for detecting dysfunction related to MS (Hendler, Squires, & Emmerich, 1990; Musiek et al., 1989). However, more testing of temporal procedures needs to be completed before a final determination regarding the value of these tests in the assessment of central auditory function in MS patients can be made.

Monaural Low Redundancy Speech Tests. Low redundancy speech tests such as filtered speech have not shown particularly notable hit rates for identifying auditory involvement in patients with MS (Musiek et al., 1989). However, in a study evaluating a mixed population of patients with MS and brainstem tumors, Karlsson and Rosenhall (1995) did demonstrate that both filtered and compressed speech tests separated the involved group from a group of normal controls. They also noted a greater deficit for the ear ipsilateral to the lesion site than for the contralateral ear in the patients with brainstem involvement. In another study, Jerger and his colleagues (1986) found that the synthetic sentence identification with ipsilateral competing message (SSI-ICM) was moderately sensitive to auditory involvement related to MS.

Binaural Interaction Tests. Two binaural interaction tests will be mentioned here: the masking level difference (MLD) test and an interaural timing task. The MLD procedure has a long history of use in patients with MS and has been shown to be reasonably sensitive to central auditory involvement (see Hendler et al., 1990; Jerger et al., 1986, Musiek et al., 1989). Although both speech and tonal stimuli can be used, low-frequency tonal stimuli (usually 500 Hz) have been more commonly utilized with patients with MS. Interaural timing tasks also have been shown to be highly sensitive to auditory involvement from MS. In fact, this procedure has been shown to be even more sensitive than the ABR in MS (Levine et al., 1994). Unfortunately, this procedure has not made its way into common clinical use.

Electrophysiologic Tests

Auditory Brainstem Response. Perhaps the most utilized audiologic test in the MS population is the ABR. Hit rates vary widely because, without detailed radiology, one cannot be sure if the auditory tracts are involved. When the brainstem auditory tracts are involved, the ABR is abnormal an extremely high percentage of the time (Levine et al., 1994). In the general MS population, ABR sensitivity hovers around 60%; however, this figure is probably somewhat artificially low as many individuals with MS do not have auditory involvement (Musiek, 1991). Compared to other central auditory tests, the ABR is one of the most sensitive measures, if not the most sensitive measure, for auditory dysfunction in patients with MS (Jerger et al., 1986, Musiek et al., 1989). When combined with other tests, however, this procedure can yield an even higher hit rate (Musiek et al., 1989). The present authors posit that the combination of an ABR and a dichotic listening procedure is the best test battery for MS as these tests assess the brainstem pathways as well as the corpus callosum — two regions of the auditory system often involved in MS.

Middle Latency Response. The MLR has been shown to be sensitive to auditory dysfunction related to MS. In fact, a 73% hit rate was reported for MS patients in a rather extensive study (Celebisoy, Aydoğdu, Ekmekçi, & Akürekli, 1996). The MLR can be easily combined with the ABR and can yield many clinical advantages. By combining the ABR and the MLR, a hit rate of 80% was noted for a group of patients with MS (Japaridze, Shakarishvili, & Kevenishvili, 2002). Although more studies need to be done, it appears that the MLR may be a valuable procedure to use in evaluating central auditory integrity in patients with MS, especially if the MLR is combined with the ABR.

Late Potentials (N1, P2, P300)

The N1, P2 waveform complex has had limited use in the evaluation of patients with MS. The studies that were available for review showed a relatively modest hit rate, which would make one ponder the utility of these potentials with this population (Boose & Cranford, 1996; Japaridze et al., 2002). However, the P300 has shown significantly delayed latencies, reduced amplitudes, and even a moderate incidence of absent waveforms for MS patients compared to control groups (Boose & Cranford, 1996; Honig, Ramsay, & Sheremata, 1992; Polich, Romine, Sipe, Aung, & Dalessio, 1992). The key question surrounding these studies is whether the P300 abnormality is related to cognitive decline, delayed (auditory) neural conduction time, or both of these conditions. It may be efficient to record both the N1, P2 wave and P300 simultaneously using a standard oddball paradigm and to compare the results of these auditory evoked potentials, as such a procedure would not significantly increase the testing time and could provide additional data for comparison and analysis.

Behavioral Test Procedures in AD

Dichotic Listening Tests. A number of studies have used the dichotic digits test to measure central auditory dysfunction in patients with AD (Gates et al., 2008; Grimes, Grady, Foster, Sunderland, & Petronas, 1985; Strouse, Hall, & Burger, 1995). Some of these studies have demonstrated significant differences between patients with AD and controls, with the AD population revealing poorer scores for both ears, whereas others have documented asymmetric performance with poorer left ear scores when compared to right ear scores in patients with AD. The dichotic sentence identification (DSI) and staggered spondaic word (SSW) tests also have shown deficits for the AD population compared to control groups (Cooper & Gates, 1991; Gates et al., 2008, Strouse et al., 1995). Given these types of findings, dichotic listening has been considered a useful procedure in evaluating auditory integrity in patients with AD (Gates et al., 2008; Iliadou & Kaprinis, 2003).

Temporal Processing Tests. Strouse and colleagues (1995) also examined the performance of patients with AD on pattern recognition tasks. The results of this study showed that the duration pattern test clearly separated patients with AD from matched controls (i.e., there was a mean difference of more than 30% between the two groups), indicating possible auditory temporal processing deficits in the study's participants with AD. Interestingly, the frequency pattern test did not yield significant differences between the patients with AD and controls in this same study. This finding points to basic differences between these two similar tests of temporal ordering, indicating that the two tests likely are assessing different underlying processes and therefore should not be used interchangeably. To date, there has been limited investigation of the application of temporal processing tests in the assessment of auditory processing in patients with AD and additional investigation in this area is warranted.

Monaural Low Redundancy Speech Tests. The SSI-ICM was one of the early tests employed in measuring central auditory function in AD. This test revealed lower scores for patients with AD when compared to a control group (see Iliadou & Kaprinis, 2003). It also has been demonstrated that for better (easier) signal-to-competition ratios this procedure was not as diagnostically sensitive as it was at poorer signal-to-noise ratios (Strouse et al., 1995).

Binaural Interaction Tests. There is some evidence that binaural interaction processes may be compromised in AD. One study clearly showed a deficit in sound localization for patients with AD compared to controls (Kurylo, Corkin, Allard, Zattore, & Growdon, 1993). This suggests that interaural timing and resolution tests may have applications in the assessment of patients with AD.

Electrophysiologic Tests

Auditory Brainstem Response. As might be expected, AD seems to have little effect on the ABR. However, few data are available in this area. In one study, Irimajiri, Golob, and Starr (2005) showed no shift in wave V latency of the ABR for patients with AD compared to normals.

Middle Latency Response. As was the case with the ABR, few data are available on the results of MLR testing in patients with AD. Based on the limited data available, AD appears to have little influence on the Na, Pa waves, but possibly some abnormalities in the later wave (P1) of the MLR (Green, Elder, & Freed, 1995; Irimajiri et al., 2005).

Late Potentials (N1, P2, P300). For many years and in many studies, the P300 has been shown to be abnormal in many patients with AD (see discussion below), but there are much less compelling data for the N1 and P2 waves. The N1 wave of the N1-P2 complex has been shown to be smaller in subjects with AD when compared to controls (Green et al., 1995; St. Clair, Blackwood, & Christie, 1985). However, there does not appear to be any influence on the latencies of these waves. The P2 also has been shown to be smaller in amplitude in patients with AD (St. Claire et al., 1985).

The P300 has been shown to reveal increased latencies and decreased amplitudes in patients diagnosed with AD (Polich & Corey-Bloom, 2005; St. Clair et al., 1995; and others). Although the P300 is clearly and systematically affected by age, it can still separate patients with AD from the normal aging population, and thus it can be a valuable tool in evaluating AD.

Case 7–3: Multiple Sclerosis

History

This young adult presented with a long-standing history of MS. He had general extremity weakness, blurred vision, ataxia, and slurred speech. He also had long-standing tinnitus on the right side and possible hearing difficulty. The clinical question posed by the patient was whether or not the auditory system was involved, and if it was, whether it was related to his diagnosed medical condition?

Audiology

This patient demonstrated normal pure-tone thresholds and excellent speech recognition ability bilaterally. His tympanograms showed normal pressure, compliance, and shape bilaterally. Contralateral acoustic reflexes were present at normal levels for the left ear, but were absent for the right ear for the frequencies tested (500 to 2000 Hz). Central auditory behavioral test results showed a left ear deficit on dichotic digits and bilateral deficits on frequency patterns, which is a common finding in people with MS—likely due to corpus callosum involvement (Figure 7–3A). Bilateral MLD for a 500 Hz tonal stimulus was 4 dB, which was abnormal (see Figure 7–3A). The ABR results demonstrated presence of the early waves (I and II), but essentially abnormal or absent later waves (III and V) bilaterally (Figure 7–3B). Low repetition rate tracings (top tracings for each ear), as well as high repetition rate tracings (bottom tracings for each ear) were of similar poor morphology. Interestingly, although the ABR was abnormal bilaterally not all of the behavioral tests were, indicating a different underlying physiology for the various tests (see Musiek et al., 1994).

Impression

Central auditory involvement secondary to MS.

Medical Management

The patient was being followed medically for MS.

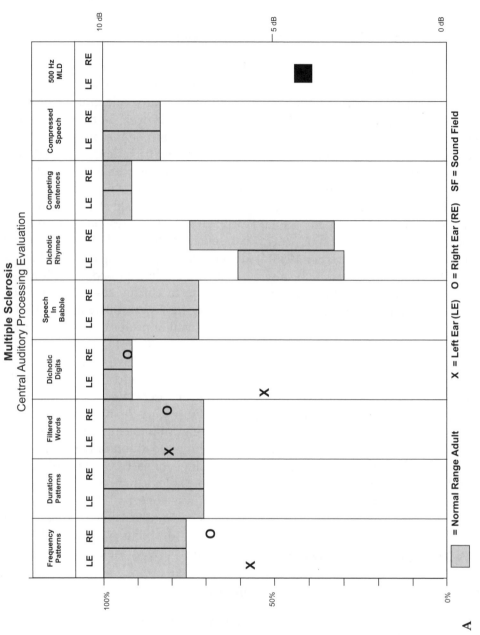

Figure 7–3. *Central behavioral test results (A) and ABR tracings (B) for a young adult with a diagnosis of MS (Case 7–3).* continues

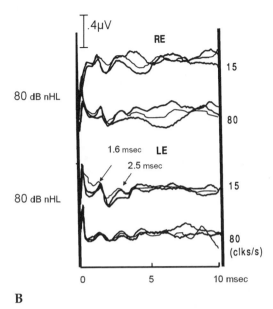

B

Figure 7–3. continued

Audiologic Management

The patient was counseled about the findings, which indicated normal peripheral hearing and likely central auditory involvement. His symptoms were discussed, but no further recommendations were made at that time.

Case 7–4: Alzheimer's Disease

History

This patient, who was in his 70s when he was seen for audiologic evaluation, presented with a previous diagnosis of early Alzheimer's dementia. The patient had complained about hearing difficulties, especially hearing in the presence of background noise, which he reportedly had experienced for a year prior to evaluation. He also complained of minor auditory hallucinations (voices), and was concerned about his hearing. He therefore sought an audiologic evaluation.

Audiology

Except for a mild high-frequency loss in both ears, this patient demonstrated a nearly normal pure-tone audiogram bilaterally. Due to this finding and his auditory complaints, a central assessment was recommended. The central auditory test results showed marked deficits, with a strong laterality effect that would argue for a specific central auditory deficit (Figure 7–4). The left ear deficits on dichotic digits and competing sentences tests, as well as bilateral deficits on a frequency patterns test, could implicate involvement of the corpus callosum (especially in light of the finding of symmetric scores for compressed speech, which is a test that does not require much interhemispheric interaction). In this case, it appeared that the central deficits identified during testing were more significant than the patient's peripheral deficit and certainly would better explain the patient's symptoms.

Impression

A likely central auditory component as a basis for the patient's auditory symptoms, with minimal peripheral involvement.

Medical Management

The patient was being followed for his Alzheimer's disease.

Audiologic Management

The patient was counseled as to the fact that there well could be an auditory component to his communication difficulties. An assistive listening device was considered.

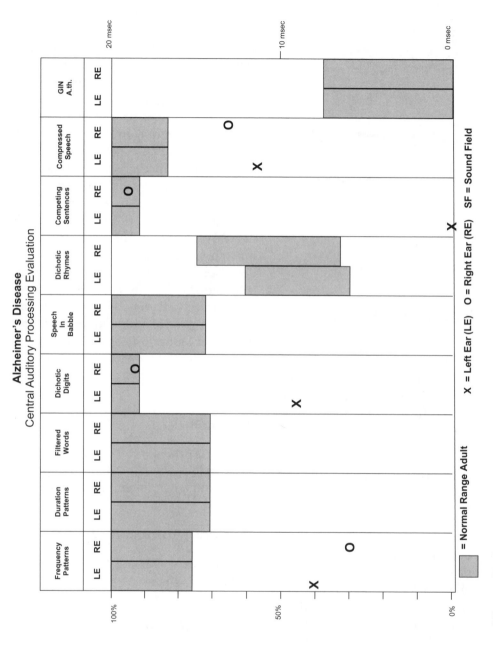

Figure 7–4. *Central behavioral test results for a patient in his mid 70s who was diagnosed with Alzheimer's disease (Case 7–4).*

NEUROTOXICITY

Introduction

Neurotoxicity disorders can affect the CANS and can be caused by both internal and external toxins. Heavy metals such as lead and mercury are commonly considered neurotoxic agents that can affect brain function and exist in the external environment. These agents are ingested or are absorbed into the body and make their way to the brain. Another agent, bilirubin, is an internal chemical agent naturally found in the body; however, high levels of this agent in the body result in a condition known as hyperbilirubinemia, which can cause damage especially to the auditory system (Markowitz, 2006). In addition, a solvent, styrene, has become a consideration in terms of compromising the CANS. In the following discussion, the heavy metals and styrene are discussed, followed by hyperbilirubinemia and kernicterus.

Heavy Metals and Solvents

Symptoms

Heavy metals such as lead and mercury can result in similar symptoms. These neurotoxins can result in hyperactivity, developmental delay, subtle sensory (including hearing problems) and cognitive deficits, ataxia, balance difficulties, and poor motor coordination. When present in children, these symptoms often lead to poor school performance (Markowitz, 2006; Needleman, 2004). Heavy metal poisoning frequently affects children; however, the symptoms may not be readily associated with a neurotoxic etiology as many of the symptoms that result are similar to those noted in other childhood disorders.

Overexposure to the agent, styrene, can affect the central auditory system and result in headache, fatigue, confusion, malaise, and drowsiness. In addition, auditory deficits have been noted in individuals who have been exposed to this particular neurotoxic agent (Campo & Lataye, 2000; Occupational Safety and Health Administration, 2003; Zamyslowska-Szmytke, Fuente, Niebudek-Bogusz, & Sliwinska-Kowalska, 2009).

Incidence and Prevalence

One of the most common age groups in which lead intoxication occurs is 1 to 5 years of age (Lanphear, Dietrich, Auinger, & Cox, 2000). The condition often is the result of children eating lead paint on walls, furniture, and/or toys. Also, children playing on the ground, sidewalks, or near streets with heavy traffic often acquire this condition as exhaust from cars leaves accumulated deposits of lead. In the 1960s, 10 to 20% of inner city children had lead blood levels of 40 µg/dl or greater (Lanphear et al., 2000). A more recent report of lead blood levels in the general school population revealed a prevalence of about 2% of the children with blood levels of higher than 10 µg/dl (Needleman, 2004). Another population exposed to significant amounts of lead includes workers employed in the lead industry, such as those who extract lead from batteries.

Mercury poisoning is rare, but still is a problem in some industrial areas where it is released into the environment from various industrial operations. Fish are exposed to mercury in certain locations, become contaminated, and are then consumed. The most famous occurrence of this was in Japan in the 1950s at Minamata Bay where the fish were contaminated by industrial mercury and consumed by people in the area, with large numbers becoming sick and/or dying from this exposure (Tsubaki & Irukayama, 1977). Today, some people still become sick from eating too much fish that is contaminated with mercury (usually sushi). Coal producing factories and power plants also release considerable amounts of mercury.

In the United States, an estimated 90,000 people are exposed to styrene working in the manufacturing of plastics, rubber, and resin (Campo & Lataye, 2000; Occupational Safety and Health Administration, 2003). These numbers indicate the need for monitoring these workers not only for hearing, but also for other potential health effects.

Etiology and Pathology

There are two kinds of mercury to consider in pathology. Dimethyl and methylmercury have different actions. Dimethyl primarily occupies fatty tissue and by 6 hours has mostly left the body. Methylmercury inhibits protein synthesis specific to certain cells, most commonly cells in the nervous system. This reduction in protein synthesis in turn upsets biochemical pathways and intercommunication among cells, blocking the uptake of calcium, zinc, and iron at nerve terminals (see Musiek & Hanlon, 1999; Ryan, 2005). Lead poisoning also can interfere with myelin formation, integrity of the blood brain barrier, collagen synthesis, and vascular permeability, with most the significant effects on the central nervous system and the kidneys (Needleman, 2004). Some reports relate that lead blood levels of 20 µg/dL are clinically significant (Markowitz, 2006); however, most

effects begin to be noticed at blood levels of 30 to 40 µg/dL.

Styrene can irritate the skin and eyes and affect hearing and vision. There also can be effects on the liver and kidneys. The etiologic actions are not well known and what is known or proposed is complex and beyond the scope of this chapter. Additional information on this topic can be accessed at http://www.cdc.gov/niosh/pdf/83-119b.pdf.

Site of Lesion

As mentioned above, the central nervous system is compromised by high levels of lead, which can slow nerve conduction velocities across multiple systems (Araki, Sato, Yokoyama, & Murata, 2000) (see later discussion in Audiology in Neurotoxic Disorders). Similar site-of-lesion indications are noted for mercury and styrene (Musiek & Hanlon, 1999; Zamyslowska-Szmytke et al., 2009).

Medical Diagnosis

A history of exposure, of course, is key in diagnosis. Beyond this, blood lead and mercury levels must be obtained as well as hair samples, which can be revealing in terms of amount of lead exposure (Mercola, 2008). These assays should be combined with careful neurologic and/or neuropsychological exams to detect subtle systemic and cognitive disorders.

Medical Management

In cases of lead or mercury poisoning, treatment is guided by the levels of lead or mercury in the blood. In cases of lead poisoning, the source of exposure must be determined and eliminated. It is helpful to optimize calcium and iron intake and place the patient on chelation therapy if blood levels are high (e.g., >45 µg/dL, for children), which aids in removing the lead from the blood. The drugs commonly used for this are versenate, succimer, British antilewisite, and penicillamine (Markowitz, 2006). For mercury poisoning, the identification of the source and the arresting of exposure is also key. Chelation therapy for mercury involves chorella, prochitosan, garlic, and cilantro, which function to help in the excretion of mercury through bowel movements. This chelation is commonly supported by mineral replacement (i.e., magnesium, sodium, zinc, etc.) (Mercola, 2008).

Hyperbilirubinemia

The third neurotoxic disorder is hyperbilirubinemia (HB), which is related to high levels of bilirubin in the blood. If left untreated, high levels of bilirubin in the blood can lead to kernicterus, a condition that may cause irreversible brain damage. Jaundice (yellowing of the skin) usually indicates high bilirubin levels and is a condition most often seen in infants. Hyperbilirubinemia (also kernicterus) can damage the central nervous system including the CANS and has a particular affinity for the cochlear nucleus (Dublin, 1976; Mollison & Walker, 1952). For many years, HB has been associated with hearing difficulties, but its mechanisms and type of associated hearing loss often have been misunderstood. In recent years, this disorder has come to the forefront because mothers and newborns often are released from the hospital before HB peaks (usually at about 4 days). If parents are not aware of the symptoms of HB and fail to seek immediate medical evaluation, valuable time can be lost in treating the problem and compromise of the central nervous system can occur.

Symptoms

The symptoms associated with HB depend on the degree of involvement, which can range from mild or subtle to severe. One of the early signs is yellowness of the face and of the whites of the eyes (i.e., jaundice). Hearing difficulties, vestibular problems, lethargy, and poor feeding habits frequently result, and in severe cases, enamel dysplasia of the teeth, hypotonia, and cerebral palsy may occur (the latter symptoms usually are associated with the medical condition known as kernicterus) (Health Topics, University of Virginia, 2008).

Incidence and Prevalence

Approximately 1 to 3 per 100,000 healthy newborns will develop kernicterus from HB if left untreated. About 2% of newborns have total serum bilirubin levels of 20 mg/dl, which is considered clinically significant for HB. However, this does not mean that all of these infants will necessarily manifest symptoms. In fact, if managed appropriately, most of these infants will not develop kernicterus or lasting effects of HB (Newman et al., 1999).

Etiology and Pathology

Shapiro (2003) overviews the etiology/pathology of HB and kernicterus. As mentioned earlier, time of hospital discharge postbirth can be a factor. In addition, infants who are breast-fed have an increased chance of developing HB, as will infants with infections and/or dehydration. Infants with uridine diphosphate glucuronosyltranferase (UDPGT) deficiencies and/or who have Rh-incompatibility may have a greater tendency to develop jaundice leading to HB. These factors can increase the amount of unconjugated bilirubin in the blood and place the infant at risk for developing HB.

The presence of unconjugated bilirubin in the blood is a more significant problem than the presence of conjugated bilirubin. Bilirubin is conjugated by the liver, specifically by the action of UDPGT (from hemoglobin). If the bilirubin is conjugated, it usually can be eliminated via the stool. However, if UDPGT is deficient, the bilirubin remains unconjugated and binds with albumin. When this occurs, the unconjugated bilirubin can cross the blood brain barrier, especially if the blood brain barrier is disrupted, resulting in jaundice and potentially kernicterus. A combination of high bilirubin levels, poor excretion, low intestinal absorption, and a high number of binding agents for albumin (skin, liver, etc.) creates a situation favorable for developing HB. During pregnancy, bilirubin is excreted by the mother, but at birth the infant's liver must assume this role. If the liver cannot effectively excrete the bilirubin, jaundice develops. For these reasons, premature infants have an increased risk of developing jaundice and kernicterus. Bilirubin problems also can affect older children and adults, but are relatively rare.

There are four common etiological bases and/or causes of jaundice. These include: (1) a physiologic condition in which the infant cannot excrete bilirubin for a few days, but then does so without problems; (2) a low calorie intake and/or dehydration condition that occurs in some infants who are fed breast milk; (3) hemolysis, which is a breakdown in red blood cells (Rh disease); and (4) standard jaundice caused by poor liver function (Shapiro, 2003).

Site of Lesion

It is important to realize that HB or kernicterus damages the central nervous system more than the peripheral nervous system (Dublin, 1986; Shapiro, 2003). A number of central nervous system structures can be involved, including the globis pallidus, the subthalamic nuclei, the brainstem nuclei (especially the auditory nuclei), the cerebellum, and the hippocampus. In regard to auditory pathology, the cochlear nuclei, the superior olivary complex, the nuclei of the lateral lemniscus, and the inferior colliculus have all shown pathology. Involvement of the auditory nerve or cochlea is seldom noted (although retrograde degeneration is possible) (Dublin, 1976, 1986).

Medical Diagnosis

A complete history of the course of the disorder with special attention to the duration of the disease and the serum levels of bilirubin are critical components of the medical evaluation. Important are blood tests for bilirubin levels and Rh-incompatibility. Bilirubin levels of 40 mg/dL are definitely too high, 30 mg/dL are of concern but many infants with this level are fine, and levels of 20 to 25 mg/dL are within the alerting range. There have been some data indicating that tissue assays of (unbound) bilirubin may be useful in diagnosis. Also helping in the diagnosis of HB can be the ABR, gaze testing (for nystagmus), tests of muscle tone, and dental abnormalities (Health Topics, University of Virginia, 2008; Shapiro, 2003).

Medical Management

It is important to diagnose the problem early. The main treatment is the use of various forms of phototherapy. Blue spectrum lights work well to degrade bilirubin and fiberoptic blankets allow long duration of light exposure. Of course, in Rh-incompatibility situations, transfusions may be necessary as these drive up the red blood cell count and reduce the bilirubin levels. It also is important to treat any underlying problems such as infections and often it may be necessary to stop breast feeding (Health Topics, University of Virginia, 2008).

AUDIOLOGY AND NEUROTOXINS

A wide variety of neurotoxic substances can compromise the CANS. It is beyond the scope of this section to discuss all of them. It is possible, however, to mention the audiologic correlates to some of the key neurotoxic substances for which there exists a reasonable amount of data. Therefore, we focus on heavy metals (lead and mercury), solvents (styrene), and the organic toxin, bilirubin. It is reasonable to assume that other neurotoxins would likely have similar effects on higher auditory function, although there is not clear evidence of this.

Audiology: Heavy Metals and Solvents

Behavioral Test Procedures

Dichotic Listening Tests. Dichotic digit results were found to be depressed for workers exposed daily to a mixture of xylene, toluene, ketone, and methyl ethyl compared to a nonexposed group of subjects (Fuente & McPherson, 2007a,

2007b). The exposed groups of subjects, however, presented with essentially normal pure-tone thresholds. Similar results on dichotic listening tasks were reported by Varney, Kubu, and Morrow (1998) in their study on workers also exposed to mixed neurotoxic solvents.

Temporal Processing Tests. In a recent study, temporal processing ability was tested using the frequency and duration pattern tests as well as the Gaps-in-Noise (GIN) test on workers exposed to styrene on a daily basis. Other workers not exposed to any solvents served as a control group. The frequency and duration pattern results were found to be reduced for the styrene-exposed group, but the GIN measures were not when pure-tone hearing loss was accounted for by using statistical procedures (Zamyslowska-Szmytke et al., 2009). Fuente and McPherson (2007a, 2007b) reported significantly lower scores for frequency patterns and random gap detection in workers exposed to solvents compared to a control group of workers.

Monaural Low Redundancy Speech Tests. The hearing in noise test (HINT), filtered speech, and interrupted speech tests have all shown lower scores for solvent exposed groups compared to controls (Dietrich, Succop, Berger, & Keith, 1992; Fuente & McPherson, 2006, 2007a, 2007b). These results and the results mentioned earlier indicate the possible use of behavioral central tests to assess central auditory function in these populations.

Electrophysiologic Tests

Auditory Brainstem Response. Perhaps the central auditory test most commonly utilized for heavy metal and solvent exposure has been the ABR. Studies have shown abnormal ABRs, primarily with extended central conduction latencies, for individuals exposed to solvents compared to control groups (see Fuente and McPherson, 2006, for review). Individuals with exposure to lead or mercury also have shown ABRs with abnormal latencies/morphology compared to control groups (Araki et al., 2000; Murata, Weihe, Budtz-Jørgenson, Jørgenson, & Grandjean, 2004; Musiek & Hanlon, 1999). However, there are data showing that abnormal central conduction times on the ABR may be related to the lead blood levels, with only the higher levels (40 ug/dL) showing an effect (Araki et al., 2000). Of interest, is the research of Allen Counter (Counter, 2002), which measured the ABR in lead-glaze workers in South America. These workers have been exposed to lead on a daily basis for years and generations; however, this population showed few, if any, abnormalities on ABRs. Some individuals did show extended central conduction times, but regression analysis showed no correlation between lead blood levels and the wave latencies obtained. Could this study show adaptive effects of the nervous system from constant exposure or do the findings simply represent variability in the neural mechanism measured via ABR? Additional studies would be needed to answer this question.

Late Potentials (N1, P2, P300). The P300 event-related potential seems to dominate the literature in regard to late potential data on heavy metal and solvent exposed individuals. In regard to solvent exposure, the P300 latency has been shown to be prolonged for those having solvent exposure versus control subjects (see Fuente & McPherson, 2006, for review). The P300 also was shown to be extended in latency for workers exposed to lead, and to be correlated with lead levels in the studies reviewed by Araki et al. (2000). In this review, there was evidence to show that, unlike findings for the ABR, even relatively low lead blood levels yielded delayed P300s. Because the P300 data on heavy metal and solvent exposure appear to be compelling, this test should be given serious consideration for inclusion in the evaluation of individuals with these types of exposures. Currently, there is a paucity of data for the N1, P2, and middle latency potentials in exposed populations. Additional data are needed before an informed recommendation regarding the applicability of these potentials in the assessment of patients exposed to toxic substances can be made.

Case 7–5: Mercury Poisoning

History

This case received national media attention when a college professor became ill from mercury poisoning during an accident in a research lab. One of the first symptoms reported following the accident was hearing difficulty, specifically difficulty understanding speech. The patient subsequently began to experience a high-pitched tinnitus in both ears, balance problems, and slurred speech. When we saw this middle-aged patient, her ability to understand speech was diminished to the point that it was necessary for individuals to resort to writing things down to be able to communicate with her.

Audiology

Interestingly, the patient's audiogram showed only a mild high-frequency hearing loss bilaterally; however, speech testing could not be carried out as she could not understand spondees or monosyllabic words at any intensity level presented in either ear (Figure 7–5A). The ABR showed poor waveform morphology for both ears, with what appeared to be severe latency delays for the right ear and essentially a loss of waveforms at high repetition rates bilaterally (Figure 7–5B). Distortion product otoacoustic emissions (DPOAEs) were essentially normal for frequencies 1000 to 4000 Hz bilaterally (Figures 7–5C and 7–5D). Clearly, this case demonstrated a greater central than peripheral effect of the mercury poisoning (see Musiek & Hanlon, 1999, for an in-depth discussion of this case).

Impression

Central auditory involvement likely secondary to mercury poisoning.

Medical Management

The patient was acutely treated for mercury poisoning, but to no avail.

Audiology: Hyperbilirubinemia

Introduction

Excess of bilirubin in the brain can be neurotoxic as mentioned earlier in this chapter. Audiologic considerations are many. One is that, most of the time, this condition occurs early in life; therefore, only limited testing can be completed. In some cases, the effect on auditory function remains and can manifest itself as an auditory processing disorder. An important consideration is that, as shown earlier, HB compromises primarily the CANS and not the auditory nerve or the cochlea

(Dublin, 1986). Therefore, with HB as an etiology, the term auditory neuropathy should be used restrictively even though many of the reports on auditory neuropathy include children with HB (see Rapin & Gravel, 2003). Because the primary effects of high bilirubin levels are on brain nuclei, it is and should be classified as a central auditory disorder. As Dublin (1986) relates, HB has a particular affinity for damaging the cochlear nucleus.

Electroacoustic and Electrophysiologic Tests

Auditory Brainstem Response. The ABR should be abnormal in patients with HB. Given the main effect is on auditory nuclei in the brainstem, early waves may be present (if peripheral hearing is adequate) and the later waves (III, IV, V) may be delayed, absent, or reduced (Shapiro & Hecox, 1988). It is possible that even the early ABR waves (I and II) could be absent if there is considerable hearing loss, or if there is retrograde degeneration of the auditory nerve from the cochlear nucleus. Therefore, it is possible that HB could yield a "no response" ABR (and as a result, be difficult to discern from auditory neuropathy). It is important to realize that not all infants with high bilirubin levels will yield abnormal ABRs as even some with severe involvement have been shown to have normal ABRs (Rhee, Park, & Jang, 1999).

Electrocochleography (ECochG). In cases of HB, the cochlear microphonic (CM) should be recordable unless there is coexisting severe damage to the cochlea. By changing polarity, the CM, if present, should reverse polarity, which is a procedure that can be used to help define the CM (Akman et al., 2004).

Disorder: Neurotoxicity (Mercury Poisoning)

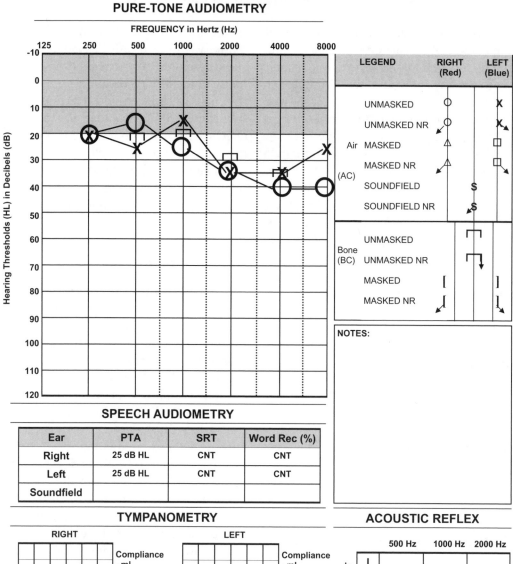

Figure 7–5. *Pure–tone thresholds and speech audiometry test results (**A**), ABR tracings (**B**), and DPOAEs (**C** and **D**) for a patient diagnosed with mercury poisoning (Case 7–5). Note: the dark lines on (C) and (D) represent the normative criteria used to differentiate normal versus abnormal DPOAE amplitude measures. (Reproduced with permission from Musiek, F. E., & Hanlon, D. P.* [1999]. *Neuroaudiological effects in a case of fatal dimethylmercury poisoning.* Ear and Hearing, *20(3), 271–275.) continues*

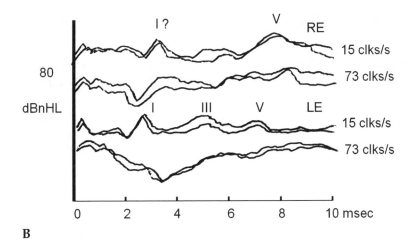

B

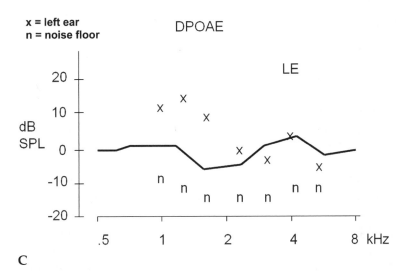

C

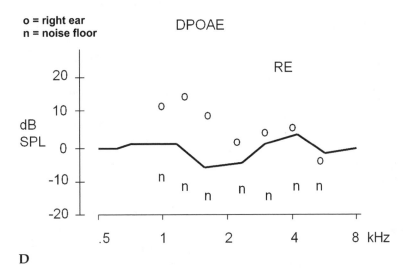

D

Figure 7–5. continued

Acoustic Reflexes and Otoacoustic Emissions. Acoustic reflex thresholds generally are absent or elevated in HB due to the brainstem involvement. Otoacoustic emissions should be normal unless there is coexisting cochlear involvement.

TRAUMA, HEAD INJURY (TRAUMATIC BRAIN INJURY, TBI)

Introduction

Earlier in this book, there were sections devoted to trauma to the peripheral auditory system. In this chapter, the focus is on trauma that may affect the CANS. The National Center for Injury Prevention and Control of the Centers for Disease Control and Prevention (2010) relates that head injury or traumatic brain injury (TBI) is caused by a jolt or blow to the head. It also can result from a penetrating head injury (i.e., a bullet wound). These injuries can result in mild to severe symptoms, which occur along a continuum with symptoms ranging from mild, brief changes in mental status to a severe alteration in mental functions where the affected individuals may experience a period of unconsciousness or amnesia. Along with these alterations are other dysfunctions that involve motor and sensory systems. Synonyms often used for head injury are head trauma, concussion, traumatic brain injury, and intracranial injury.

Symptoms

As noted above, the symptoms related to head injury can range from subtle to severe. In some cases, the symptoms related to a head injury will not appear until days or even weeks after the injury. Some of the more common symptoms are headaches and a neck pain that does not subside after a reasonable period of time. Also, difficulty remembering and/or concentrating, slowness in speaking, thinking, acting, and reading, and confusion are symptoms of concern following a head injury. In addition, after hitting one's head, extreme tiredness, mood changes, and poor sleep patterns may evolve. Sensory symptoms such as dizziness, poor balance, hypersensitivity to sounds and light, and decreased sensitivity for smell and taste can occur secondary to head injury. In addition, difficulty hearing in background noise and tinnitus, can be symptoms related to head injury (National Center for Injury Prevention and Control, Centers for Disease Control and Prevention, 2010). Of course, the nature of these symptoms is related to the specific locus of the head injury's effects on the brain. One has to consider that, in most cases of head injury, it is possible that more than one system may be involved and therefore multiple symptoms often appear.

Incidence and Prevalence

Head injury is a common disorder. Approximately 1.4 million cases of head injury are reported per year in the United States. Of these 1.4 million, 1.1 million are treated and released from the emergency rooms around the country (National Center for Injury Prevention and Control, Centers for Disease Control and Prevention, 2010). The same source relates that approximately 50,000 individuals per year die from head injury in the United States. An at-risk population to consider is our service men and women in the Middle East where blast injuries are unfortunately all too common. In regard to the general population, head injury is a result of falls in about 28% of the cases, with motor vehicle accidents following at 20%. Events that result in a person being struck by or thrown against something or someone, such as in sports, have a 19% incidence, and assaults make up 11% of the total head injuries in the United States (National Center for Injury Prevention and Control, 2010).

Etiology and Pathology

In head injuries, several stages of pathologic activity can unfold after the incident. The immediate insult is one that is mechanical, that is, direct tissue damage as a result of the brain being accelerated and decelerated quickly, which means the tissue can be expanded. These mechanical mechanisms can cause tearing and/or stretching of neural tissue and may contribute to tissue displacement and shearing forces, which can result in hemorrhage. Impaired cerebral blood flow (CBF) and altered tissue metabolism are likely actions in head injury. From a vascular perspective, there can be a series of events that can create problems. There can be hemorrhage and hyperfusion or hypofusion to involved tissue. Often, CBF autoregulation is impaired and cerebral vasospasm can occur. Additionally, oxygen and glucose metabolism can be affected by head injury, which can result in a host of problems. Soon after the injury, edema and inflammation can evolve causing serious symptoms. If these conditions are not ameliorated, necrosis and apoptosis (cell death) ensues (Werner & Engelhard, 2007).

Analysis of head injuries from blasts have revealed that diffuse axonal injury often happens in the frontotemporal areas, the internal capsule, the deep gray matter, the upper brainstem, and the corpus callosum. Contusions of the brain commonly happen in the superficial gray matter, and can affect the inferior, lateral, and anterior frontal and temporal lobes. Subdural hematomas seem to occur at the convexities of the frontal and parietal lobes (Taber, Warden, & Hurley, 2006). From the information just presented, it is obvious that, from an anatomic perspective, the auditory system often is involved and therefore requires careful assessment.

Medical Diagnosis

Medical diagnosis is dependent on report of the actual incident, quick assessment of mental status, and whether or not consciousness was lost and for how long. For more involved cases, such measures as the Glasgow Coma Scale (GCS), which yields mild, moderate, or severe classifications, may be used. The GCS grades the level of consciousness on scale ranging from 3 to 15 using verbal, motor, and eye-opening responses to stimuli as an index (13–15 = mild, 9–12 = moderate, 3–8 = severe). There also are classifications for posttraumatic amnesia from less than an hour to more than a day and for loss of consciousness related to the duration of unconsciousness from less than 30 minutes to more than 24 hours (Saatman et al., 2008; Valadka, 2004). Use of evoked potentials can also contribute to diagnosis (see discussion below).

Medical Management

Medical management of patients with head injuries can be highly varied depending on the type and severity of the injury, making it difficult to cover in a concise fashion. Acutely, neurosurgical procedures to release intracranial pressure, arrest bleeding, and repair tissue are all possibilities. Less acute management may include management of symptoms (i.e., seizure, pain, etc.). Rest is often key as well as specialized therapies of all types. Also important is patient and family education for overall optimum management and accommodation (Martin, Lu, Helmick, French, & Warden, 2008).

Audiology

Head injury or traumatic brain injury (TBI) are terms that by their core meaning indicate possible damage to the central nervous system. The CANS therefore must be considered a potential site of involvement in patients presenting with head injuries. Although this seems obvious, many who evaluate patients with head injuries seem to ignore this obvious fact. Head injury, like other disorders that affect the CANS such as strokes, tumors, and degenerative and developmental disorders, is more likely to compromise the higher auditory system, although involvement of the lower CANS can result. Although head injury has its own unique set of circumstances in the onset and evolution of the problem, it has many similarities to other CANS disorders. Disruption of appropriate neural function in the CANS in head injury is secondary to pathophysiologic factors such as immediate mechanical displacement and torquing of tissue, stretching and tearing of neurons and blood vessels, and, later, edema, reduced circulation, demyelination, and overall degeneration of affected neural substrate (Musiek et al., 1994). The degree of involvement depends on the severity and nature of the blow, the areas affected, and the subsequent care received. There has been a recent increase in the interest

in head injury because of its incidence in veterans returning with such injuries from the Middle East.

The degree of central auditory involvement depends on whether or not the auditory tracts are involved. There are data showing a relatively high incidence of either peripheral or central deficits (68%) in head injury populations (Bergemalm & Borg, 2001). It must also be realized that many individuals with head injury have a number of other nonauditory problems such as attention, memory, and emotional factors that can influence auditory assessment.

Behavioral Test Procedures

Dichotic Listening Tests. There is a reasonable amount of data on dichotic listening and head injury. It appears that left ear deficits on dichotic listening tests are common among patients with head injury. This is likely related to the stress placed on the corpus callosum during head trauma (Levin et al., 1989). Meyers and associates (Meyers et al., 2002) reported a 60% sensitivity and a 100% specificity for a population with mild brain injury using a dichotic word test. Significant ear asymmetry with left ear performance poorer than right ear performance also was reported for school-age children with head injury compared to normal data. In the normal population, the difference between ears yielded a modest right ear advantage, whereas the head injury population revealed nearly a 40% performance advantage for the right ear (Benavidez et al., 1999). Ear asymmetry appears to be related to the severity of the injury as noted on radiology (Levin et al., 1989). It appears that both cortical and brainstem damage from trauma can yield abnormal dichotic listening results; however, only a few cases of brainstem involvement have been reported (Musiek et al., 1994; Pinheiro, Jacobson, & Boller, 1982).

Temporal Processing Tests. There is a paucity of reports on various temporal processing tests and head injury. Pinheiro et al. (1982) showed deficits for brainstem involvement on auditory patterns, and deficits have been shown for cortical injury (Musiek et al., 1994, Musiek, Baran, & Shinn, 2004). However, normal findings have also been reported for patients with head injury on an auditory pattern perception test (Musiek et al., 2004). The results reported above were essentially based on the assessment of individual cases; therefore, the findings must be interpreted with proper caution. With timing being critical for temporal tests, logically, it would be appealing to utilize these procedures for patients with head injury; however, more investigation is required before a recommendation of routine application of these procedures to the head injury population can be made.

Binaural Interaction Tests. Similar to temporal processing tests, little data are available on head injury and binaural interaction tests. However, a critically important study completed many years ago may provide some insights in terms of the kinds of procedures that may be useful. Lackner and Teuber (1973) employed a binaural click fusion task with subjects with head injury. Two clicks, with one presented to the right ear and one to the left ear, were separated by a varying interstimulus interval. When the clicks were perceived as one stimulus, the result was considered as the subject's fusion threshold. Click fusion thresholds were significantly higher for the head injury group than for the control group. This group difference was especially noted for individuals with left hemisphere involvement.

Based on the available evidence, this procedure seems both valid and powerful and should be reintroduced in clinical audiology.

Electrophysiologic Tests

Auditory Brainstem Response. The ABR has been a key test for individuals with head injury. The generators of the ABR are the auditory nerve and brainstem tracts. Therefore, these anatomic loci are best evaluated by this test. The brainstem is commonly involved in head trauma from blast injuries (Taber et al., 2006). Three key investigations have shown approximately a 50% hit rate for ABR and head injury of a mild degree (Bergemalm & Borg, 2001; Gaetz & Bernstein 2001; Rowe & Carlson, 1980). Other studies have reported a slightly poorer hit rate (McClelland, Fenton, & Rutherford, 1994; Schoenhuber, Gentilini, & Orlando, 1988). The ABR diagnostic index that shows the highest sensitivity is the I–V interwave interval reflecting mostly central conduction time (Bergemalm & Borg, 2001). Although high repetition rate ABRs have not always reflected a diagnostic advantage for many clinical populations with CANS compromise, in patients with head injury, it appears that they could be worthwhile (Soustiel, Hafner, Chistyakov, Barzilai, & Feinsod, 1995). If the value of the ABR for assessment of patients with head injury is established, maximum length sequences (MLS) techniques, which permit high rates of stimulation using the ABR, could be of value and should be investigated.

Middle Latency Response. Generators of the MLR are located in the thalmocortical auditory tracts of the CANS. This is rostral to the ABR generators and, hence, an important supplement to the

ABR for investigating the effects of head injury. The MLR can be recorded simultaneously with the ABR, which provides an efficient diagnostic advantage in determining the site of involvement. The MLR has not been investigated as much as the ABR in patients with head injury. However, significant differences for Na, Pa amplitude and latency between controls and mild head injury groups have been reported (Drake, Weate, & Newell, 1996; Soustiel et al., 1995). In addition, totally absent MLRs (6 out of 20) have been shown in subjects with head injury. Certainly, more research on the MLR and head injury is indicated, especially when it is combined with the ABR, which could yield a powerful diagnostic index.

Late Evoked Potentials (N1, P2, P300). The N1 and P2 late potentials are generated by the primary auditory cortex and regions close to it in humans. The P300 likely is generated by a number of areas in the brain including the primary auditory areas. The N1, P2 track record for use in head injury is somewhat mixed. Drake, Weat, Andrews, and Castleberry (1996) reported N1 to be significantly delayed for patients with mild head injuries compared to controls. Jones et al. (2000) found that almost 90% of postcomatose patients with head injury demonstrated abnormal N1, P2 responses. Conversely, Harris and Hall (1990) and Segalowitz, Bernstein, and Lawson (2001) related that the N1 and P2 late responses from patients with head injury did not differ significantly from those of their control group. Other studies have also shown this variance in findings for TBI. The findings for the P300; however, do not appear to have this variability.

The P300 has been shown to be significantly sensitive to mild head injury in a number of studies (see Segalowitz et al., 2001). It may be the most useful evoked potential procedure for defining head injury and can be applied across modalities, which can be useful in identifying the site of lesion (Lew, Lee, Pan, & Date, 2004).

Case 7–6: Head Injury

History

This teenager was referred by his pediatrician for an audiologic evaluation. About 3 weeks before he was seen for his audiologic appointment he fell while snowboarding, hitting the back of his head and rendering him unconscious for several minutes. He was taken to a local hospital and released after medical evaluation. However, in a day or two he began noticing difficulty hearing. During his audiologic evaluation, he reported that music sounded strange and distorted (described as being "robotic in nature") and that he was experiencing trouble understanding speech. He claimed his right ear was poorer than his left ear, but that neither ear was "normal." An MRI done at the hospital was normal.

Audiology

A pure-tone audiogram showed normal hearing thresholds at the octave frequencies from 250 to 8000 Hz bilaterally, and speech recognition scores were 100% and 96% for left and right ears, respectively. Tympanograms were of normal pressure, shape, and compliance bilaterally.

Central auditory testing included dichotic digits, frequency patterns, compressed speech, and dichotic rhymes and test results were all within normal limits bilaterally (Figure 7–6A). The ABR, however, was clearly abnormal (Figure 7–6B).

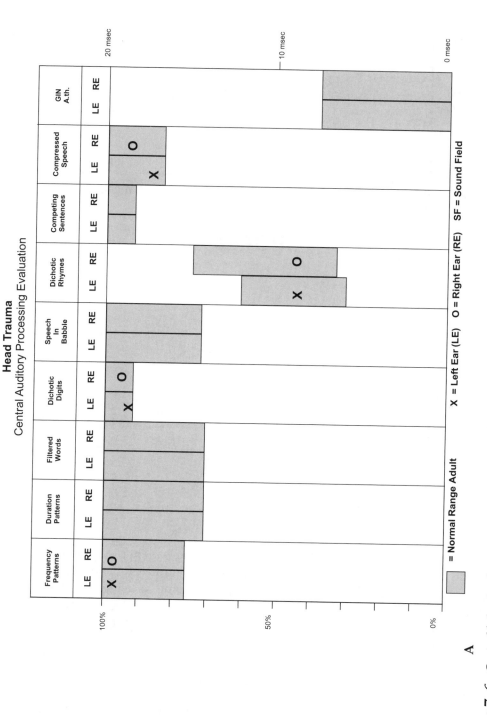

Head Trauma
Central Auditory Processing Evaluation

Figure 7–6. *Central behavioral test results (A), ABR tracings (B), and DPOAEs (C) for a teenager who sustained a head injury (Case 7–6). Key for (B): HR = high repetition rate of 79.3 clicks per second, top tracing shows latencies for waves I, III, V in msec., 4th tracing shows latency of wave V in msec. Key for (C): X = left ear, O = right ear, n = averaged noise floor for both the right and left ears, dark line = normative criteria used to differentiate normal versus abnormal DPOAE amplitude measures. continues*

ABR

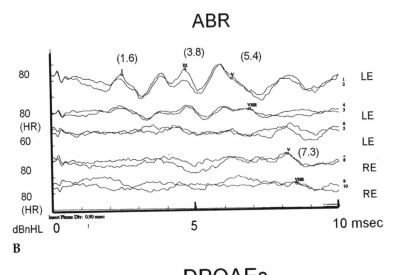

B

DPOAEs

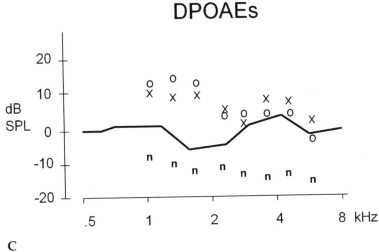

C

Figure 7–6. continued

The left ear showed normal findings at both low and high repetition rates, but was abnormal at 60 dB nHL with a questionable response being observed. In the right ear, the early waves were absent with a severely delayed wave V noted at a low repetition rate. At a high repetition rate, there was essentially no response for the right ear. Distortion product otoacoustic emissions were essentially normal bilaterally (Figure 7–6C). Although many of the tests were normal, the ABR was con-

sistent with the patient's symptoms and revealed poor auditory function. This case portrays the value of using both behavioral and electrophysiologic approaches to diagnostic testing in patients at risk for CANS disorders.

Impression

This patient likely had central auditory involvement secondary to head trauma. He steadily improved following his audiologic evaluation and in about a month all symptoms had disappeared and an ABR test administered at that time showed essentially normal waveforms bilaterally.

TEMPORAL LOBE EPILEPSY

Introduction

Temporal lobe epilepsy (TLE) is a specific type of epilepsy. The reason TLE is addressed here is that it is a seizure of the temporal lobe that is located in an anatomic region of the brain, which is likely to lead to dysfunction of the central auditory system. Of the various seizure disorders, one that is especially relevant here is Landau-Kleffner syndrome, again because it often manifests auditory symptoms.

Epilepsy, in general, is considered a brain disorder. This disease is characterized by the abnormal firing of clusters of nerve cells, which results in unusual sensations, perceptions, behaviors, and motor activity. Temporal lobe epilepsy can broadly be divided into two major anatomic areas: (1) the mesial temporal lobe, which includes the hippocampus and amygdala; and (2) the lateral temporal lobe, which is the surface of the temporal lobe. A seizure focus in either of these sites may affect the auditory areas as the abnormal firing of cells often spreads to adjacent areas resulting in symptoms.

Symptoms

Three classifications of epilepsy are defined by Commission on Classification and Terminology of International League Against Epilepsy (1981). One classifica-

tion is simple partial seizures, which are defined by involvement of small areas of the brain with seizures that do not result in the loss of consciousness. This type is associated with sensations that are dependent on the area affected (i.e., sounds, images, unusual tastes and smells, etc., or focal motor activity). A second category is complex partial seizures, which impair consciousness to some extent. The area involved here is larger than in the previous classification. This category often is characterized by motionless staring, automatic movements of the hands, mouth, and unusual speech utterances. The third category is generalized tonic clonic seizures, which involve the loss of consciousness, the stiffening of the trunk, and subsequent jerking movements involving much of the body. This type of seizure has a large spread of activity to adjacent and even remote regions of the brain.

If the seizure activity affects auditory areas, often auras (sensations preceding the seizure) of sounds occur. Seizures do damage underlying neural substrate; hence, if auditory tissue is damaged, then auditory symptoms such as trouble hearing in noise can evolve.

Of special interest is Landau-Kleffner syndrome. This is where the seizure focus is at or near the auditory cortex. It is notable for mild, simple, absence (very subtle) seizures that often go unnoticed. It is characterized by an arrest of language development and a deterioration of speech often secondary to auditory compromise. It usually manifests at 1½ to 3 years of age, but can occur at any age. Toddlers with Landau-Kleffner syndrome usually have inconsistent responses to sound and some are even thought to be "deaf." Older individuals who have this disorder are more easily diagnosed due to their obvious communication difficulties (Sotero de Menezes, 2007).

Incidence and Prevalence

Almost 3 million people in the United States have epilepsy (Epilepsy Foundation of America, 2010). About 50% have partial epilepsy and most of these have TLE; however, the true prevalence (or incidence) is not known. It has been reported that about 10 new cases of Landau-Kleffner syndrome (in the United States) are documented each year; however, many more cases are believed to exist which are not documented (Berg, Shinnar, Levy, & Testa, 1999; Bronen, 2000; Perkins, 2002).

Etiology and Pathology

Epilepsy can have many causes, including genetic mutations in ion channels, focal brain injuries (due to prior insults such as stroke or infection), and metabolic disease, although the cause is not known in many cases. As stated earlier, epilepsy results in the abnormal firing of nerve cells. Heredity also may play a role in regard to susceptibility of the disease. Other conditions associated with this disorder are meningitis, encephalitis (such as herpes encephalitis), vascular malformations, head injury, and mass lesions. It is fair to say that the greater the involvement of a given lesion, the great the possibility of seizure disorder (Berg et al., 1999; Bronen, 2000; Perkins, 2002). Sclerosis (scarring) of the medial temporal lobe often is seen in TLE but it is unclear if this is a cause or an effect of the epilepsy.

Medical Diagnosis

Temporal lobe epilepsy or epilepsy in general is medically diagnosed by using some key procedures. Besides an in-depth neurologic and family history, EEGs and EEG monitoring over a 24- to 48-hour period will determine if there are aberrant neural discharges from the brain and where the main epileptic focus is located if aberrant discharges are detected. The EEG also can provide insight as to the spread of epileptic activity. This is especially important if the seizure activity spreads across the corpus callosum to the opposite hemisphere. Radiologic procedures such as CT, PET, MRI, fMRI, and SPECT are commonly used to document other possible factors that may have contributed to the epilepsy. Other factors could include temporal lobe sclerosis, trauma, vascular problems, and so forth that could be triggering the seizure disorder. A variety of blood tests can be done to check for heavy metal poisoning, anemia, and diabetes, which also can be linked to epilepsy. In addition, developmental and genetic testing for children, as well as a host of neurologic and behavioral tests can be used (Perkins, 2002). Finally, individuals with TLE should undergo central auditory testing to determine if the auditory system has been compromised (Kwan & Brodie, 2000; Perkins, 2002).

Medical Management

Medical management of TLE falls into two main categories: medical and surgical. Medications are commonly used in an attempt to decrease the excitation level of the neurons in the brain by blocking sodium or calcium channels. Examples of some of these drugs include: phenytoin, carbamazepine, valpoate, phenobarbital, and some newer drugs such as gabapentin, lamotrigine, and topiramate. The newer drugs have a better side effect profile; hence, they recently have gained popularity (Perkins, 2002).

Surgery usually is reserved for cases where medications fail. The essence of the surgical procedures is to excise the area of the brain that is responsible for the abnormal EEG activity. Temporal lobectomies are performed for TLE, and of course, there is a possibility of central auditory compromise that should be checked. If the TLE has or could spread to the other hemisphere, commissurotomy or split-brain surgery can be considered. This may prevent the spread of epilepsy, but can have consequences for proper interhemispheric interaction, including the interaction between the important areas of the auditory system (Musiek et al., 1994; Perkins, 2002).

Audiology

In terms of anatomic locus, the temporal lobe is a common site for the focus of epilepsy. Because it also is the key lobe involved in auditory processing, there is a probable relationship between central hearing deficits and epilepsy. Seizure disorders can damage underlying neural tissue resulting in degeneration and even sclerosis (see earlier comments). If the seizure focus is in auditory regions, it is likely that central auditory dysfunction may result. An even bigger issue is that sometimes epilepsy requires surgery of the underlying tissue, such as temporal lobectomy and/or commissurotomy. When surgery is to be done, it is critical that the CANS be tested before and after this surgery, especially when significant auditory neural tissue is to be removed.

Behavioral Test Procedures

Dichotic Listening Tests. Dichotic speech tests generally demonstrate sig-

nificant deficits for TLE when compared to controls (Gramstad, Engelsen, & Hugdahl, 2006; Roberts, Varney, Paulsen, & Richardson, 2004). Another trend is that, when the epilepsy is confined to one hemisphere, the contralateral ear is most often affected (Gramstad et al., 2006). Various kinds of dichotic tests including dichotic digits, staggered spondaic words (SSW), and CVs have been administered to patients with epilepsy, with the results documenting poorer scores in the experimental group than in controls and left ear scores that are poorer than right ear scores (Collard, 1984). Dichotic listening has been shown to reflect improvement when patients are given anticonvulsant therapies or when the seizure activity was reduced (Musiek, Bromley, Roberts, & Lamb, 1990; Roberts et al., 1990).

Temporal Processing Tests. Brief tone audiometry, using Békésy tracking procedures, did not show any significant shift in thresholds between patients with seizures and controls. However, there was a difference in the excursions noted for brief tones (20 ms) compared to long duration tones (500 ms) between the two groups (Collard, 1984). Duration patterns were found to be reduced bilaterally for patients with seizure disorders compared to controls in a recent study (Meneguello, Leonhardt, & Pereira, 2006).

Electrophysiologic Tests

Some important evoked potential studies have been performed on patients with TLE. Soysal and colleagues (2002) demonstrated that P2, N2, and P3 (P300) waves were all delayed in latency for a large group of patients diagnosed with epilepsy compared to a control group. Interestingly, amplitudes were also lower for the epileptic group, but the differences did not reach statistical significance. Verma, Twitty, and Fuerst (1993) were interested in using evoked potentials for lateralizing the seizure focus. They concluded that N1 and P2 were better than the P3 (P300) for lateralizing information, but even these potentials were not consistently accurate for lateralization of the epileptic focus. Other studies have not shown the N1 and P2 or P3 (P300) to be sensitive to seizure lesions (Boutras, Elger, Kurthen, & Rosburg, 2006; Chayasirisobhon et al., 2007). The P50 response has been shown to exhibit delayed latencies and smaller amplitudes for seizure patients compared to controls in one large study (Drake et al., 1995), but not so in another investigation (Boutros et al., 2006).

Case 7–7: Temporal Lobe Epilepsy

History

This young adult had a long history of seizure disorder with its locus in the right temporal lobe near Heschl's gyrus. There were minimal hearing complaints. The patient was being considered for possible surgery to control seizures and therefore was being seen for a preoperative audiologic evaluation.

Audiology

Pure-tone thresholds were within the normal range for the octave frequencies between 250 to 8000 Hz and speech recognition scores were excellent bilaterally. Behavioral central auditory tests, including dichotic digits and dichotic rhyme tests, revealed reduced scores in the ear contra-lateral to the lesioned hemisphere when compared to the scores noted in the ear ipsilateral to the lesion site (Figure 7–7A). The late auditory evoked potentials (N1 and P2; traced from the originals) showed poor morphology except for the right ear at C3 (Figure 7–7B). The next best recordings were from the left ear also at the C3 electrode site (this electrode site was over the healthy or unaffected hemisphere), and the poorest recordings were from the C4 site over the involved hemisphere (see Figure 7–7B). As can be seen, all of these recordings are noisy with poor replicability.

Medical Management

At last contact with the patient he had not undergone surgery as he and his parents were still considering various options for the control of the seizure disorder.

SURGICAL INTERVENTION THAT ALTERS CENTRAL AUDITORY FUNCTION

Temporal lobe epilepsy leads into another topic of interest. As mentioned earlier, epilepsy sometimes is treated by temporal lobectomy or commissurotomy (i.e., sectioning the corpus callosum). These procedures can have rather marked consequences for central auditory function. Considerable data have been generated on central auditory deficits associated with temporal lobectomy and split-brain surgery. The closer the surgical sectioning to the primary auditory areas, the greater the deficit and vice versa, and this needs to be kept in mind when reviewing these types of studies (see Oxbury & Oxbury, 1969).

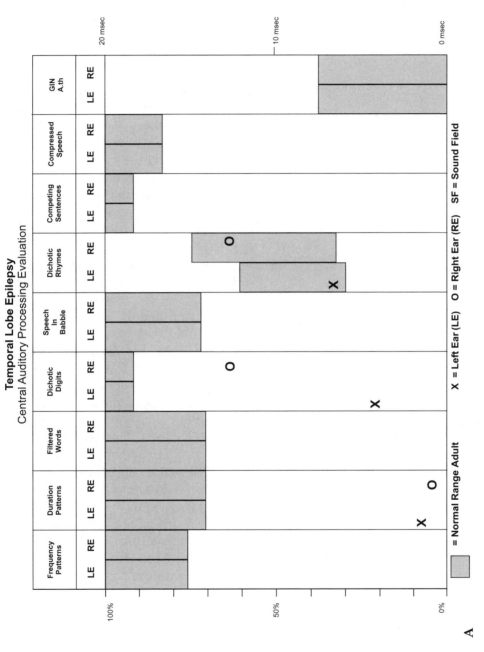

Figure 7–7. *Central behavioral test results (A) and P1, N1, and P2 cortical auditory evoked potentials (smoothed and retraced) (B) for a young adult with temporal lobe epilepsy (Case 7–7). (Note: C3 and C4 = electrode sites). continues*

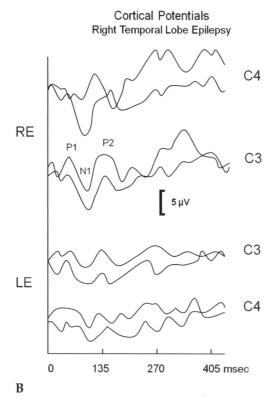

Cortical Potentials
Right Temporal Lobe Epilepsy

RE

P1 P2

N1

C4

C3

5 µV

C3

LE

C4

0   135   270   405 msec

B

Figure 7–7. continued

Temporal Lobectomy

Behavioral Tests

Dichotic Listening Tests. In temporal lobectomy, dichotic listening results showed deficits (often severe) in the ear opposite the side of the temporal lobectomy (Oxbury & Oxbury, 1969). In some situations, excision of part of the temporal lobe does not create large deficits. In one study utilizing the SSW and dichotic CVs, there were no significant differences between pre- and postoperative results for the left ear, but there were for the right ear and for the difference between ears (Collard et al., 1986). There is some evidence that left temporal lobe excisions result in

greater deficits than those in the right hemisphere (Bougeard & Fischer, 2002). These types of comparisons, however, suffer from the high probability that the lesions studied were not equivalent and therefore the results must be cautiously interpreted.

Temporal Processing Tests. There is a paucity of information on temporal processing functions and temporal lobectomy. There was, however, a key study reported on anterior temporal lobectomy (ATL) and gap detection. In this study, gap intervals in noise were significantly longer for those with ATL than for the control group. In addition, it appeared that the greater deficit was contralateral to the lesioned hemisphere (Efron et al., 1985). This study raises the issue that these patients may have temporal resolution problems and that the anterior temporal lobe possibly may play a role in auditory processing. Another study revealed problems in musical timbre perception in general, and more specifically on a subtest of multidimensional scaling, among patients with temporal lobotomies compared to controls. This procedure was complex and a full description of the procedure is beyond the scope of what can be reported here. However, it is interesting to note that, depending on which particular subtest was given, the right hemisphere (when compromised) seemed to have considerable influence on performance (Samson, Zatorre, & Ramsey, 2002).

Electrophysiologic Tests

Like temporal processing, there is limited information on the results of evoked potential testing in individuals who have undergone temporal lobectomies. The MLR Na wave has been shown to be delayed across Cz, C5, and C6 electrode sites in patients with ATL compared to controls. Also, interestingly, the NaPa amplitude was found to be greater after surgery (at the same electrode positions) than it was prior to surgery (Jacobson, Privitera, Neils, Grayson, & Yeh, 1990). In a case study, P300 amplitude was decreased after temporal lobectomy, but returned to near preoperative values 2 weeks after surgery (Hirayasu, Ohta, Fukao, Ogura, & Mukawa, 1995). In another case study, N1, P2, and P3 (P300) evoked potentials actually increased in amplitude and decreased in latency after surgery (Musiek, Bromley, et al., 1990). In this case, it was hypothesized that reducing the seizure disturbance allowed the evoked potential responses to become more synchronous, allowing more of the generators to respond appropriately.

Commissurotomy

The next major surgical intervention, also for intractable seizures, is commissurotomy or split-brain surgery. This surgical procedure is done to prevent epilepsy from spreading from one hemisphere to the other. Much has been written about these cases and their deficits, but only a thumbnail sketch is offered here. Of note is that only certain audiologic tests will show deficits in these kinds of patients. The most heralded is dichotic listening. The other, although not as profound, is certain types of pattern perception. Other diagnostic tests, which do not engage (at least to a high degree) the corpus callosum, do not show deficits and can be utilized to rule in or out hemispheric or subcortical involvement (see Baran & Musiek, 1999).

Behavioral Tests

Dichotic Listening Tests. As is now well known, commissurotomy results in severe left ear deficits in these patients. Although not a consistent finding, in some patients, the right ear performance actually improves after surgery (Musiek et al., 1984). Auditory deficits can be demonstrated only if the posterior half of the corpus callosum is sectioned as that is where the auditory fibers cross from one hemisphere to the other (Baran, Musiek, & Reeves, 1986). Severe dichotic left ear deficits and normal performance on other central tests such as filtered speech and speech in noise help make the diagnosis of callosal involvement.

Temporal Processing Tests. The frequency pattern perception test yields a bilateral deficit (for verbal report) in split-brain patients (Musiek et al., 1980). This is because both hemispheres are needed to decode and verbally report the pattern. Often, there can be asymmetry, but both ears will yield performance below the normal range.

Monaural Low Redundancy Speech Tests. Tests such as filtered speech, compressed speech, and speech in noise are typically not affected by sectioning of the corpus callosum. These tests usually yield normal or near-normal performance bilaterally. This is important to know because these kinds of tests help in determining if left ear deficits are related to right hemisphere involvement or corpus callosum compromise. That is, if the monaural speech test (as well as dichotic tests) shows a left ear deficit, then it is likely that the right hemisphere is involved. However, if the monaural speech test is normal and the dichotic test shows a left ear deficit, then it is likely that the corpus callosum is not transferring information appropriately.

Electrophysiologic Tests

Few studies have been conducted in patients with commissurotomy. Probably the most cited is a study by Kutus, Hillyard, Volpe, and Gazzaniga (1990). This study showed that, for N2 and P3 (P300) evoked potentials, split-brain patients showed smaller potentials over the left hemisphere compared to the right for the P3 (P300). Also, when compared to the control subjects, the evoked potentials were smaller for the patients who had undergone commissurotomy. However, as mentioned previously, these smaller responses also could be related to damage to other auditory areas of the brain in these subjects. In our own experience using tonal stimuli, there has been essentially little or no change in N1, P2, or P3 (P300) potentials before compared to after commissurotomy. Of course, the utilization of speech stimuli, especially in some type of dichotic paradigm, may result in much different results.

Case 7–8: Commissurotomy

History. This young adult underwent surgical commissurotomy for intractable grand mal seizures. This patient had previously been under a neurologic protocol for seizure management as daily activities were becoming difficult to carry out.

Audiology. Pure-tone thresholds were normal with excellent speech recognition bilaterally before and after surgery. Presurgery, central auditory tests were within the normal range bilaterally. How-

ever, postsurgery, there was a marked left ear deficit for the dichotic digits and the staggered spondaic word (SSW) tests (Figure 7–8). Speech in babble scores were normal bilaterally and frequency patterns were abnormal for both ears (see Figure 7–8). These results were consistent with expected postcommissurotomy audiologic results.

Medical Examination and Management. The focus of the seizure activity was localized by EEG in both hemispheres. Computerized tomography scans were normal except for slightly enlarged lateral ventricles. There was no history of any auditory problems. The surgery went well and the patient was able to resume many normal everyday activities due to a marked decrease in the number of seizures. Tasks requiring interhemispheric interaction were, of course, difficult for the patient.

CENTRAL AUDITORY DISORDER ASSOCIATED WITH LEARNING PROBLEMS

Introduction

One of the most popular uses of central auditory tests is to identify individuals (mostly children) with auditory processing disorder that may either precipitate or coexist with learning difficulties. Although the basis for this kind of problem is not known, there are several good leads as to what may cause these problems. Children with normal hearing and intelligence, but who complain of hearing difficulties and

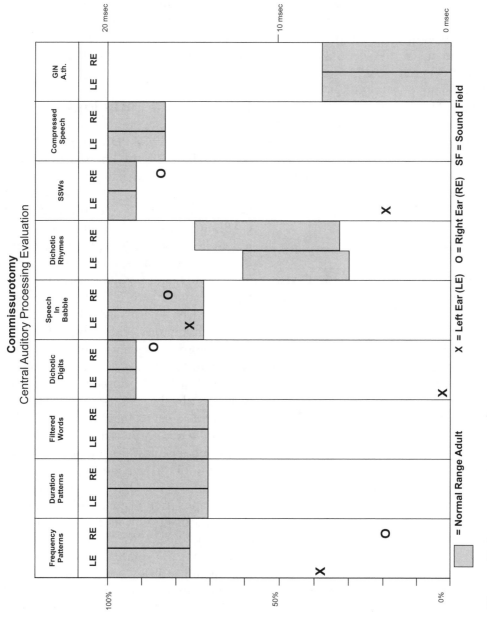

Figure 7–8. *Central behavioral test results for a young adult who underwent a commissurotomy to control intractable grand mal seizures (Case 7–8).*

who also have difficulty with learning (especially in the verbally related subjects such as reading and spelling) are candidates for this diagnosis. Other factors, such as language proficiency and attention, often enter into this complex picture. However, many cases of central auditory processing disorder (CAPD) do not have either language or attention issues. The combining of behavioral and electrophysiologic tests of central auditory function is a prudent approach to defining this problem. Evaluation of speech-language and attention also is key in making an accurate diagnosis.

Symptoms

As with other disorders of the CANS, children with learning-related central auditory disorder complain of difficulty hearing in background noise, trouble understanding people who talk fast, problems hearing in highly reverberant rooms, problems following multistep directions, difficulty in interpreting verbal messages, and sometimes even having trouble localizing sound sources. Academically, these individuals often have trouble reading and spelling, but do fine in math and science. At times, some students appear to be inattentive, whereas others seem to attend closely in watching people speak (see Chermak & Musiek, 1997, pp. 91–108).

Incidence and Prevalence

The incidence or prevalence of CAPD associated with learning disability is unknown. There are some "educated guesses" that place the prevalence around 2 to 3% of the school-age population (Chermak & Musiek, 1997, pp. 20–23). Of

course, this is not based on any prevalence study, but does seem to be a reasonable estimate based on our experience in seeing large numbers of school-age children with this type of problem and reviewing the prevalence of related problems such as learning disabilities, ADHD, and so on.

Etiology and Pathology

The etiology of CAPD related to learning problems is not known, but more information is emerging that supports our early theoretical categories of what may cause or play a role in this type of CAPD (Chermak & Musiek, 2011; Musiek, Gollegly, & Ross, 1985). One category is neurologic. That is, a small percentage have CAPD (and possibly learning problems) secondary to a frank neurologic problem (see Chermak & Musiek, 2011). Although any of a wide range of neurologic disorders, such as those discussed earlier in this chapter, can play a role in this kind of CAPD, absence seizure disorder may be the most common. Another category is delayed maturation of myelin within the auditory system. Myelination of the higher auditory regions does not mature until the teenage years (Yakovlev & LeCours, 1967). This long maturational course lends itself to great variability over the years of growth and some children may "lag" behind in the maturation of their CANS. This maturational lag means less myelin and slower transfer velocities and potential central deficits that may manifest as CAPD. The third category is that of neuromorphological abnormalities (see Galaburda, Sherman, Rosen, Aboitz, & Geschwind, 1985). Polymicrogyri, heterotopias, and ectopic areas of the brain have been shown to exist primarily in the left hemisphere and in the auditory regions in individuals with dyslexia. In addition, the planum temporale, which is usually larger on the left than right side, often is symmetrical in children with dyslexia/learning disabilities. These abnormalities are anatomic abnormalities that could easily disrupt appropriate functions, especially auditory functions. In fact, a recent report has shown this to be the case in children with polymicrogyri who do poorly on central auditory tests (Boscariol et al., 2009).

Site of Lesion

Depending on what may be the underlying condition that results in the CAPD related to learning disability, the site of lesion will vary. However, it seems that most individuals with this problem have auditory cortex or corpus callosum dysfunction (normal ABRs are common in this particular population). If heterotopias and polymicrogyri are players, then obviously the auditory cortex will be involved. Myelination of the corpus callosum is the last to mature within the auditory system; hence, this could be a site for "delayed" maturation. Recent work from Skoe and Kraus (2010) indicates that abnormalities on speech ABRs possibly could implicate the brainstem as a site for dysfunction in these kinds of cases, but further work must be done to solidify this possibility.

Medical Diagnosis

Central auditory processing disorder related to learning disability is primarily an audiologic diagnosis. Only when there is an underlying medical condition is there medical input to the diagnosis. The same can be said for treatment.

Audiology

In the assessment of learning problems linked with CAPD, tests with reasonable sensitivity and specificity (based on cases of confirmed lesions of the central auditory system) should be considered first. Consistent with this thinking, behavioral tests of dichotic listening, temporal processing, and degraded monaural speech tests are useful. Also, binaural interaction procedures such as masking level differences can be of value. In addition, auditory evoked potentials like the combination of ABR-MLR (or others) are suggested. It is important to attempt to evaluate as many processes as possible without making the test battery too long and tiring.

Audiologic Management

Treatment can include several approaches. One is auditory training (AT), which capitalizes on auditory plasticity. By training on tasks that are related to the deficit, in many cases the deficit can be ameliorated (see Chermak & Musiek, 2007). Assistive listening devices, which provide improved signal-to-noise ratios in settings such as the classroom, can help with the problem. These approaches, as well as metacognitive strategies, can well serve those with learning disabilities and associated auditory processing difficulties (see Musiek & Chermak, 2007, for an in-depth review).

Case 7–9: Learning Problems

History

This was a 13-year-old who had a long history of learning problems especially in the verbally related subjects in school. He was having difficulty in school despite investing many study hours a week. He also had problems hearing in noise and following directions for many years (likely for most of his school years) as noted by teachers and his parents. After years of considering an auditory processing problem, he was referred for evaluation.

Audiology

This student demonstrated normal puretone thresholds and excellent speech recognition scores bilaterally. As can be seen in Figure 7–9, he demonstrated a left ear deficit on dichotic listening (digits, sentences, and staggered spondees) and a mildly depressed score for the left ear on filtered speech.

Audiologic Management

Given this was essentially a dichotic problem, the student was enrolled in dichotic interaural intensity difference training (DIID) (see Musiek, Weihing, & Lau, 2008; Weihing & Musiek, 2007). This auditory training involves dichotic listening with an intensity (or temporal) advantage provided to the poorer ear. As can be seen by the arrows in the illustration, after a couple of months of training, the left ear deficit noted during his central auditory evaluation improved on each of the three dichotic speech tests that initially showed left deficits. Within the next school year, both his parents and teachers reported that his performance in school had improved.

SUMMARY

This chapter highlighted selected disorders that can and do affect the CANS. Mass lesions, vascular lesions, degenerative dis-

orders, neurotoxic agents, head trauma, temporal lobe epilepsy, and learning problems are among the more common disorders that can compromise the CANS. However, the reader should be aware that many other central nervous system disorders not mentioned in this chapter can cause central auditory deficits. Each of these disorders could not be elaborated on here due to the scope of this chapter. Among the disorders not addressed, but deserving of comment, is central presbycusis. Both the peripheral and central auditory systems undergo normal aging processes. In some people, there is more central aging; in others, there is greater peripheral auditory system aging. Therefore, whenever possible, it is important to evaluate both the peripheral and central auditory systems when evaluating an elderly patient. A common central deficit noted in many older individuals is a left ear deficit on dichotic listening tests that is secondary to compromise of the corpus callosum due to normal aging effects (Bellis & Wilbur, 2001).

Other central trends are not as obvious, but should be pursued clinically. Hydrocephalus is another disorder that should be mentioned. Third, fourth, and lateral ventricle hydrocephalus can easily compromise the CANS due the close proximity of these ventricles to central auditory nuclei and tracts (Musiek et al., 1994). Leukodystrophies are a category of degenerative disorders often inherited that can result in myelin damage. The auditory evoked potentials often are abnormal in this category of disease (De Meirleir, Taylor, &nd Logan, 1988). Recently, Bamiou and colleagues (2007) have shown auditory interhemispheric processing difficulties in children with congenital aniridia due to PAX6 genetic mutations. Auditory deprivation from

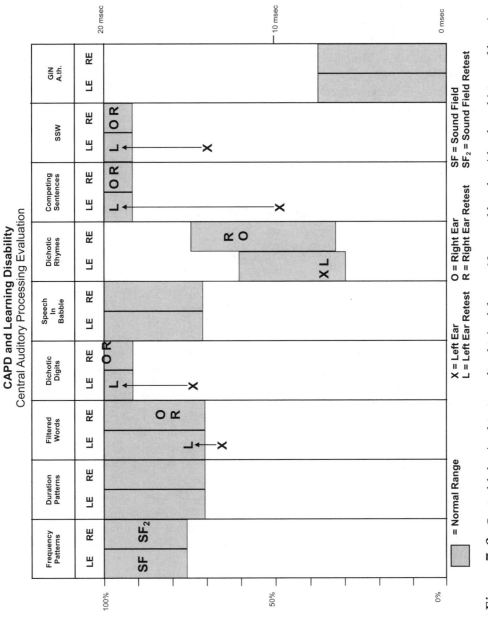

Figure 7–9. *Central behavioral test results obtained from a 13-year-old male with a long history of learning problems (Case 7–9). Test results obtained both before and after therapy are displayed.*

long-standing peripheral hearing loss is a condition that can also result in central auditory deficits. Research in animals with peripheral hearing deficits has demonstrated trans-synaptic degeneration and altered cortical organization due to a lack of auditory stimulation (Morest, 1983). The foregoing are some of the additional types of central nervous system disorders that can affect the central auditory structures. As we learn more about central mechanisms, we undoubtedly will uncover other disorders that can compromise the CANS.

Acknowledgment. The authors gratefully acknowledge the contributions of Erik Musiek, MD, PhD, Department of Neurology, Washington University School of Medicine to this chapter.

REFERENCES

Akman, I., Ozek, E., Kulekci, S., Türkdogan, D., Cebeci, D., & Akdaş, F. (2004). Auditory neuropathy in hyperbilirubinemia: Is there a correlation between serum bilirubin, neuron-specific enolase levels and auditory neuropathy? *International Journal of Audiology, 43*(9), 516–522.

Araki, S., Sato, H., Yokoyama, K., & Murata, K. (2000). Subclinical neurophysiological effects of lead: A review of peripheral, central, and autonomic nervous system effects in lead workers. *Amercian Journal of Industrial Medicine, 37*(2), 193–204.

Bamiou, D. E., Free, S. L., Sisodiya, S. M., Chong, W. K., Musiek, F., Williamson, K. A., . . . Luxon, L. M. (2007). Auditory interhemispheric transfer deficits, hearing difficulties, and brain magnetic resonance imaging abnormalities in children with congenital aniridia due to PAX6 mutations. *Archives of Pediatric and Adolescent Medicine, 161*(5), 463–469.

Bamiou, D. E., Musiek, F. E., Stow, I., Stevens, J., Cipolotti, L., Brown, M. M., & Luxon, L. M. (2006). Auditory temporal processing deficits in patients with insular stroke. *Neurology, 67*(4), 614–619.

Baran, J. A., Bothfeldt, R. W., & Musiek, F. E. (2004). Central auditory deficits associated with compromise of the primary auditory cortex. *Journal of the American Academy of Audiology, 15*(2), 106–116.

Baran, J. A., & Musiek, F. E. (1999). Behavioral assessment of the central auditory nervous system. In F. E. Musiek & W. F. Rintelmann (Eds.), *Contemporary perspectives in hearing assessment* (pp. 375–413). Boston, MA: Allyn & Bacon.

Baran, J. A., Musiek, F. E., & Reeves, A. G. (1986). Central auditory function following anterior sectioning of the corpus callosum. *Ear and Hearing, 7*(6), 359–362.

Baru, A. V., & Karaseva, T. A. (1972). *The brain and hearing: Hearing disturbances associated with local brain lesions.* New York, NY: Consultants Bureau.

Bellis, T. J., & Wilber, L. A. (2001). Effects of aging and gender on interhemispheric function. *Journal of Speech, Language, and Hearing Research, 44*(2), 246–263.

Benavidez, D. A., Fletcher, J. M., Hannay, H. J., Bland, S. T., Caudle, S. E., . . . Song, J. (1999). Corpus callosum damage and interhemispheric transfer of information following closed head injury in children. *Cortex, 35*(3), 315–336.

Berg, A. T., Shinnar, S., Levy, S. R., & Testa, F. M. (1999). Childhood-onset epilepsy with and without preceding febrile seizures. *Neurology, 53*(8), 1742–1748.

Bergemalm, P. O., & Borg, E. (2001). Long-term objective and subjective audiologic consequences of closed-head injury. *Acta Otolaryngologica, 121*(6), 724–734.

Bocca, E., Calearo, C., & Cassinari, V. (1954). A new method for testing hearing in temporal lobe tumours: Preliminary report. *Acta Otolaryngologica, 44*(3), 219–221.

Boose, M. A., & Cranford, J. L. (1996). Auditory event-related potentials in multiple sclerosis. *American Journal of Otology, 17*(1), 165–170.

Boscariol, M., Garcia, V. L., Guimarães, C. A., Hage, S. R., Montenegro, M. A., Cendes, F., & Guerreiro, M. M. (2009). Auditory processing disorders in twins with perisylvian polymicrogyria. *Arquivos de Neuropsiquiatria, 67*(2B), 499–501.

Bougeard, R., & Fischer, C. (2002). The role of the temporal pole in auditory processing. *Epileptic Disorders, 4*(1), S29–S32.

Boutros, N. N., Trautner, P., Korzyukov, O., Grunwald T., Burroughs, S., . . . Rosburg, T. (2006). Mid-latency auditory-evoked responses and sensory gating in focal epilepsy: A preliminary exploration. *Journal of Neuropsychiatry and Clinical Neurosciences, 18*(3), 409–416.

Bronen, R. A. (2000).The status of status: Seizures are bad for your brain's health. *American Journal of Neuroradiology, 21*(10), 1782–1783.

Calabresi, P. (2006). Multiple sclerosis. In R. T. Johnson, J. W. Griffin, & J. C. McAurthur (Eds.), *Current therapies in neurologic disease* (7th ed., pp. 221–223). London, UK: Mosby.

Campo, P., & Lataye, R. (2000). Noise and solvent, alcohol and solvent: Two dangerous interactions on auditory function. *Noise and Health, 3*(9), 49–57.

Celebisoy, N., Aydoğdu, I., Ekmekçi, O., & Akürekli, O. (1996). Middle latency auditory evoked potentials (MLAEPs) in (MS). *Acta Neurologica Scandinavica, 93*(5), 317–321.

Centers for Disease Control and Prevention, National Center for Injury Prevention and Control. (2010). Traumatic brain injury. Retrieved 6/15/11 from http://www.cdc.gov/TraumaticBrainInjury/index.html.

Chaves, C. J., & Jones, H. R. (2005). Ischemic stroke. In H. R. Jones (Ed.), *Netter's neurology* (pp. 195–217). Teterboro, NJ: Icon Learning Systems.

Chayasirisobhon, W. V., Chayasirisobhon, S., Tin, S. N., Leu, N., Tehrani, K., & McGuckin, J. S. (2007). Scalp-recorded auditory P300 event-related potentials in new-onset un-treated temporal lobe epilepsy. *Clinical EEG and Neuroscience, 38*(3), 167–171.

Chermak, G. D., & Musiek, F. E. (1997). *Central auditory processing disorders: New perspectives.* San Diego, CA: Singular Publishing.

Chermak, G. D., & Musiek, F. E. (Eds.). (2007). *Handbook of (central) auditory processing disorder: Comprehensive intervention* (Vol. 2). San Diego, CA: Plural Publishing.

Chermak, G. D., & Musiek, F. E. (2011) Neurological substrate of central auditory processing deficits in children. *Current Pediatric Reviews, 7*(3), 241–251.

Chiappa, K. H. (1988). Use of evoked potentials for diagnosis of multiple sclerosis. *Neurology Clinics, 6*(4), 861–880.

Cohen, M., Hynd, G., & Hugdahl, K. (1992). Dichotic listening performance in subtypes of developmental dyslexia and a left temporal lobe brain tumor contrast group. *Brain and Language, 42*(2), 187–202.

Collard, M. E. (1984). Central auditory tests in patients with intractable seizures. *Seminars in Hearing, 3*(5), 277–295.

Collard, M. E., Lesser, R. P., Lüders, H., Dinner, D. S., Morris, H. H., Hahn, J. F., & Rothner, A. D. (1986). Four dichotic speech tests before and after temporal lobectomy. *Ear and Hearing, 7*(6), 363–369.

Commission on Classification and Terminology of the International League Against Epilepsy. (1981). Proposal for revised clinical and electrographic classification of epileptic seizures. *Epilepsia, 22*(4), 489–501.

Cooper, J. C., Jr., & Gates, G. A. (1991). Hearing in the elderly—the Framingham cohort, 1983–1985: Part II. Prevalence of central auditory processing disorders. *Ear and Hearing, 12*(5), 304–311.

Counter, S. A. (2002). Brainstem neural conduction biomarkers in lead-exposed children of Andean lead-glaze workers. *Journal of Occupational and Environmental Medicine, 44*(9), 855–864.

Cranford, J., Diamond, I. T., Ravizza, R., & Whitfield, L. C. (1971). Unilateral lesions of the auditory cortex and the "precedence effect." *Journal of Physiology, 213*(2), 24P–36P.

Cranford, J. L., Stream, R. W., Rye, C. V., & Slade, T. L. (1982). Detection v discrimination of brief duration tones: Findings in patients with temporal lobe damage. *Archives of Otolaryngology, 108*(6), 350–356.

De Meirleir, L. J., Taylor, M. J., & Logan, W. J. (1988). Multimodal evoked potential studies in leukodystrophies of children. *Canadian Journal of Neurological Sciences, 15*(1), 26–31.

Dietrich, K. N., Succop, P. A., Berger, O. G., & Keith, R. W. (1992). Lead exposure and the central auditory processing abilities and cognitive development of urban children: The Cincinnati Lead Study cohort at age 5 years. *Neurotoxicology and Teratology, 14*(1), 51–56.

Drake, M. E., Weate, S. J., Andrews, J. M., & Castleberry C. J. (1995). P50 auditory evoked potentials in epilepsy. *Journal of Epilepsy, 8*(3), 197–200.

Drake, M. E., Weate, S. J., & Newell, S. A. (1996). Auditory evoked potentials in postconcussive syndrome. *Electromyography and Clinical Neurophysiology, 36*(8), 457–462.

Dublin, W. B. (1976). The combined correlated audiohistogram. Incorporation of the superior ventral cochlear nucleus. *Annals of Otology, Rhinology, and Laryngology, 85*(6, Pt. 1), 813–819.

Dublin, W. B. (1986). Central auditory pathology. *Otolaryngology-Head and Neck Surgery, 95*(3, Pt. 2), 363–424.

Efron, R., Yund, E. W., Nichols, D., & Crandall, P. H. (1985). An ear asymmetry for gap detection following anterior temporal lobectomy. *Neuropsychologia, 23*(1), 43–50.

Fallis-Cunningham, R., Keith, R. W., & Warnick, R. E. (1998). Central auditory processing in a patient with bilateral temporal lobe tumors: Case report. *Journal of the American Academy of Audiology, 9*(4), 299–304.

Fuente, A., & McPherson, B. (2006). Organic solvents and hearing loss: The challenge for audiology. *International Journal of Audiology, 45*(7), 367–381.

Fuente, A., & McPherson, B. (2007a). Central auditory damage induced by solvent exposure. *International Journal of Occupational Safety and Ergonomics, 13*(4), 391–397.

Fuente, A., & McPherson, B. (2007b). Central auditory processing effects induced by solvent exposure. *International Journal of Occupational Medicine and Environmental Health, 20*(3), 271–279.

Gadea, M., Marti-Bonmatí, L., Arana, E., Espert, R., Salvador, A., & Casanova, B. (2009). Corpus callosum function in verbal dichotic listening: Inferences from a longitudinal follow-up of relapsing-remitting multiple sclerosis patients. *Brain and Language, 110*(2), 101–105.

Gaetz, M., & Bernstein, D. M. (2001). The current status of electrophysiologic procedures for the assessment of mild traumatic brain injury. *Journal of Head Trauma Rehabilitation, 16*(4), 386–405.

Galaburda, A. M., Sherman, G. F., Rosen, G. D., Aboitz, F., & Geschwind, N. (1985). Developmental dyslexia: Four consecutive cases with cortical anomalies. *Annals of Neurology, 18*(2), 222–233.

Gates, G. A., Anderson, M. L., Feeney, M. P., McCurry, S. M., & Larson, E. B. (2008). Central auditory dysfunction in older persons with memory impairment or Alzheimer's dementia. *Archives of Otolaryngology-Head and Neck Surgery, 134*(7), 771–777.

Gramstad, A., Engelsen, B. A., & Hugdahl, K. (2006). Dichotic listening with forced attention in patients with temporal lobe epilepsy: Significance of left hemisphere cognitive dysfunction. *Scandinavian Journal of Psychology, 47*(3), 163–170.

Green, J. B., Elder, W. W., & Freed, D. M. (1995). The P1 component of the middle latency auditory evoked potential predicts a practice effect during clinical trials in Alzheimer's disease. *Neurology, 45*(5), 962–966.

Grimes, A. M., Grady, C. L., Foster, N. L., Sunderland, T., & Patronas, N. J. (1985). Central auditory function in Alzheimer's disease. *Neurology, 35*(3), 352–358.

Harris, D. P., & Hall, J. W. (1990). Feasibility of auditory event-related potential measurement in brain injury rehabilitation. *Ear and Hearing, 11*(5), 340–350.

Health Topics, University of Virginia Health System. (2009). Hyperbilirubinemia. Retrieved 6/15/11 from http://www.hsc.virginia.edu/uvahealth/peds_hrnewborn/hyperb.cfm.

Hendler, T., Squires, N. K., & Emmerich, D. S. (1990). Psychophysical measures of central auditory dysfunction in multiple sclerosis: Neurophysiological and neuroanatomical correlates. *Ear and Hearing, 11(6)*, 403–416.

Hirayasu, Y., Ohta, H., Fukao, K., Ogura, C., & Mukawa, J. (1995). Transient P300 abnormality of event-related potentials following unilateral temporal lobectomy. *Psychiatry and Clinical Neurosciences, 49(4)*, 223–226.

Honig, L. S., Ramsay, R. E., & Sheremata, W. A. (1992). Event-related potential P300 in multiple sclerosis: Relation to magnetic resonance imaging and cognitive impairment. *Archives of Neurology, 49(1)*, 44–50.

Hreib, K. K., & Jones, H. R. (2005). Intracerebral hemorrhage. In H. R. Jones (Ed.), *Netter's neurology* (pp. 195–217). Teterboro, NJ: Icon Learning Systems.

Iliadou, V., & Kaprinis, S. (2003). Clinical psychoacoustics in Alzheimer's disease central auditory processing disorders and speech deterioration. *Annals of General Hospital Psychiatry, 2(1)*, 12.

Ilvonen, T. M., Kujala, T., Tervaniemi, M., Salonen, O., Näätänen, R., & Pekkonen, E. (2001). The processing of sound duration after left hemisphere stroke: Event-related potential and behavioral evidence. *Psychophysiology, 38(4)*, 622–628.

Irimajiri, R., Golob, E. J., & Starr, A. (2005). Auditory brainstem, middle- and long-latency evoked potentials in mild cognitive impairment. *Clinical Neurophysiology, 116(8)*, 1917–1929.

Jacobson, G. P., Privitera, M., Neils, J. R., Grayson, A. S., & Yeh, H. S. (1990). The effects of anterior temporal lobectomy (ATL) on the middle-latency auditory evoked potential (MLAEP). *Electroencephalography and Clinical Neurophysiology, 75(3)*, 230–241.

Japaridze, G., Shakarishvili, R., & Kevanishvili, Z. (2002). Auditory brainstem, middle-latency, and slow cortical responses in multiple sclerosis. *Acta Neurologica Scandinavica, 106(1)*, 47–53.

Jerger, J., & Jerger, S. (1974). Auditory findings in brain stem disorders. *Archives of Otolaryngology, 99(5)*, 342–350.

Jerger, J. F., Oliver, T. A., Chmiel, R. A., & Rivera, V. M. (1986). Patterns of auditory abnormality in multiple sclerosis. *Audiology, 25(4–5)*, 193–209.

Jerger, S., & Jerger, J. (1981). *Auditory disorders: A manual for clinical evaluation.* Boston, MA: Little, Brown.

Jones, S. J., Vaz Pato, M., Sprague, L., Stokes, M., Munday, R., & Haque, N. (2000). Auditory evoked potentials to spectro-temporal modulation of complex tones in normal subjects and patients with severe brain injury. *Brain, 123*(Pt. 5), 1007–1016.

Karlsson, A. K., & Rosenhall, U. (1995). Clinical application of distorted speech audiometry. *Scandinavian Audiology, 24(3)*, 155–160.

Katz, J., Basil, R. A., & Smith, J. M. (1963). A staggered spondaic word test for detecting central auditory lesions. *Annals of Otology, Rhinology, and Laryngology, 72*, 907–917.

Kaufman, D. (1990). *Clinical neurology for psychiatrists.* Philadelphia, PA: W. B. Saunders.

Kileny, P., Paccioretti, D., & Wilson, A. F. (1987). Effects of cortical lesions on middle-latency auditory evoked responses (MLR). *Electroencephalography and Clinical Neurophysiology, 66(2)*, 107–120.

Kimura, D. (1961). Some effects of temporal-lobe damage on auditory perception. *Canadian Journal of Psychology, 15*, 156–165.

Knight, R. T., Hillyard, S. A., Woods, D. L., & Neville, H. J. (1980). The effects of frontal and temporal-parietal lesions on the auditory evoked potential in man. *Electroencephalography and Clinical Neurophysiology, 50(1–2)*, 112–124.

Knight, R. T., Scabini, D., Woods, D. L., & Clayworth, C. (1988). The effects of lesions of superior temporal gyrus and inferior parietal lobe on temporal and vertex components of the human AEP. *Electroencephalography and Clinical Neurophysiology, 70(6)*, 499–509.

Knight, R. T., Scabini, D., Woods, D. L., & Clayworth, C. C. (1989). Contributions of temporal-parietal junction to the human auditory P3. *Brain Research, 502(1)*, 109–116.

Kurylo, D. D., Corkin, S., Allard, T., Zatorre, R. J., & Growdon, J. H. (1993). Auditory function in Alzheimer's disease. *Neurology, 43*(10), 1893–1899.

Kutas, M., Hillyard, S. A., Volpe, B. T., & Gazzaniga, M. S. (1990). Late positive event-related potentials after commissural section in humans. *Journal of Cognitive Neuroscience, 2*(3), 257–271.

Kwan, P., & Brodie, M. J. (2000). Early identification of refractory epilepsy. *New England Journal of Medicine, 342*(5), 314–319.

Lackner, J. R., & Teuber, H. L. (1973). Alterations in auditory fusion thresholds after cerebral injury in man. *Neuropsychología, 11*(4), 409–415.

Lanphear, B. P., Dietrich, K., Auinger, P., & Cox, C. (2000). Cognitive deficits associated with blood lead concentrations <10 microg/dL in US children and adolescents. *Public Health Reports, 115*(6), 521–529.

Larjavaara, S., Mäntylä, R., Salminen, T., Haapasalo, H., Raitanen, J., Jääskeläinen, J., & Auvinen, A. (2007). Incidence of gliomas by anatomic location. *Neuro-oncology, 9*(3), 319–325.

Levin, H. S., High W. M., Williams, D. H., Eisenberg, H. M., Amparo, E. G., . . . Ewert, J. (1989). Dichotic listening and manual performance in relation to magnetic resonance imaging after closed head injury. *Journal of Neurology, Neurosurgery, and Psychiatry, 52*(10), 1162–1169.

Levine, R. A., Gardner, J. C., Fullerton, B. C., Stufflebeam, S. M., Furst, M., & Rosen, B. R. (1994). Multiple sclerosis lesions of the pons are not silent. *Brain, 117*(Pt. 5), 1127–1141.

Lew, H. L., Lee, E. H., Pan, S. S., & Date, E. S. (2004). Electrophysiologic abnormalities of auditory and visual information processing in patients with traumatic brain injury. *American Journal of Physical Medicine and Rehabilitation, 83*(6), 427–433.

Luxon, L. M. (1980). Hearing loss in brainstem disorders. *Journal of Neurology, Neurosurgery, and Psychiatry, 43*(6), 510–515.

Lynn, G. E., & Gilroy, J. (1972). Neuro-audiological abnormalities in patients with temporal lobe tumors. *Journal of the Neurological Sciences, 17*(2), 167–184.

Lynn, G. E., & Gilroy, J. (1975). Effects of brain lesions on the perception of monotic and dichotic speech stimuli. In M. D. Sullivan (Ed.), *Central auditory processing disorders* (pp. 47–83). Proceedings of a Conference at the University of Nebraska, Omaha.

Lynn, G. E., Gilroy, J., Taylor, P. C., & Leiser, R. P. (1981). Binaural masking-level differences in neurological disorders. *Archives of Otolaryngology, 107*(6), 357–362.

Markowitz, M. E. (2006). Management of lead poisoning in children. In R. T. Johnson, J. W. Griffin, & J. C. McAurthur (Eds.), *Current therapies in neurologic disease* (7th ed., pp. 352–353). London, UK: Mosby.

Martin, E. M., Lu, W. C., Helmick, K., French, L., & Warden, D. L. (2008). Traumatic brain injuries sustained in the Afghanistan and Iraq Wars. *Journal of Trauma Nursing, 15*(3), 94–99.

McClelland, R. J., Fenton, G. W., & Rutherford, W. (1994). The postconcussional syndrome revisited. *Journal of the Royal Society of Medicine, 87*(9), 507–510.

McLeod, J. G., & Lance, J. W. (1989). *Introductory neurology*, Oxford, UK: Blackwell.

Meneguello, J., Leonhardt, F. D., & Pereira, L. D. (2006). Auditory processing in patients with temporal lobe epilepsy. *Brazilian Journal of Otorhinolaryngology, 72*(4), 496–504.

Mercola, J. (2008). Mercury detox diet. Retrieved 6-15-11 from http//:heartspring.net .

Merritt, H., & Antunes, J. (1979). Tumors. In H. Merritt (Ed.), *A textbook of neurology* (6th ed., pp. 214–217). Philadelphia, PA: Lee & Febiger.

Meyers, J. E., Roberts, R. J., Bayless, J. D., Volkert, K., & Evitts, P. E. (2002). Dichotic listening: Expanded norms and clinical application. *Archives of Clinical Neuropsychology, 17*(1), 79–90.

Mollison, P. L., & Walker, W. (1952). Controlled trials of the treatment of haemolytic disease of the newborn. *Lancet, 1*(6705), 429–433.

Morales-Garcia, C., & Poole, J. P. (1972). Masked speech audiometry in central deafness. *Acta Otolaryngologica, 74*(5), 307–316.

Morest, K. (1983). Degeneration in the brain following exposure to noise. In R. Hamernik, D. Henderson, & R. Salvi (Eds.), *New per-*

spectives on noise-induced hearing loss (pp. 87–89). New York, NY: Raven Press.

Murata, K., Weihe, P., Budtz-Jørgensen, E., Jørgensen, P. J., & Grandjean, P. (2004). Delayed brainstem auditory evoked potential latencies in 14-year-old children exposed to methylmercury. *Journal of Pediatrics, 144*(2), 177–183.

Muriello, M. A., Jones, H. R., & Chaves, C. J. (2005). Multiple sclerosis and acute disseminated encephalomyelitis. In H. R. Jones (Ed.), *Netter's neurology* (pp. 537–559). Teterboro, NJ: Icon Learning Systems.

Musiek, F. E. (1983a). Assessment of central auditory dysfunction: The dichotic digit test revisited. *Ear and Hearing, 4*(2), 79–83.

Musiek, F. E. (1983b). Results of three dichotic speech tests on subjects with intracranial lesions. *Ear and Hearing, 4*(6), 317–323.

Musiek, F. E. (1991). Auditory evoked responses in a site of lesion assessment. In W. F. Rintelmann (Ed.), *Hearing assessment* (2nd ed., pp. 383–428). Austin, TX: Pro-Ed.

Musiek, F. E., & Baran, J. A. (2004). Audiological correlates to a rupture of a pontine arteriovenous malformation. *Journal of the American Academy of Audiology, 15*(2), 161–171.

Musiek, F. E., Baran, J. A., & Pinheiro, M. L. (1990). Duration pattern recognition in normal subjects and patients with cerebral and cochlear lesions. *Audiology, 29*(6), 304–313.

Musiek, F. E., Baran, J. A., & Pinheiro, M. L. (1992). P300 results in patients with lesions of the auditory areas of the cerebrum. *Journal of the American Academy of Audiology, 3*(1), 5–15.

Musiek, F. E., Baran, J. A., & Pinheiro, M. L. (1994). *Neuroaudiology: Case studies*. San Diego, CA: Singular Publishing.

Musiek, F. E., Baran, J. A., & Shinn, J. (2004). Assessment and remediation of an auditory processing disorder associated with head trauma. *Journal of the American Academy of Audiology, 15*(2), 117–132.

Musiek, F. E., Bromley, M. E., Roberts, D. W., & Lamb, L. (1990). Improvement of central auditory function after partial temporal lobectomy in a patient with seizure disorder.

Journal of the American Academy of Audiology, 1(3), 146–150.

Musiek, F., Charette, L., Kelly, T., Lee, W. W., & Musiek, E. (1999). Hit and false-positive rates for the middle latency response in patients with central nervous system involvement. *Journal of the American Academy of Audiology, 10*(3), 124–132.

Musiek, F. E., & Geurkink, N. A. (1982). Auditory brain stem response and central auditory test findings for patients with brain stem lesions: A preliminary report. *Laryngoscope, 92*(8, Pt. 1), 891–900.

Musiek, F. E., Gollegly, K. M., Kibbe, K. S., & Reeves, A. G. (1989). Electrophysiologic and behavioral auditory findings in multiple sclerosis. *American Journal of Otology, 10*(5), 343–350.

Musiek, F. E., Gollegly, K. M., & Ross, M. K. (1985). Profile of types of central auditory processing disorders in children with learning disabilities. *Journal of Childhood Communication Disorders, 9*(1), 43–63.

Musiek, F. E., & Hanlon, D. P. (1999). Neuroaudiological effects in a case of fatal dimethylmercury poisoning. *Ear and Hearing, 20*(3), 271–275.

Musiek, F. E., Kibbe, K., & Baran, J. A. (1984). Neuroaudiological results from split-brain patients. *Seminars in Hearing, 5*(3), 219–229.

Musiek, F. E., & Lee, W. W. (1995). The auditory brain stem response in patients with brain stem or cochlear pathology. *Ear and Hearing, 16*(6), 631–636.

Musiek, F. E., & Lee, W. W. (1998). Neuroanatomical correlates to central deafness. *Scandinavian Audiology, 27*(Suppl. 49), 17–25.

Musiek, F. E., & Lee, W. W. (1999). Auditory middle and late potentials. In F. E. Musiek & W. F. Rintelmann (Eds.), *Contemporary perspectives in hearing assessment* (pp. 243–260). Boston, MA: Allyn & Bacon.

Musiek, F. E., & Pinheiro, M. L. (1987). Frequency patterns in cochlear, brainstem, and cerebral lesions. *Audiology, 26*(2), 79–88.

Musiek, F. E., Pinheiro, M. L., & Wilson, D. H. (1980). Auditory pattern perception in 'split brain' patients. *Archives of Otolaryngology, 106*(10), 610–612.

Musiek, F. E., Shinn, J. B., Jirsa, R., Bamiou, D. E., Baran, J. A., & Zaidan, E. (2005). GIN (Gaps-In-Noise) test performance in subjects with confirmed central auditory nervous system involvement. *Ear and Hearing, 26*(6), 607–618.

Musiek, F., Weihing, J., & Lau, C. (2008). Dichotic interaural intensity difference (DIID). *Journal of the Auditory Rehabilitation Association, 41,* 51–65.

National Cancer Institute. (2000). National Cancer Institute Brain Tumor Study: Fact sheet, 2000. Retrieved 6/15/11 from http://nci.nih.gov/cancertopics/factsheet/Risk/Fs3_88.pdf.

Needleman, H. L. (2004). Low level lead exposure and the development of children. *Southeast Asian Journal of Tropical Medicine and Public Health, 35*(2), 252–254.

Newman, T. B., Escobar, G. J., Gonzales, V. M., Armstrong, M. A., Gardner, M. N., & Folck, B. F. (1999). Frequency of neonatal bilirubin testing and hyperbilirubinemia in a large health maintenance organization. *Pediatrics, 104*(5, Pt. 2), 1197–1203.

Obert, A. D., & Cranford, J. L. (1990). Effects of neocortical lesions on the P300 component of the auditory evoked response. *American Journal of Otology, 11*(6), 447–453.

Occupational Safety and Health Administration, Department of Labor. (2003). Styrene. Retrieved from 6/15/11 from: http://www.osha.gov/SLTC/styrene/index.html.

Oxbury, J. M., & Oxbury, S. M. (1969). Effects of temporal lobectomy on the report of dichotically presented digits. *Cortex, 5*(1), 3–14.

Perkins, D. (2002). *Neurology* (2nd ed.). London, UK: Mosby.

Pinheiro, M. L., Jacobson, G., & Boller, F. (1982). Auditory dysfunction following a gunshot wound to the pons. *Journal of Speech and Hearing Disorders, 47*(3), 296–300.

Pinheiro, M. L., & Tobin, H. (1969). Interaural intensity difference for intracranial lateralization. *Journal of the Acoustical Society of America, 46*(6), 1482–1487.

Polich, J., & Corey-Bloom, J. (2005). Alzheimer's disease and P300: Review and evaluation of task and modality. *Current Alzheimer Research, 2*(5), 515–525.

Polich, J., Romine, J. S., Sipe, J. C., Aung, M., & Dalessio, D. J. (1992). P300 in multiple sclerosis: A preliminary report. *International Journal of Psychophysiology, 12*(2), 155–163.

Poser, C. M. (1979). Multiple sclerosis. *Medical Clinics of North America, 63*(4), 729–743.

Raeder, M. B., Helland, C. A., Hugdahl, K., & Wester, K. (2005). Arachnoid cysts cause cognitive deficits that improve after surgery. *Neurology, 64*(1), 160–162.

Rapin, I., & Gravel, J. (2003). "Auditory neuropathy:" Physiologic and pathologic evidence calls for more diagnostic specificity. *International Journal of Pediatric Otorhinolaryngology, 67*(7), 707–728.

Reeves, A. (1981). *Disorders of the nervous system.* Chicago, IL: Yearbook Medical.

Rhee, C. K., Park, H. M., & Jang, Y. J. (1999). Audiological evaluation of neonates with severe hyperbilirubinemia using transiently evoked otoacoustic emissions and auditory brainstem responses. *Laryngoscope, 109*(12), 2005–2008.

Ries, L. A. G., Melbert, D., Krapcho, M., Mariotto, A., Miller, B. A., Feuer, E. J., . . . Edwards, B. K. (Eds.). (2007). SEER Cancer Statistics Review, 1975–2004, National Cancer Institute. Bethesda, MD, http://seer.cancer.gov/csr/1975_2004/, based on November 2006 SEER data submission, posted to the SEER Web site, 2007.

Rintelmann, W. F. (1985). Monaural speech tests in the detection of central auditory disorders. In Musiek, F. E. & Pinheiro, M. L. (Eds.), *Assessment of central auditory dysfunction: Foundations and clinical correlates* (pp. 173–200). Baltimore, MD: Williams & Wilkins.

Roberts, R. J., Varney, N. R., Paulsen, J. S., & Richardson, E. D. (1990). Dichotic listening and complex partial seizures. *Journal of Clinical and Experimental Neuropsychology, 12*(4), 447–458.

Rowe, M. J., & Carlson, C. (1980). Brainstem auditory evoked potentials in postconcussion dizziness. *Archives of Neurology, 37*(11), 679–683.

Rubens, A. B., Froehling, B., Slater, G., & Anderson, D. (1985). Left ear suppression on verbal dichotic tests in patients with multiple sclerosis. *Annals of Neurology, 18*(4), 459–463.

Ryan, M. M. (2005). Neuromuscular junction anatomy and physiology. In H. R. Jones (Ed.), *Netter's neurology* (pp. 850–857). Teterboro, NJ: Icon Learning Systems.

Saatman, K. E., Duhaime, A. C., Bullock, R., Maas, A. I., Valadka, A., & Manley, G. T. (2008). Classification of traumatic brain injury for targeted therapies. *Journal of Neurotrauma, 25*(7) 719–738.

Samson, S., Zatorre, R. J., & Ramsay, J. O. (2002). Deficits of musical timbre perception after unilateral temporal-lobe lesion revealed with multidimensional scaling. *Brain, 125*(Pt. 3), 511–523.

Sanchez-Longo L. P., Forster, F. M., & Auth T. L. (1957). A clinical test for sound localization and its applications. *Neurology, 7*(9), 655–663.

Scherg, M., & Von Cramon, D. (1986). Evoked dipole source potentials of the human auditory cortex. *Electroencephalography and Clinical Neurophysiology, 65*(5), 344–360.

Schoenhuber, R., Gentilini, M., & Orlando, A. (1988). Prognostic value of auditory brainstem responses for late postconcussion symptoms following minor head injury. *Journal of Neurosurgery, 68*(5), 742–744.

Segalowitz, S. J., Bernstein, D. M., & Lawson, S. (2001). P300 event-related potential decrements in well-functioning university students with mild head injury. *Brain and Cognition, 45*(3), 342–356.

Shapiro, S. M. (2003). Bilirubin toxicity in the developing nervous system. *Pediatric Neurology, 29*(5), 410–421.

Shapiro, S. M., & Hecox, K. E. (1988). Development of brainstem auditory evoked potentials in heterozygous and homozygous jaundiced Gunn rats. *Brain Research, 469*(1–2), 147–157.

Skoe, E., & Kraus, N. (2010). Auditory brain stem response to complex sounds: A tutorial. *Ear and Hearing, 31*(3), 302–324.

Sotero de Menezes, M. Landau-Kleffner syndrome. *eMedicine* 20 Mar 2007 26 Apr 2007.

Retrieved 6/15/11 from http://www.emedicine.com/neuro/topic182.htm .

Soustiel, J. F., Hafner, H., Chistyakov, A. V., Barzilai, A., & Feinsod, M. (1995). Trigeminal and auditory evoked responses in minor head injuries and post-concussion syndrome. *Brain Injury, 9*(8), 805–813.

Soysal, A., Atakli, D., Atay, T., Altintas, H., Baybas, S., & Arpac, B. (2002). Auditory event-related potentials (P300) in partial and generalized epileptic patients. *Seizure, 8*(2), 107–110.

Speaks, C., Gray, T., & Miller, J. (1975). Central auditory deficits and temporal-lobe lesions. *Journal of Speech and Hearing Disorders, 40*(2), 192–205.

Starr, A., & Achor, J. (1975). Auditory brain stem responses in neurological disease. *Archives of Neurology, 32*(11), 761–768.

Steel, J. G., Thomas, H. A., & Strollo, P. J. (1982). Fusiform basilar aneurysm as a cause of embolic stroke. *Stroke, 13*(5), 712–716.

St. Clair, D. M., Blackwood, D. H., & Christie, J. E. (1985). P3 and other long latency evoked potentials in presenile dementia Alzheimer type and alcoholic Korsakoff syndrome. *British Journal of Psychiatry, 14*, 702–706.

Strouse, A. L., Hall, J. W., & Burger, M. C. (1995). Central auditory processing in Alzheimer's disease. *Ear and Hearing, 16*(2), 230–238.

Sung, G. (2006). Intracerebral hemorrhage. In R. T. Johnson, J. W. Griffin, & J. C. McArthur (Eds.), *Current therapies in neurologic disease* (7th ed., pp. 221–223). London, UK: Mosby.

Taber, K. H., Warden, D. L., & Hurley, R. A. (2006). Blast-related traumatic brain injury: What is known? *Journal of Neuropsychiatry and Clinical Neurosciences, 18*(2), 141–145.

Toole, J. (1979). Vascular diseases of brain and spinal cord. In H. Merritt (Ed.), *A textbook of neurology* (6th ed., pp. 149–209). Philadelphia, PA: Lee & Febiger.

Tsubaki, T., & Irukayama, K. (1977). *Minamata disease: Methylmercury poisoning in Minamata and Nigata, Japan.* New York, NY: Elsevier Science.

Valadka, A. (2004). Injury to the cranium. In E. Moore, D. Feleciano, & K. Mattox (Eds.), *Trauma* (pp. 385–406). New York, NY: McGraw-Hill.

Varney, N. R., Kubu, C. S., & Morrow, L. A. (1998). Dichotic listening performances of patients with chronic exposure to organic solvents. *Clinical Neuropsychology, 12*(1), 107–112.

Verma, N. P., Twitty, G. R., & Fuerst, D. R. (1993). Event-related potentials in complex partial seizures. *Brain Topography, 6*(1), 35–41.

WebMD. (2009). *Alzheimer's disease guide.* Retrieved 6/15/11 from http://www.webmd.com/alzheimers/guide/default.htm.

Weihing, J. A., & Musiek, F. E. (2007). Dichotic interaural intensity difference (DIID) training. In D. Geffner & D. Ross-Swain (Eds.), *Auditory processing disorders: Assessment, management, and treatment* (pp. 281–300). San Diego, CA: Plural Publishing.

Werner, C., & Engelhard, K. (2007). Pathophysiology of traumatic brain injury. *British Journal of Anesthesia, 99,* 4–9.

Yakovlev, P., & LeCours, A. (1967). Myelogenetic cycles of regional maturation of the brain. In A. Minkiniwski (Ed.), *Regional development of the brain in early life* (pp. 3–70). Oxford, UK: Blackwell Press.

Young, H. (1983). Brain tumors. In R. Rosenber (Ed.), *The clinical neurosciences, Section 2, Neuro-surgery* (pp. 1141–1204). New York, NY: Churchill Livingstone.

Zabar, Y. (2005). Memory and cognitive disorders. In H. R. Jones (Ed.), *Netter's neurology* (pp. 322–365). Teterboro, NJ: Icon Learning Systems.

Zamyslowska-Szmytke, E., Fuente, A., Niebudek-Bogusz, E., & Sliwinska-Kowalska, M. (2009). Temporal processing disorder associated with styrene exposure. *Audiology and Neurotology, 14*(5), 296–302.

8

Tinnitus, Hyperacusis, and Auditory Hallucinations

INTRODUCTION

The topics covered in this chapter (tinnitus, hyperacusis, and auditory hallucinations) easily could have been included as segments in other chapters. However, it was difficult to determine in which chapter to include these topics as these common auditory disorders can have a number of different etiologies and a variety of sites of lesion and origins. Given this challenge, as well as the keen general interest in these disorders, the decision was made to include a separate chapter for coverage of these three entities.

Tinnitus has been written about for many years in the fields of otology, psychology, and audiology and it has been the focus of considerable research; however, in spite of these efforts, a cure for this malady remains elusive. Awareness of this problem and a better understanding of the nature and origins of this auditory symptom, including interventions that may help moderate the severity of a patient's tinnitus and/or the individual's ability to cope with the symptom have

been enhanced by the many contributions of the late Jack Vernon. In addition, the fine work of the American Tinnitus Association has done much to inform the public about this common and bothersome disorder. In this regard, public information has played, and can continue to play, a major role in reducing one of the main causes of tinnitus (i.e., exposure to high intensity sounds). Without a doubt, there have been advances in the understanding of tinnitus and certain treatments have been shown to help some individuals. Interestingly, most treatment approaches have been nonmedical in nature with their roots anchored in the early approaches introduced by Jack Vernon.

Hyperacusis, or the increased sensitivity to sounds caused by abnormal loudness perception, is often associated with tinnitus, but not all individuals with this auditory condition will report experiencing tinnitus. The abnormal loudness perception noted in hyperacusis frequently is related to the presence of a sensorineural hearing loss and the lack of an acoustic reflex (Møller, 2000). Damage to outer hair cells in the cochlea has been linked to the recruitment phenomenon and the lack of an acoustic reflex disallows the natural attenuation of incoming loud sounds. It is understandable how these two dysfunctions of hearing can be a basis for hyperacusis; however, it should be noted that not all individuals with hyperacusis have hearing loss and absent acoustic reflexes.

Hyperacusis has not been studied as long or as extensively as tinnitus. However, in many patients, tinnitus and hyperacusis coexist and are treated together. As was the case with tinnitus, no definitive cure for hyperacusis has been identified, but through counseling and various treatments approaches (e.g., desensitization therapy) this disorder can be managed successfully in many individuals. Procedures such as these can be a critical factor in restoring or establishing the ability of patients to function normally in their everyday activities despite the continued presence of aversions to many common, everyday sounds.

Auditory hallucinations are new to audiology here in the United States. Although new to audiology, this disorder has been studied by psychologists and psychiatrists for some time as many individuals with auditory hallucinations present with psychiatric conditions, such as schizophrenia. However, many people without comorbid diagnoses of psychologic and/or psychiatric conditions also experience auditory hallucinations, and these are the individuals who have stirred the interest of audiologists. The elderly with histories of long-standing severe hearing loss are one group of patients who seem to be prone to auditory hallucinations. Another group that experiences auditory hallucinations includes patients with neurologic damage involving the central auditory structures. As you will read later in this chapter, the definitions

of subjective tinnitus and auditory hallucinations are quite similar—both involve the perception of sound in the absence of an external sound stimulus.

The research surrounding tinnitus, hyperacusis, and auditory hallucinations is indeed interesting and will be pursued more in the future. Similarities as well as differences in these three hearing disorders will likely herald advances in both the understanding and treatment of these problems. However, it is important to keep in mind that not all patients who experience one or more of these "hearing" symptoms will necessarily have an auditory basis for their disorder and referrals to other professionals will be critical for those cases where psychologic, psychiatric, or emotional problems are suspected either as a primary or a comorbid condition.

TINNITUS

Introduction

Tinnitus can be defined as the perception of sound in the absence of an environmental stimulus (Chan, 2009). It is derived from the Latin word *tinnire* meaning ringing. Many people are bothered by tinnitus, with some experiencing debilitating tinnitus. Despite being a common disorder and the focus of considerable research, a cure for this disorder remains elusive. However, some treatments do provide relief from tinnitus for at least some patients.

Tinnitus generally is classified into two main categories, subjective and objective. Subjective tinnitus can be heard only by the person who experiences it. It is often described as a ringing, hissing, humming, chirping (as in the sounds made by crickets and/or cicadas), whistling, blowing, or roaring sound. Objective tinnitus, on the other hand, can be measured if a probe microphone, or stethoscope (even a hearing aid stethoscope) is placed in the ear canal or on the pinna. It also may be heard by others who are in close proximity to the individual if the tinnitus is loud enough to be perceived. This type of tinnitus is commonly described by sufferers as being a pulsatile, clicking, or rushing type of sound (Marion & Cevette, 1991).

Symptoms

Tinnitus is a symptom. Hence, this section title is redundant, but it provides an opportunity to discuss the various characteristics of tinnitus. As mentioned earlier, the perceptual experience of tinnitus can be quite diverse, and in some individuals, more than one type of sound can be experienced. The tinnitus can be constant, intermittent, fluctuating, triggered by external and/or internal stimuli, and unilateral or bilateral. In addition, it may be accompanied by hearing loss or normal hearing, vestibular symptoms, and a variety of other ear symptoms. The tinnitus and other ear symptoms may vary in severity from essentially unnoticeable to intolerable (Chan, 2009; Marion & Cevette, 1991).

Incidence and Prevalence

Tinnitus is a common disorder of the auditory system with some reports relating that 10% of the general population has this problem (Chan, 2009). The incidence does increase with age and one in 200 cases with tinnitus is considered to be

severely bothered by it (Tyler & Erlandsson, 2003).

Etiology and Pathology

Objective tinnitus usually is pulsatile and often has a vascular basis. This vascular involvement is usually located around the temporal bone. Arteriovenous shunts, venous hum, paragangliomas, neoplasms, hypertension, and elevated intercranial pressure are some of the etiologic bases for objective tinnitus (Chan, 2009; Møller, 2000).

Subjective tinnitus is often a result of noise exposure (18%), trauma (8%), otologic infections and illness (8%), and drugs (2%) (Henry, Dennis, & Schecter, 2005), and it can be associated with general sensorineural hearing loss, Ménière's disease, strokes of the central nervous system, vascular loops, and aging (Henry et al., 2005; Møller, 2000). In the remainder of the cases (64%), the subjective experiences of tinnitus being reported possibly could be attributed to psychological or non-auditory factors, such as negative counseling or other undetermined factors or events.

The pathophysiology of tinnitus is not well understood, and although interesting theories abound, only a few of these will be mentioned here. It is well known that, if tinnitus is present, there is likely to be damage, or a substantial change to the auditory system's function. This damage may not be measurable or diagnosed as the compromise may be subclinical (i.e., it is not detected by routine audiologic procedures), but the damage still is present and is likely the generator or the origin of the tinnitus. One commonly accepted theory posits that tinnitus is caused by increased spontaneous auditory activity involving the "in phase" firing of a sufficient number of nerve fibers to result in the perception of sound (Møller, 2000; Tyler & Erlandsson, 2003). Also advanced is the theory that damage to the auditory system results in an alteration of the normal firing rates of the inhibitory and excitatory fibers within the auditory nerve or the brain. In this case, the firing of excitatory fibers that are normally suppressed by the inhibitory circuits results in the experience of tinnitus (Møller, 2000). A third theory suggests that the decoupling of hair cells secondary to damage of the cochlea and/or related structural damage to other inner ear structures involving the hair cells (e.g., a collapsing tectorial membrane) could cause the hair cells to fire without sound stimulation (Tonndorf, 1980). It also has been proposed that defects in the reticular lamina may cause a random depolarization of hair cells resulting in the perception of tinnitus (Feldmann, 1988). Finally, Eggermont (2007) advances the notion that the pathophysiology of tinnitus depends on the particular disorder associated with it. He discusses how ion channel alteration for particular disorders could trigger the tinnitus response. He also discusses various neurotransmitters and drugs that can affect the auditory system and how these could play a role in tinnitus. All of these theories are based on the concept that there is structural or biochemical damage to the cochlea, which in turn creates improper function of the structures within the organ of Corti giving rise to the tinnitus. What this means is that, when the cochlea is damaged, there are multiple sites at which processing changes can occur, and various types of dysfunction can occur that may lead to the experience of tinnitus.

Due to the likely presence of multiple pathophysiologic factors in many tinnitus sufferers, it is difficult to determine which one actually triggers the tinnitus. It may be possible that a constellation of factors needs to exist to create the perception of tinnitus. Although the previous discussion has focused on pathophysiologic alterations or compromise in the cochlea, it also is important to realize that compromise of the auditory pathways in the brain can additionally result in tinnitus (Møller, 2000). There currently is compelling evidence of a centrally mediated basis for tinnitus (Lockwood, Salvi, & Burkard, 2002).

Site of Lesion

Objective tinnitus is most often related to dysfunction of the middle ear or its immediate area (Chan, 2009). Muscular or vascular problems often give rise to pulsatile or clicking-type sounds that are heard by the patient. Seldom does this type of tinnitus originate from the cochlea or more central auditory structures.

For many years, subjective tinnitus was believed primarily to be a cochlear problem. However, periodic reports have suggested that this may not always be the case. Most startling were reports of individuals with severe tinnitus and hearing loss who underwent surgical sectioning of the auditory nerve only to have the tinnitus either remain or become worse (see Møller, 2000). This kind of finding indicated that the central auditory pathways may be responsible for the generation of tinnitus in some cases. This is not to say that cochlear damage cannot cause tinnitus. It is highly likely that damage to the cochlea from such insults as high intensity noise or Ménière's disease will result in the cochlea generating subjective tinnitus. However, a study by Lockwood et al. (2002) indicates that neural activity within the brain also can generate tinnitus (at least some of the time). Functional imaging studies have demonstrated that tinnitus activates the auditory cortex on only one side of the brain, whereas an external tonal stimulus activates both cortices. In addition, changes in functional imaging measures have been documented for individuals who can increase the loudness of their tinnitus by gazing in a certain direction or by clenching their teeth. In these cases, the changes in functional imaging measures revealed increased cortical activity that correlated with the tinnitus-provoking maneuvers (see Lockwood et al., 2002, and Møller, 2000, for reviews).

One other observation that is worth mentioning relates to what appears to be a disconnect between the apparent anatomic site of abnormality and the site of physiologic abnormality. This "disconnect" could add to the difficulty of interpreting the triggers and nature of tinnitus in many patients. Additional research is needed to delineate the nature and exact site of physiologic abnormalities in individuals for whom there may be a discrepancy between the apparent anatomic site of pathology and the actual physiologic site of abnormality.

At this point in time, it is probably best to keep an open mind and entertain the possibility that subjective tinnitus can be localized in the cochlea, the auditory nerve, and/or the central pathways. Currently, there is little in terms of test procedures that allow the accurate localization of tinnitus within the peripheral and/or central auditory system. Tinnitus often can be localized by the patient to one ear,

both ears, or the head. If localized to one or both ears, it is commonly assumed that the tinnitus arises from a peripheral auditory structure. On the other hand, it is inviting to think that tinnitus located in the head or midline may have a central origin. Although there is little, if any, evidence to support this assumption at this time, it does remain a possibility.

Medical and Audiologic Evaluation

One of the most important steps in the medical evaluation of tinnitus is obtaining a thorough history from the patient in order to begin the process of making a correct diagnosis of the etiology (Perry & Gantz, 2000). Closely listening to the patient's reported symptoms is key. It is important to determine if the reported tinnitus is the chief complaint, or if this symptom is secondary to other issues (hearing loss, vertigo, etc.). In addition, the characterization of the tinnitus, such as whether it is symmetric (often reported to be "in the head") or lateralized to one ear or the other, is of utmost importance.

Following a thorough case history, a full head and neck examination is necessary. Included in this examination should be a comprehensive otologic examination, including otomicroscopy, and an audiologic evaluation, including tympanometry. Additionally, each cranial nerve should be examined as some otologic disorders (such as a mass lesion) may affect primarily the auditory nerve, resulting in tinnitus, but they also may affect one or more of the adjacent nerves. An examination of all of the cranial nerves can provide insight as to the basis of the underlying problem (Fortune, Haynes, & Hall,

1999). An audiologic evaluation also is often warranted to rule out significant retrocochlear involvement as a contributory factor to the symptom. Although nonpulsatile, bilateral tinnitus often does not require any further medical examination, individuals who present with unilateral tinnitus or pulsatile tinnitus, as well as those with asymmetric hearing loss, should be seen for a magnetic resonance imaging (MRI) with gadolinium contrast procedure (Schwaber, 2003). In particular, the internal auditory canals should be examined. For those patients who cannot undergo an MRI, an auditory brainstem response (ABR) or computed tomography (CT) scan should be considered. In addition to traditional imaging, patients with pulsatile tinnitus should evaluated for a variety of vascular disorders, such as acquired arterial alteration, stenosis, tutosisty, dissection, or aneurysm (Perry & Gantz, 2000), and they should undergo additional examinations, as appropriate. These may include magnetic resonance angiography (MRA) or arteriorgrams. The benefit of MRA is that it is essentially noninvasive and it is helpful in determining both arterial and venous involvement. Laboratory testing also may be indicated for some patients. Patients may be evaluated for a variety of disorders, which may include endocrinopathies, metabolic disorders, autoimmune diseases, and syphilis (House & Derebery, 1995).

A complete audiologic evaluation is an important early step in the diagnosis and treatment of tinnitus. Classic puretone and speech audiometric procedures along with immittance testing and otoacoustic emissions should be completed. If indicated, a workup for auditory nerve or central involvement should be carried out (Marion & Cevette, 1991). For puretone thresholds, the use of pulsed tones

may make it easier for the patient to identify the stimuli accurately. It also is helpful to have the patient indicate how much the tinnitus bothers him or her. Møller (2000) advocates using three categories for this purpose. These categories include: (1) mild—doesn't interfere with daily living; (2) moderate—annoying and unpleasant; and (3) severe—interferes with daily living in major ways. A number of self-assessment scales have been developed for the purpose of documenting the effects of tinnitus on the patient's daily activities. A listing of some of the more common self-assessment scales is provided later.

An audiologic or sometimes termed a psychoacoustic assessment of tinnitus can prove valuable in a number of ways and should be included in the evaluation of the patient who presents with tinnitus. Tyler and Erlandsson (2003) mention five ways that the evaluation of tinnitus can be used. These include: (1) to confirm that the patient has tinnitus, (2) to monitor changes in the tinnitus over time, (3) to provide insights as to underlying mechanisms, (4) to help in the fitting of devices for tinnitus treatment, and (5) to render a determination of the reliability of the patient's report of tinnitus, which may be important, especially in legal cases. Although such testing is often desirable, many patients will find tinnitus assessments to be challenging and often difficult to complete. Therefore, it is important that the audiologist's rationale for conducting the psychophysical testing be well thought out and made clear to the patient.

The evaluation of tinnitus is indeed difficult and not as accurate or precise as most would like it to be. This fact should be understood by those undertaking this challenging task. Despite various psychoacoustic strategies that have been invoked to complete tinnitus matching procedures in the clinical setting, the results remain quite variable as tinnitus has many components and it often changes quickly in pitch and loudness rendering it difficult to measure.

The key aspects of tinnitus assessment center around pitch and loudness matching (see Marion & Cevette, 1991; Tyler & Erlandsson, 2003). In tinnitus matching procedures, the patient is asked to match the pitch and loudness of his or her tinnitus to external sounds presented under earphones. Multiple replications usually are required to reach stable values. In cases of unilateral tinnitus, matching can be performed with the external sound presented to the ipsilateral ear (ear with the tinnitus) or the contralateral ear (ear without the tinnitus). If bilateral tinnitus is present, each ear must be evaluated separately, which can be challenging. In addition to the matching procedure, a masking procedure can be used in which the sound pressure level (SPL) of a broadband noise needed to mask out perception of the tinnitus is determined. This procedure, as well as the loudness matching procedure, can give some indication of the perceived loudness of the tinnitus. It has been reported that most people match their tinnitus to an external stimulus that is in the 10 to 30 dB sensation level (SL) range (Møller, 2000). However, a more recent study has shown that the average intensity match for tinnitus was under 10 dB SL for patients with histories of noise exposure (Nageris, Attius, & Raveh, 2010), and clinical experience has shown that the intensity match for the majority of patients is below 10 dB SL (Vernon & Meikle, 2000). It is important to note that the measurement of tinnitus loudness is affected considerably by the frequency at which the measure is obtained. The SL values typically are lower when loudness is measured at the pitch (i.e., the frequency) of the tinnitus than when it is measured at a lower frequency (see Vernon & Meikle, 2000, for additional information on loudness matching procedures and findings).

In regard to pitch-matching procedures, tinnitus is usually matched to high frequencies. Vernon and Meikle (1988) reported that tinnitus in their subjects was matched to frequencies above 3000 Hz 83% of the time. Similar findings have been reported by others (Nageris et al., 2010). It is important to note that the pitch, quality, and loudness of tinnitus may vary together or they may vary independently (which can complicate the pitch-matching procedure). Also many patients with tinnitus experience more than one tinnitus sound. In these cases, efforts to determine the perceived pitch of the tinnitus may require multiple assessments to fully appreciate the nature of the tinnitus that the patient is experiencing. This type of information can have important implications for treatment decisions, especially if sound maskers, hearing aids, or tinnitus instruments (i.e., devices that combine both of these technologies) are being considered (see Meikle, Creedon, & Griest, 2004).

Sometimes the frequency of the tinnitus is related to particular otologic problems. For example, the tinnitus experienced by patients with Ménière's disease often is matched to a low-frequency stimulus, whereas the tinnitus experienced by patients with noise-induced loss is more commonly matched to a high-frequency stimulus (Douek & Reid, 1968). Even the recent report from Nageris et al. (2010) reflected this trend in individuals with noise-induced hearing losses. However, from the present authors' view, the strength of these relationships has not always been highly reliable or specific. Therefore, it is important that one does not limit testing to a particular frequency range when assessing patients, even if one anticipates a likely match within a specific frequency range based on the patient's presenting symptoms and/or otologic diagnosis.

The masking of a patient's tinnitus has been discussed for many years, both as a diagnostic procedure and as a management tool. In most cases, tinnitus can be effectively masked using a broadband noise stimulus. In fact, 91% of the patients in an investigation conducted by Vernon and Meikle (1988) achieved complete masking of the tinnitus. If a patient's tinnitus can be easily masked with a broadband stimulus, it may indicate that a masking device may work well as a treatment option for that patient. In a large number of subjects with tinnitus, Savastano (2008) reported that slightly more than 50% of the patients had their tinnitus masked by broadband noise in the 31 to 60 dB range, whereas slightly more than 30% required levels in excess of 60 dB (although not specified in this study, these levels were assumed to be effective masking levels and not SL measures). Savastano (2008) also related that individuals with hearing loss required higher levels of noise to mask their tinnitus than those with normal hearing (see qualifying comment offered above).

In assessing tinnitus, perhaps one of the most interesting measures is that of residual inhibition (RI). This measure is accomplished by using a masking noise (usually a broadband noise, but narrowband noise or tones can also be used) that is presented above the intensity level needed to mask the tinnitus (usually 10 dB) for a period of time (usually 1 minute). After the exposure time has lapsed, the patients are asked if they still hear the tin-

nitus, and if they do, they are asked if the tinnitus sounds as loud as it did before the presentation of the masker, or whether it appears that the intensity of the tinnitus has been reduced. If the patients report hearing no tinnitus, it is considered positive or complete RI, and the period of time required for the tinnitus to return is measured. If the tinnitus is the same after the presentation of the masker, it is considered a negative result, and if the tinnitus is present but reduced in loudness it is classified as a partial RI (Meikle et al., 2004).

Residual inhibition (the time period without tinnitus) can last from seconds to several minutes. Most people with tinnitus have some degree of RI (Meikle et al., 2004), but some (10% to 15%) note complete abolition of the tinnitus signal (Savastano, 2008). In a large data set, between 2 and 3% of individuals who experienced RI had durations of greater than 10 minutes (Meikle et al., 2004). Residual inhibition does not have strong clinical implications for routine clinical application at this time, but it is a phenomenon of great interest and should be studied much more than it is. Therefore, the present authors believe that measures of RI should be included in the evaluation of tinnitus.

Medical and Audiologic Treatment

As outlined above, numerous disorders are associated with tinnitus and treatment of these associated disorders varies significantly. Perhaps one of the most common medical approaches to tinnitus is pharmacologic management. This is partially related to the strong psychological component associated with tinnitus, which is discussed below.

Psychological Treatment

When a nonotologic or nonaudiologic etiology for tinnitus is uncovered, referrals to other specialists, such as dentists, neurologists, and psychologists may be necessary. Psychological treatment plays a critical role for many patients with tinnitus as there is a high comorbidity between tinnitus and associated psychological disorders. These often include anxiety, depression, sleep disturbance, and general social impairment. As a result, tinnitus is often diagnosed as a psychological disorder with psychological consequences (Wilson & Henry, 2000). In conjunction with audiologic management, cognitive behavioral therapy may prove beneficial for patients with significant tinnitus. Tinnitus is often compared to and treated in a manner similar to chronic pain (Tonndorf, 1987). Patients with tinnitus, not unlike patients with chronic pain, have extreme difficulty coping with the symptom and often feel as though they have no control over it. As a result, several treatment approaches have been suggested to help alleviate the psychological impact of tinnitus on the patient's life. In addition to pharmacologic agents, these include approaches such as biofeedback, cognitive therapy, and relaxation training.

There are numerous assessments related to the psychological impact of tinnitus. Examples of these include the Tinnitus Reaction Questionnaire (Wilson, Henry, Bowen, & Haralambous, 1991), the Tinnitus Handicap Inventory (Newman, Jacobson, & Spitzer, 1996), the Tinnitus Effects Questionnaire (Hallam, 1996), the Tinnitus Severity Scale (Halford & Anderson, 1991), the Tinnitus Handicap Questionnaire (Kuk, Tyler, Russell, & Jordan, 1990), and the Tinnitus Coping Style Questionnaire (Budd & Pugh, 1996). These types of questionnaires have proven to be very beneficial to clinicians as they can be used to determine the psychological impact of tinnitus on a patient's everyday functioning. In addition to providing an initial assessment of the impact of the tinnitus on the patient's functioning, these questionnaires can be used to monitor the efficacy of treatment as well.

Relaxation methods are a form of biofeedback that have been employed with patients who have chronic tinnitus. Some of the first psychological approaches to the treatment or management of tinnitus used similar techniques. The most common form of training is progressive muscular relaxation as described by Bernstein and Borkovec (1973). Through a series of exercises, the patient learns to tense and relax muscle groups. Although this approach alone may not demonstrate significant benefit, it may prove beneficial when used in conjunction with other therapeutic techniques. It also may be effective in treating or managing some of the other disorders/symptoms that are often experienced by the tinnitus sufferer. For example, many patients with tinnitus suffer from severe sleep disturbance and this particular approach has proven to be helpful in assisting patients with general sleep disorders (Morin, Culbert, & Schwartz, 1994).

Due to the strong psychological component associated with tinnitus, cognitive behavioral therapy (CBT) for use in tinnitus patients was first recommended by Sweetow in 1980. A CBT approach can be defined as an attempt to change negative thoughts and behaviors by applying strategies designed to change the unproductive thoughts. The following systematic 10-step approach is the recommended procedure for implementing CBT with tinnitus patients (Sweetow, 2000).

1. Define the problem in terms of a framework that allows for amenable solutions.
2. Identify the behaviors and thoughts affected by the tinnitus.
3. List the maladaptive strategies and cognitive distortions currently employed.
4. Distinguish between the tinnitus experience and the maladaptive behavior.
5. Identify alternative thoughts, behaviors, and strategies.
6. Encourage the patient to formulate and prioritize attainable target goals.
7. Collaboratively devise and rehearse strategies that can be measured.
8. Regularly assess success or failure of coping strategies.
9. Question and challenge unsubstantiated statements.
10. Lay a framework for maintenance of positive change.

Although CBT has been found to be a helpful therapeutic approach for the tinnitus patient, care must be taken to counsel the patient that tinnitus generally is an incurable condition. As is the case in many of the current therapies and/or interventions for tinnitus, this approach is designed to help in the management of the condition, but will not result in the elimination of the tinnitus.

Pharmacologic Treatment

Numerous drugs have been investigated for the treatment of tinnitus (Elgoyhen & Langguth, 2010); however, there are no standardized protocols for the use of medications to treat tinnitus at this time. These drugs include antiarrhythmics, anticonvulsants, anxiolytics, glutamate receptor antagonists, antidepressants, and miscellaneous other pharmaceuticals or homeopathic agents, including both controlled and over-the-counter medications.

Perhaps the most routinely prescribed drugs are antidepressants (Darlington & Smith, 2007). This is likely a result of the high comorbidity between tinnitus and psychological involvement. Additionally, anxiolytics have been prescribed with success in managing tinnitus. Both antidepressents and anxiolytics have been shown to result in statistically significant improvements in tinnitus patients when evaluated using a double-blind, placebo-controlled investigations (Johnson, Brummett, & Schleuning, 1993; Sullivan, Katon, Russo, Dobie, & Sakai, 1992). Intravenous lidocaine also has proven effective; however, the effect is short lived and there can be notable side effects; hence, the use of intravenous lidocaine is not a practical approach to the treatment of tinnitus. Although a number of drug treatments are available, no drug has proven to be sufficient in treating all tinnitus patients. Such treatments should be closely monitored by a physician and will likely prove most beneficial if used in conjunction with other nonpharmaceutical management strategies.

Sound Generators and Maskers

One of the earliest forms of treatment for tinnitus was the use of sound generators and maskers. This form of management can be dated to the early 1820s when the famous French physician Jean Itard described trying to "cover up the internal noise" by using various environmental noises. The first attempt to use ear-level devices to mask the tinnitus was initiated in the early to mid-1970s (see Vernon, 1975). These devices have been termed tinnitus maskers and tinnitus instruments and are officially classified by the Food and Drug Administration as therapeutic devices. Tinnitus maskers can be worn as both behind-the-ear and in-the-ear devices.

Nonwearable devices are often used to assist in masking tinnitus, particularly in an effort to improve sleep disturbance. Reports indicate that nearly 70% of patients with tinnitus suffer from sleep problems (Meikle et al., 2004). As a result, many patients use items such as fans, televisions, mistuned radios, and commercially available sound generators to "mask" their tinnitus and promote sleep.

Traditional hearing aids also have been used in the management of tinnitus patients. Amplification devices such as hearing aids have proven successful because, when these devices are worn by the tinnitus sufferer, ambient noise in the environment is amplified and the patient's tinnitus is masked. Kochlin and Tyler (2008) have reported that approximately 60% of individuals with tinnitus who were fitted with hearing aids have reported improvement in their tinnitus symptoms. There have been many significant developments in signal processing since the time that tinnitus maskers were first introduced. At the present time, devices that combine both a traditional hearing aid and a tinnitus masker in one unit are commercially available. These instruments are appropriate for patients who may need additional tinnitus masking beyond that provided by a hearing aid alone (see Folmer, Martin, Shi, & Edlefsen, 2006, and Searchfield, 2006, for additional discussion).

Although ear-level maskers continue to be used, they are limited as a therapeutic approach in that, when they are not being worn, the tinnitus typically continues to be problematic for the patient. It is important for the clinician fitting such devices to be keenly aware of the importance of appropriate fitting techniques. This includes assessments of the patient's tinnitus, including pitch and loudness matching, minimum masking level, and residual inhibition as outlined above. Additionally, one must understand that there is a distinct difference between an effective versus an acceptable level of masking (Vernon & Meikle, 2000). Effective masking or "complete masking" refers to the ability to successfully cover the tinnitus so that the patient can no longer hear it, whereas an acceptable level of masking or "partial masking" refers to a situation in which the patient is provided a masking sound which offers some relief from the tinnitus. In the latter situation, the tinnitus is still present, although it is perceived by the patient to be of lower intensity and less of an annoyance. There are a number of factors that determine whether complete masking can be achieved for a given patient. These include such variables as the level of the tinnitus, the frequency of the tinnitus (e.g., if the tinnitus is matched to a speech frequency, it may be difficult to provide sufficient masking without affecting speech understanding), and the presence of multiple tinnitus sounds (for additional information, see Vernon & Meikle, 2000).

Neurophysiologic Rehabilitation

Neurophysiologic rehabilitation relies on the plasticity of the brain to create neural changes, which can alleviate the tinnitus. Plasticity can be defined as the alteration of nerve cells to better conform to immediate environmental influences, with this alteration often associated with behavioral change (Musiek & Berge, 1998). It has been theorized, that tinnitus is driven not only by a dysfunction of the auditory system, but also by involvement of the limbic and autonomic nervous systems as well (Jastreboff, 1998). The strong emotional and often physical response exhibited by many tinnitus sufferers would suggest that there are non-auditory areas within the central nervous system that contribute to tinnitus. The limbic system is responsible for behavioral responses including mood state and emotion. The autonomic nervous system, on the other hand, provides for motor innervations. As many patients report issues associated with sleep, anxiety, and tension, this would suggest that both systems may somehow play a role in tinnitus. The theory behind the neurophysiologic rehabilitative approach is that, if both the audiologic (central auditory nervous system) and the psychological (limbic system) aspects can be addressed, improvement in symptoms will be observed.

In the most simplistic terms, it is theorized that the "central gain" produced within the brain is enhanced because of lack of inhibitory neural control, which leads to enhanced excitatory activity. Tinnitus is believed to be a result of such activity. Neurophysiologic rehabilitation theoretically aims to decrease the central gain by reorganizing the auditory inhibitory and excitatory balance within the brain (Hanley, Davis, Paki, Quinn, & Bellekom, 2008). One such approach has been Tinnitus Habituation Therapy (THT), which was introduced on a theoretical basis by Hallum and colleagues (Hallam, Rachman, & Hinchcliffe, 1984). The goal of this therapy is not to cure tinnitus, but rather to filter and block tinnitus-related activity within the brain, thus reducing awareness and disturbance

(Jastreboff, 2000). In recent years, several THT approaches have been relatively successful in achieving this goal.

Tinnitus Retraining Therapy (TRT) is a multicomponent program that utilizes both sound therapy along with counseling to achieve habituation of tinnitus. Tinnitus patients are categorized along a 4-point scale with 0 suggesting a low impact on life and 4 a high impact on life with significant hyperacusis and prolonged sound-induced exacerbation (Jastreboff, 1998). The intent of TRT is to remove the negative association attached to tinnitus perception and to help the patient to habituate to the tinnitus so that it becomes less aversive (Jastreboff, 2008). This is achieved by presenting low level, broadband acoustic stimulation, which is used to initiate and encourage tinnitus habituation. This process takes approximately 12 to 18 months. The effectiveness of TRT has been reported to be significant, with improvement in symptoms reported for up to 80% of patients (Jastreboff, Gray, & Gold, 1996).

Another therapeutic technique is one described by Davis in the 1990s. Davis developed a device (Neuromonics Oasis) and program intended to address the audiologic, psychological, and neurologic aspects of tinnitus (see Davis, Wilde, Steed, & Hanley, 2008). The patient wears a small device (similar to a personal listening device), which presents precisely designed music that has been tailored spectrally to account for the patient's auditory thresholds and loudness tolerance. The theory behind this device is that, over time, plasticity will occur through which the negative conscious association with tinnitus will be reduced and its disturbance decreased. This is a multistage treatment program that takes approximately 6 to 9 months for the patient to complete.

Several reports have demonstrated the efficacy of treatment with this approach (Davis et al., 2008; Hanley et al., 2008).

A variety of therapeutic tools are available to assist clinicians with today's tinnitus patients. The previous expression "you'll just have to live with it" rarely applies to today's patients. What is important to understand is that, although treatment approaches are available that may help alleviate the "symptom," there are still no cures for the disorder.

HYPERACUSIS

Introduction

Hyperacusis is a disorder related to loudness perception. Specifically, it is defined as the "consistently exaggerated or inappropriate responses to sounds that are neither threatening nor uncomfortably loud to a typical person" (Klein, Armstrong, Greer, & Brown, 1990). It is not to be confused with phonophobia (i.e., a fear of sounds) or misophonia (i.e., a dislike for particular sounds). Phonophobia and misophonia differ from hyperacusis in that they typically have strong emotional links related to particular sounds, whereas hyperacusis, which also may have emotional links, tends to be generalized to nearly all loud sounds (Baguley & Andersson, 2007). Hyperacusis also varies from recruitment, which is associated with an abnormally rapid growth of loudness perception as intensity increases—a symptom typically found in individuals with cochlear impairment. For example, a patient with recruitment typically would have some degree of senorineural hearing loss and would perceive a moderately loud sound as uncomfortable (i.e., sounds that are not perceived as uncomfortable by normal hearers are perceived by patients with recruitment as being uncomfortably loud), whereas a patient with hyperacusis usually presents with normal hearing and is disturbed even by low-intensity sounds.

Symptoms

Hyperacusis, like tinnitus, is a symptom and not a disorder. Patients who experience hyperacusis often will demonstrate some overt behaviors that reflect their aversion to sounds that are perceived as being "too loud." Such behaviors include the avoidance of sounds that are perceived to be too loud, covering the ears with the hands when anticipating an aversive sound may occur, and grimacing when exposed to offending sounds, and so forth.

Incidence and Prevalence

There is a paucity of data related to the incidence and prevalence of hyperacusis. European reports suggest anywhere from 8% (Andersson, Lindvall, Hursti, & Carlbring, 2002) to 15% (Fabijanska, Rogowski, Bartnik, & Skarzynski, 1999) incidence rates, whereas rates among children are reported to be around 3.2% with 9% of children experiencing phonophobia (Coelho, Sanchez, & Tyler, 2007). Of note is that there is a high comorbidity of hyperacusis (approximately 40%) in patients whose primary complaint is tinnitus (Jastreboff & Jastreboff, 2000; Sood & Coles, 1988). However, according to Anari, Axelsson, Eliasson, and Magnusson (1999), the comorbidity of these two conditions is reported to be even higher, with 86% of patients in their sample who presented with hyperacusis as their primary complaint also reporting experiencing tinnitus.

Etiology and Pathology

Given the commonality between hyperacusis and tinnitus, one would be led to speculate that there is a shared mechanism(s) underlying the etiology and pathology of the two disorders. Although in some cases of hyperacusis, an underlying etiology can be found, in the majority of cases no specific etiology can be identified (Baguley, 2003). Several peripheral and central conditions often result in hyperacusis. Table 8–1 lists some of the common peripheral and central conditions that may be associated with hyperacusis.

Although the exact mechanism(s) underlying hyperacusis is unknown, there are several hypotheses which attempt to explain this phenomenon. It is believed that there is a strong link between hyperacusis and the neurotransmitter 5-HT. This is a serotonin receptor that regulates the modulation of many neurotransmitters, including those responsible for aggression, anxiety, appetite, cognition, learning, memory, mood, nausea, and sleep. Marriage and Barnes (1995) have suggested that when 5-HT becomes disordered the result is not only hyperacusis, but also other disorders as outlined in Table 8–1. It also has been hypothesized that there are enhanced cortical responses secondary to poor regulation of GABAergic neurons. GABAergic neurons are responsible for inhibition of central activity. Recent studies of hyperacusis have demonstrated a reduction in neuronal activity in the auditory cortex (see Wang, Luo, Huang, Zhou, & Chen, 2008). However, a recent report has demonstrated that individuals with hyperacusis have increased amplitude for late auditory evoked potentials compared to control subjects (Norris & Ceranic,

Table 8–1. Examples of Peripheral and Central Conditions as Well as Other Hormonal and Infectious Diseases That Can Result in Hyperacusis (Based on Katzenell & Segal, 2001)

Peripheral	*Central*	*Hormonal and Infectious Disease*
Bell's Palsy	Headache	Addison's Disease
Stapedectomy	Depression	Lyme Disease
Ramsey Hunt Syndrome	Minor Head Injury	
Recruitment	Williams Syndrome	
Noise-Induced Hearing Loss	Learning Disabilities	
Acoustic Trauma	Tinnitus	
Ménière's Disease	Spinal Involvement	
	Brain Lesions (i.e., Multiple Sclerosis, Stroke, Tumor)	
	Stuttering	

2011). Although there are many theories related to the mechanism(s) underlying hyperacusis, there is no consensus regarding its etiology or its specific site of origin at this time.

Site of Lesion

As mentioned above, many theories have been proposed in an attempt to define the potential mechanisms underlying hyperacusis, and hyperacusis has been noted in patients with a variety of peripheral and central system disorders (see Table 8–1). Therefore, it is likely that there may be both peripheral and/or central system involvement; however, as noted above, at the present time there is no definitive information on the origin(s) of this symptom, and additional research is needed.

Medical and Audiologic Evaluation

As hyperacusis has been linked to both neurologic and hormonal pathologies, it is important to fully examine the patient to rule out any serious disease process. One of the most important components of the examination of the patient with hyperacusis is a careful history. As with any audiologic complaint, a careful description of the presenting complaint and any important features and/or characteristics of the reported symptom such as the degree, length, and frequency of disturbance, are important to obtain and document. A careful history also includes any history of otologic (ear pathology, tinnitus, vertigo, etc.), neurologic (migraine, stroke, muscle numbness or weakness, head injury, etc.), or audiologic (hearing loss, noise exposure, etc.) involvement. Additionally, it is important to determine the presence of any other medical or psychological condition.

The physical examination should include a careful head and neck examination. In addition, general physical health measurements such as pulse, blood pressure, and weight should be considered. A neurologic examination should include a screening of the cranial nerves and both the motor and sensory systems (Katzenell & Segal, 2001). Additional laboratory tests should include a complete blood count. In addition, electrolyte, cortisol, and thyroid stimulating hormone levels should be measured (Katzenell & Segal, 2001).

The audiologic evaluation should be complete and comprehensive. This should include both pure-tone air conduction (and bone if warranted) and speech audiometry. Additionally, loudness discomfort levels for both tones and speech are important in determining the degree of involvement. As there have been reports of abnormal acoustic reflex measures in hyperacusic patients (Gordon, 1986), the assessment of acoustic reflex thresholds should also be considered. The sequence of audiologic tests for patients with hyperacusis is an important consideration. Tests that require high intensity levels could exacerbate this symptom. This in turn could influence test results. Therefore, it may be prudent to administer any audiologic tests requiring high intensity stimuli (e.g., acoustic reflex testing) at the end of the test battery.

Results from the patient's reported history, otologic examination, and audiologic testing may result in referral to a variety of other medical professionals. This may range from neurologists to psychiatrists. It is important for both audiologists and otolaryngologists to have referral sources who have experience in working with these types of patients so that they can readily refer their patients to these professionals when necessary.

Medical and Audiologic Treatment

There is no consensus regarding the best treatment approach for patients who present with hyperacusis. If, after the audiologic examination, the patient is found to present with an underlying disease, then management of such disease may lead to resolution of the hyperacusis. For many patients suffering from hyperacusis, an initial flight response often occurs in which the patient desires to protect his or her hearing through the use of hearing protection. However, there is no evidence to support such practice, and in fact, many individuals would argue that this may in fact exacerbate the condition (Baguley, 2003).

It has been suggested that therapeutic approaches to tinnitus may provide benefit to tinnitus patients who also suffer from hyperacusis. In this regard, both TRT (Jastreboff & Jastreboff, 2000) and commercially available programs such as Neuromonics (as described above) have been proposed as alternative therapies for hyperacusis. The theory behind these therapeutic approaches is that the use of low-level sound stimulation acts to promote cortical reorganization and desensitization. However, although these therapies have been proposed as "off-label" uses for the treatment of hyperacusis, to the authors' knowledge, there are no published data to support the efficacy of these approaches.

Perhaps one of the best treatment approaches for many patients with hyper-

acusis is reassurance that there are no pathologic clinical conditions contributing to the symptoms once these have in fact been ruled out. Both tinnitus and hyperacusis have a strong psychological component, which must be considered when managing these patients. In conjunction with this, CBT has been advocated in the management and treatment of the hyperacusic patient using a multidisciplinary team to address the sensitivity, annoyance, and fear associated with the condition. This is a complicated condition about which we know very little, but perhaps with future research both at the basic science and clinical levels we will be able to unravel the etiology and pathophysiologic mechanisms underlying this auditory condition and uncover efficacious approaches to the treatment and/or management of this condition.

AUDITORY HALLUCINATIONS

Introduction

For many years, auditory hallucinations were considered the domain of the psychiatrist or clinical psychologist. However, recently there has been a growing interest among professionals in the field of audiology perhaps related to two factors: (1) auditory hallucinations are not just seen in people with psychiatric problems, but also in those with auditory difficulties, and (2) the experience of auditory hallucinations can be viewed as an auditory disturbance for which there is an anatomic and physiologic correlate. Individuals who suffer from auditory hallucinations without any comorbid psychiatric illness have to be considered to have a form of auditory dysfunction. It also seems reasonable that, even in patients with psychiatric illness, the auditory system is involved in generating the hallucinations. Individuals with auditory hallucinations do perceive sound in some form; therefore, the auditory perceptual mechanism must be activated in some manner. This activation is supported by functional imaging studies as will be discussed later.

Auditory hallucinations are auditory perceptions that are experienced in the absence of corresponding external acoustic stimuli (Evers & Ellger, 2004). They can be perceived as whistles, bangs, clapping, ticks, screams, voices, intelligible or unintelligible speech, singing, and instrumental music, as well as other permutations of sound (Bentall, 1990). The definition and many of the examples of the perceived sounds in auditory hallucinations could, in part, be confused with tinnitus; although most would agree that tinnitus, as it is commonly recognized, would seldom take the form of voices, singing, speech, or music. In addition, there can be auditory hallucinations that are perceived as multiple sounds simultaneously or as different sounds that are perceived at different times. In many cases, however, the sounds heard are similar for each instance of an auditory hallucination (Musiek et al., 2007).

Symptoms

Like tinnitus, an auditory hallucination is a symptom. It could be associated with a peripheral or central auditory problem and/or a psychiatric disturbance. In some cases, hallucinations in other sensory modalities (primarily visual) can co-occur with auditory hallucinations. The experience of auditory hallucinations can be quite disturbing to the individual. As a result, the individual may become nervous, tense, irritated, and worried (Tien, 1991). This psychological "baggage" makes the hallucinations much worse.

Incidence and Prevalence

Studies on the prevalence of auditory hallucinations show statistics that are higher than one might expect. In a large sample of adults, ranging in age from young to old, between 2 and 3% reported experiencing auditory hallucinations (Remschmidt, 2002). Tien (1991) reported the incidence of auditory hallucinations also to be in the 2 to 3% range and the prevalence to be between 10 to 15%, with little influence of age until the 8th decade of life. This same study showed more women than men experiencing auditory hallucinations and that visual hallucinations were most often experienced, followed by auditory, somatic, and olfactory hallucinations. A factor potentially influencing the incidence and prevalence of auditory hallucinations is tinnitus. Tinnitus is sometimes difficult to discern from auditory hallucinations—especially in its more complex forms. It therefore may be mistakenly identified as an auditory hallucination rather than as tinnitus.

Etiology and Pathology

As already stated, auditory hallucinations frequently are associated with psychiatric illness, but they also can be related to peripheral and central auditory disorders. In regard to psychiatric disorders, schizophrenia is the psychiatric condition most commonly associated with auditory hallucinations (60–80%) (Shergill, Murray, & McGuire, 1998). Depression, compulsive disorder, and a host of other psychiatric symptoms also have been linked with auditory hallucinations, but the coincidence is extremely small. Long-standing moderate to severe hearing loss could be the basis for some auditory hallucinations, especially in the elderly population (Berios, 1990). This is likely related to what can be a long duration of auditory deprivation secondary to the hearing loss. There also have been many reports linking focal brain lesions (epilepsy, tumors, strokes) and degenerative diseases to the occurrence of auditory hallucinations (Evers & Ellger, 2004; see Musiek et al., 2007).

The pathophysiologic mechanisms underlying auditory hallucinations are not known. However, the leading theory seems to be one of reduced neural connectivity and the existence of random neural discharges in the auditory regions of the brain. In brief, the reduced neural connectivity is presumed to be related to a loss of neural connections as a consequence of deprivation, damage, aging, and other mechanisms, which results in regions of the brain functioning in isolation (i.e., not appropriately connected to other brain regions) and randomly creating perceived sounds. The neural discharge theory supposes that (damaged) neural generators in the auditory cortex similar to epileptic foci give rise to the firing of neuron groups that results in the auditory hallucination (David, 1994; Musiek et al., 2007).

Site of Lesion

It is logical and likely that auditory hallucinations are caused by compromise of the auditory cortex and other related brain regions. The classic human neurosurgical study performed by Wilder Penfield and his colleague (Penfield & Perot, 1963) demonstrated that auditory perceptions can be triggered by electrical stimulation of the auditory cortex. This finding opened the door to the likelihood that auditory cortex could play an integral part in the occurrence of auditory hallucinations. As was alluded to earlier, damage to the central auditory nervous system has been linked to auditory hallucinations in a temporal manner, with these perceptions occurring at the time of or shortly after the event. However, perhaps the most compelling evidence for a central nervous system locus for auditory hallucinations comes from functional imaging studies (Shergill et al., 2004). Functional magnetic resonance imaging (fMRI) studies have shown a relationship between increased cortical activity in auditory regions of the brain and the occurrence of auditory hallucinations. There also have been reports that argue that the brain activity related to an auditory hallucination could be subcortical, but is likely to involve complex interactions between the brainstem and cortex (see Musiek et al., 2007).

Medical and Audiologic Evaluation

The medical evaluation of hallucinations requires a psychiatric and/or neurologic consult. If the patient has no psychiatric problems, focus should be on neurology; however, if the patient is at risk for a psychiatric condition, then the psychiatrist becomes the key professional. The focus of both of these professionals is to find the underlying cause. For example, if a person suffered a temporal lobe stroke and auditory hallucinations appeared in the same time period, the objective following evaluation would be to treat the stroke. Often, however, there is no clear underlying cause, especially in psychiatric cases. A thorough medical and psychiatric history is essential. It is important that drug use be ruled in or out as a cause of the auditory hallucination. Long-standing, severe hearing loss can also be a factor that needs to be considered, especially in the elderly. Details of the medical evaluation of auditory hallucinations are beyond the scope of this chapter. For more information on the medical evaluation of patients with auditory hallucination, see http://auditory hallucinations/Mayo Clinic.com/.

There is a paucity of data on the audiologic assessment of auditory hallucinations. Clearly, the direct evaluation of auditory hallucinations is difficult. Perhaps the most direct approach would be to try to mask the auditory hallucinations. In one of the author's (FM) experience, masking of an auditory hallucination can be accomplished, but much depends on the specific type of auditory hallucination that the patient is experiencing and how well the masker matches the type of sound(s) composing the auditory hallucination(s). Perhaps the most useful audiologic evaluation of auditory hallucinations is not the evaluation of the hallucination itself but rather the audiologic evaluation of the integrity of the central auditory nervous system. This approach assumes the auditory hallucinations are related to dysfunction of the central auditory system. There have been some studies of dichotic listening, speech-in-noise recognition performance, and auditory evoked potential assessments that have demonstrated differential performance for individuals with auditory hallucinations and controls, as well as for individuals who have a history of auditory hallucinations who are assessed while they are experiencing a hallucination and then again when they are free of auditory hallucinations (Løberg, Jørgensen, & Hugdahl, 2004; Musiek et al., 2007; Tiihonen et al., 1992). A factor in the audiologic evaluation of auditory hallucinations is that many people with this condition are schizophrenic, and schizophrenics, even those who do not experience auditory hallucinations, often do poorly on tests of central auditory function. This is likely related to the degenerative neural process that accompanies schizophrenia (see Musiek et al., 2007).

Medical and Audiologic Treatment

Treating underlying medical disorders is the first route to help those with auditory hallucinations. These underlying causes could encompass a large range of disorders, ranging from high fevers to trauma. Medical intervention is key if the underlying cause is found. Although one of the most common provoking causes is the illicit use of hallucinatory drugs, several prescribed medications can trigger auditory hallucinations. Treatment for auditory hallucinations in these cases typically involves the cessation of the use of the drug or medication, and in some cases, the prescription of an alternative medication. Such approaches often reduce and/or arrest the auditory hallucinations. There are also pharmacologic agents that are used to treat auditory hallucinations. For example, dopamine cholinesterase inhibitors have been shown to be useful in treating hallucinations in some patients (Korczyn, 2001). However, in many cases the cause of the auditory hallucination cannot be determined, and in other cases, the origins of the hallucination may be identified, but no medical treatment is available. In these cases, other forms of therapy have been tried with varying degrees of success.

Shergill et al. (1998) reviews a number of nonmedical therapies for auditory hallucinations. Counseling and education of the patient seem to have positive results for some patients. In addition, relaxation therapy, distraction techniques, mood monitoring, and discussion classes have all been tried, but have not proven to be highly successful. More studies on the effectiveness of these therapies are needed before these approaches are routinely recommended.

One treatment that seems to hold some promise for controlling auditory hallucinations is transcranial magnetic stimulation (TMS). This procedure is a noninvasive technique used to stimulate various regions of the brain. A magnetic coil applied to the scalp generates a current that passes through the scalp and stimulates brain tissue (Haraldsson, Ferrarelli, Kalin, & Tononi, 2004). This technique has approximately a 50% success rate. However, many investigators feel its full potential in the treatment of hallucinations has not been realized (Haraldsson et al., 2004).

Interestingly, acoustic treatments have been tried with patients with auditory hallucinations with mixed results (Collins, Cull, & Sireling, 1989; Nelson, Thrasher, & Barnes, 1991). The use of sounds of various types to distract the patient's attention from the hallucination has been employed as an intervention strategy. In some cases, this intervention has worked to a moderate degree but, in other patients, this approach was not effective. Masking is also a consideration that could potentially help some patients. In individuals with long-standing hearing loss, deprivation is potentially a key factor and the fitting of amplification could be a major help.

SUMMARY

Tinnitus, hyperacusis, and auditory hallucinations are all auditory disorders that affect many people and are of concern to the hearing health professional. None of these disorders has a cure at this time, but they all can be managed to some extent. Theories abound regarding their underlying pathophysiology. However, none account for the myriad differences between patient reports and persistent difficulties. Nonetheless, progress is being made in these areas, especially with the use of functional imaging techniques. As a result of the progress that has been made, it has become increasingly clear that the brain is more involved in these disorders than has been previously appreciated. This understanding, coupled with further research, could lead to advances in both the diagnosis and management of these three auditory disorders. The importance of careful and insightful audiologic, otologic, and neurologic evaluations of patients with tinnitus, hyperacusis, and/ or auditory hallucinations cannot be overstated. This triad of hearing disorders/ symptoms highlights the importance of the ear–brain relationship and the need to have several professionals involved in the assessment and management of patients with these disorders.

REFERENCES

Anari, M., Axelsson, A., Eliasson, A., & Magnusson, L. (1999). Hypersensitivity to sound —questionnaire data, audiometry and classification. *Scandinavian Audiology, 28*(4), 219–230.

Andersson, G., Lindvall, N., Hursti, T., & Carl-bring, P. (2002). Hypersensitivity to sound (hyperacusis): A prevalence study conducted via the Internet and post. *International Journal of Audiology, 41*(8), 545–554.

Baguley, D. M. (2003). Hyperacusis. *Journal of the Royal Society of Medicine, 96*(12), 582–585.

Baguley, D. M., & Andersson, G. (2007). *Hyperacusis: Mechanisms, diagnosis, and therapies.* San Diego, CA: Plural Publishing.

Bentall, R. P. (1990). The illusion of reality: A review and integration of psychological research on hallucinations. *Psychological Bulletin, 107*(1), 82–95.

Bernstein, D. A., & Borkovec, T. D. (1973). *Progressive relaxation training: A manual for the helping professions.* Champaign, IL: Research Press.

Berrios, G. E. (1990). Musical hallucinations: A historical and clinical study. *British Journal of Psychiatry, 156,* 188–194.

Budd, R. J., & Pugh, R. (1996). Tinnitus coping style and its relationship to tinnitus severity and emotional distress. *Journal of Psychosomatic Research, 41*(4), 327–335.

Chan, Y. (2009). Tinnitus: Etiology, classification, characteristics, and treatment. *Discovery Medicine, 42,* 133–136.

Coelho, C. B., Sanchez, T. G., & Tyler, R. S. (2007). Hyperacusis, sound annoyance, and loudness hypersensitivity in children. *Progress in Brain Research, 166,* 169–178.

Collins, M. N., Cull, C. A., & Sireling, L. (1989). Pilot study of treatment of persistent auditory hallucinations by modified auditory input. *British Journal of Medicine, 299*(6696), 431–432.

Darlington, C. L., & Smith, P. F. (2007). Drug treatments for tinnitus. *Progress in Brain Research, 166,* 249–262.

David, A. S. (1994). The neuropsychological origin of auditory hallucinations. In A. S. David & J. C. Cutting (Eds.), *The neuropsychology of schizophrenia* (pp. 269–313). London, UK: Lawrence Erlbaum.

Davis, P. B., Wilde, R. A., Steed, L. G., & Hanley, P. J. (2008). Treatment of tinnitus with a customized acoustic neural stimulus: A controlled clinical study. *Ear, Nose, and Throat Journal, 87*(6), 330–339.

Douek, E., & Reid, J. (1968). The diagnostic value of tinnitus pitch. *Journal of Laryngology and Otology, 82*(11), 1039–1042.

Eggermont, J. J. (2007). Pathophysiology of tinnitus. *Progress in Brain Research, 166,* 19–35.

Elgoyhen, A., & Langguth, B. (2010). Pharmacological approaches to the treatment of tinnitus. *Drug Discovery Today, 15,* 300–305.

Evers, S., & Ellger, T. (2004). The clinical spectrum of musical hallucinations. *Journal of the Neurological Sciences, 227*(1), 55–65.

Fabijanska, A., Rogowski, M., Bartnik, G., & Skarzynski, H. (1999). *Epidemiology of tinnitus and hyperacusis in Poland.* Paper presented at the Proceedings of the Sixth International Tinnitus Seminar, London, UK.

Feldmann, H. (1988). Pathophysiology of tinnitus. In M. Kitahara (Ed.), *Tinnitus: Pathophysiology and management* (pp. 7–35). Tokyo, Japan: Igaku-Shoin.

Folmer, R. L., Martin, W. H., Shi, Y., & Edlefsen, L. L.(2006). Tinnitus sound therapies. In R. S. Tyler (Ed.), *Tinnitus treatments: Clinical protocols* (pp. 176–186). New York, NY: Thieme.

Fortune, D. S., Haynes, D. S., & Hall, J. W., 3rd. (1999). Tinnitus: Current evaluation and management. *Medical Clinics of North America, 83*(1), 153–162.

Gordon, A. G. (1986). Abnormal middle ear muscle reflexes and audiosensitivity. *British Journal of Audiology, 20*(2), 95–99.

Halford, J. B., & Anderson, S. D. (1991). Tinnitus severity measured by a subjective scale, audiometry and clinical judgement. *Journal of Laryngology and Otology, 105*(2), 89–93.

Hallam, R. (1996). *Manual of the Tinnitus Questionnaire.* London, UK: Psychological Corporation, Harcourt Brace.

Hallam, R. S., Rachman, S., & Hinchcliffe, R. (1984). Psychological aspects of tinnitus. In S. Rachman (Ed.), *Contributions to medical psychology* (Vol. 3, pp. 31–53). London, UK: Pergamon Press.

Hanley, P. J., Davis, P. B., Paki, B., Quinn, S. A., & Bellekom, S. R. (2008). Treatment of tinnitus with a customized, dynamic acoustic neural stimulus: Clinical outcomes in general private practice. *Annals of Otology, Rhinology, and Laryngology, 117*(11), 791–799.

Haraldsson, H. M., Ferrarelli, F., Kalin, N. H., & Tononi, G. (2004). Transcranial magnetic stimulation in the investigation and treatment of schizophrenia: A review. *Schizophrenia Research, 71*(1), 1–16.

Henry, J. A., Dennis, K. C., & Schechter, M. A. (2005). General review of tinnitus: Prevalence, mechanisms, effects, and management. *Journal of Speech, Language and Hearing Research, 48*(5), 1204–1235.

House, J., & Derebery, M. (1995). Tinnitus: Evaluation and treatment. In F. Lucente (Ed.), *Highlights of the instructional courses* (pp. 293–297). St. Louis, MO: Mosby.

Jastreboff, P. J. (1998). Tinnitus; the method of. In G. A. Gates (Ed.), *Current therapy in otolaryngology-head and neck surgery* (pp. 90–95). St. Louis, MO: Mosby.

Jastreboff, P. J. (2000). Tinnitus Habituation Therapy (THT) and Tinnitus Retraining Therapy (TRT). In R. S. Tyler (Ed.), *Tinnitus handbook* (pp. 357–376). San Diego, CA: Singular Publishing.

Jastreboff, P. J. (2008). Tinnitus and hyperacusis center. Retrieved 6/15/11 from http://www.tinnitus-pjj.com/.

Jastreboff, P. J., Gray, W. C., & Gold, S. L. (1996). Neurophysiological approach to tinnitus patients. *American Journal of Otology, 17*(2), 236–240.

Jastreboff, P. J., & Jastreboff, M. M. (2000). Tinnitus Retraining Therapy (TRT) as a method for treatment of tinnitus and hyperacusis patients. *Journal of the American Academy of Audiology, 11*(3), 162–177.

Johnson, R. M., Brummett, R., & Schleuning, A. (1993). Use of alprazolam for relief of tinnitus. A double-blind study. *Archives of Otolaryngology-Head and Neck Surgery, 119*(8), 842–845.

Katzenell, U., & Segal, S. (2001). Hyperacusis: Review and clinical guidelines. *Otology*

& Neurotology, 22(3), 321–326; discussion 326–327.

Klein, A. J., Armstrong, B. L., Greer, M. K., & Brown, F. R. (1990). Hyperacusis and otitis media in individuals with Williams syndrome. *Journal of Speech and Hearing Disorders, 55*(2), 339–344.

Kochkin, S., & Tyler, R. (2008). Tinnitus treatment and the effectiveness of hearing aids: Hearing care professional perceptions. *Hearing Review, 15*(13), 4–18.

Korczyn, A. D. (2001). Hallucinations in Parkinson's disease. *Lancet, 358*(9287), 1031–1032.

Kuk, F. K., Tyler, R. S., Russell, D., & Jordan, H. (1990). The psychometric properties of a tinnitus handicap questionnaire. *Ear and Hearing, 11*(6), 434–445.

Løberg, E. M., Jørgensen, H. A., & Hugdahl, K. (2004). Dichotic listening in schizophrenic patients: Effects of previous vs. ongoing auditory hallucinations. *Psychiatry Research, 128*(2), 167–174.

Lockwood, A. H., Salvi, R. J., & Burkard, R. F. (2002). Tinnitus. *New England Journal of Medicine, 347*(12), 904–910.

Marion, M., & Cevette, M. (1991). Tinnitus. *Mayo Clinic Proceedings, 66,* 614–620.

Marriage, J., & Barnes, N. M. (1995). Is central hyperacusis a symptom of 5-hydroxytryptamine (5-HT) dysfunction? *Journal of Laryngology and Otology, 109*(10), 915–921.

Meikle, M. B., Creedon, T. A., & Griest, S. E. (2004). *Tinnitus archive* (2nd ed.). Retrieved 6-15-11 from http://www.tinnitusarchive.org/.

Møller, A. R. (2000). *Hearing and its physiology and pathophysiology.* New York, NY: Academic Press.

Morin, C. M., Culbert, J. P., & Schwartz, S. M. (1994). Nonpharmacological interventions for insomnia: A meta-analysis of treatment efficacy. *American Journal of Psychiatry, 151*(8), 1172–1180.

Musiek, F., Ballingham, R., Liu, B., Paulovicks, J., Swainson, B., Tyler, K., . . . Weihing, J. (2007). Auditory hallucinations: An audiological perspective. *Hearing Journal, 60,* 32–52.

Musiek, F. E., & Berge, B. E. (1998). Neuroscience, auditory training and CAPD. In M. G. Masters, N. A. Stecker & J. Katz (Eds.), *Central auditory processing disorders: Mostly management* (pp. 15–32). Boston, MA: Allyn & Bacon.

Nageris, B. I., Attius, J., & Raveh, E. (2010). Test-retest tinnitus characteristics in patients with noise-induced hearing loss. *American Journal of Otolaryngology, 31*(3), 181–184.

Nelson, H. E., Thrasher, S., & Barnes, T. R. (1991). Practical ways of alleviating auditory hallucinations. *British Medical Journal, 302*(67722), 327.

Newman, C. W., Jacobson, G. P., & Spitzer, J. B. (1996). Development of the Tinnitus Handicap Inventory. *Archives of Otolaryngology-Head and Neck Surgery, 122*(2), 143–148.

Norris, A., & Ceranic, B. (2011). Is adaptation of cortical evoked responses impaired in patients with hyperacusis? *Journal of Hearing Science, 1*, 57.

Penfield, W., & Perot, P. (1963). The brain's record of auditory and visual experience. A final summary and discussion. *Brain, 86*, 595–696.

Perry, B. P., & Gantz, B. J. (2000). Medical and surgical evaluation and management of tinnitus. In R. S. Tyler (Ed.), *Tinnitus handbook* (pp. 221–242). San Diego, CA: Singular Publishing.

Remschmidt, H. (2002). Early-onset schizophrenia as a progressive-deteriorating developmental disorder: Evidence from child psychiatry. *Journal of Neural Transmission, 109*(1), 101–117.

Savastano, M. (2008). Tinnitus with or without hearing loss: Are characteristics different? *European Archives of Oto-rhino-laryngology, 265*(11), 1295–1300.

Schwaber, M. K. (2003). Medical evaluation of tinnitus. *Otolaryngologic Clinics of North America, 36*(2), 287–292, vi.

Searchfield, G. D.. (2006). Hearing aids and tinnitus. In R. S. Tyler (Ed.), *Tinnitus treatments: Clinical protocols* (pp. 165–175). New York, NY: Thieme.

Shergill, S. S., Brammer, M. J., Amaro, E., Williams, S. C., Murray, R. M., & McGuire, P. K. (2004). Temporal course of auditory hallucinations. *British Journal of Psychiatry, 185*, 516–517.

Shergill, S. S., Murray, R. M., & McGuire, P. K. (1998). Auditory hallucinations: A review of psychological treatments. *Schizophrenia Research, 32*(3), 137–150.

Sood, S. K., & Coles, R. R. A. (1988). Hyperacusis and phonophobia in tinnitus patients. British *Journal of Audiology, 22*, 228.

Sullivan, M., Katon, W., Russo, J., Dobie, R., & Sakai, C. (1993). A randomized trial of nortriptyline for severe chronic tinnitus. Effects on depression, disability, and tinnitus symptoms. *Archives of Internal Medicine, 153*(19), 2251–2259.

Sweetow, R. (1980). Cognitive aspects of tinnitus patient management. *Ear and Hearing, 7*(6), 390–396.

Sweetow, R. (2000). Cognitive-behavior modification. In R. S. Tyler (Ed.), *Tinnitus handbook* (pp. 297–311). San Diego, CA: Singular Publishing.

Tien, A. Y. (1991). Distributions of hallucinations in the population. *Social Psychiatry and Psychiatric Epidemiology, 26*(6), 287–292.

Tiihonen, J., Hari, R., Naukkarinen, H., Rimón, R., Jousmäki, V., & Kajola, M. (1992). Modified activity of the human auditory cortex during auditory hallucinations. *American Journal of Psychiatry, 149*(2), 255–257.

Tonndorf, J. (1980). Acute cochlear disorders: The combination of hearing loss, recruitment, poor speech discrimination and tinnitus. *Annals of Otology, Rhinology, and Laryngology, 89*(4, Pt. 1), 353–358.

Tonndorf, J. (1987). The analogy between tinnitus and pain: A suggestion for a physiological basis of chronic tinnitus. *Hearing Research, 28*(2–3), 271–275.

Tyler, R. S., & Erlandsson, S. (2003). Management of the tinnitus patient. In L. Luxon, J. M. Furman, A. Martini, & D. Stephens (Eds.), *Audiological medicine: Clinical aspects of hearing and balance* (pp. 571–578). London, UK: Martin Dunitz.

Vernon, J. A. (1975). Tinnitus. *Hearing Aid Journal, 13*, 82–83.

Vernon, J. A., & Meikle, M. B. (1988). Measurement of tinnitus: An update. In M. Kitahara (Ed.), *Tinnitus: Pathophysiology, diagnosis, and treatment* (pp. 36–52). Tokyo, Japan: Igaku-Shoin.

Vernon, J. A., & Meikle, M. B. (2000). Tinnitus masking. In R. S. Tyler (Ed.), *Tinnitus handbook* (pp. 313–356). San Diego, CA: Singular Publishing.

Wang, H. T., Luo, B., Huang, Y. N., Zhou, K. Q., & Chen, L. (2008). Sodium salicylate suppresses serotonin-induced enhancement of GABAergic spontaneous inhibitory post-synaptic currents in rat inferior colliculus in vitro. *Hearing Research, 236*(1–2), 42–51.

Wilson, P. H., & Henry, J. (2000). Psychological management of tinnitus. In R. S. Tyler (Ed.), *Tinnitus handbook* (pp. 263–279). San Diego, CA: Singular Publishing.

Wilson, P., Henry, J. A., Bowen, M., & Haralambous, G. (1991). Tinnitus reaction questionnaire: Psychometric properties of a measure of distress associated with tinnitus. *Journal of Speech and Hearing Research, 34*(1), 197–201.

9

Hereditary and Congenital Hearing Loss

Genetics is emerging as a very important topic in the field of audiology today. It is particularly valuable for the audiologist and health care professional to have knowledge of genetics when discussing disorders of the auditory system, because many conditions have strong genetic associations. Although the purpose of this book is not to provide the reader with a comprehensive coverage of the genetic disorders that can result in hearing loss, we felt that we could not write a book on auditory disorders without dedicating some time to a review of basic genetic principles and disorders. It is beyond the scope of this book to discuss these topics in great depth; however, we provide the reader with some of the more critical concepts associated with genetics, along with a brief overview of the more common genetically based hearing disorders. For those interested in learning more about these topics, the following resources are recommended:

➤ GeneTests (http://www.ncbi.nlm.nih.gov/sites/GeneTests/)
➤ Genetics Home Reference: Your Guide to Understanding Genetic Conditions (http://www.ghr.hlm.hih.gov)
➤ *Hereditary Hearing Loss and Its Syndromes* (Toriello, Reardon, & Gorlin, 2004)
➤ Hereditary Hearing Loss homepage (http://hereditaryhearingloss.org/) (Van Camp & Smith)
➤ *Medical Genetics: Its Applications to Speech, Hearing, and Craniofacial Disorders* (Genetics and Communication Disorders) (Robin, 2008)

GENETICS OVERVIEW

The normal human being has 23 pairs of chromosomes, including 22 pairs of autosomes and a pair of sex chromosomes (i.e., XX in females and XY in males). These chromosomes contain genetic material composed of deoxyribonucleic acid (DNA) that is arranged on chromosomes in units called genes. DNA is inherited from one's parents and is composed of four chemical bases or nucleotides.[1] These include adenine, thymine, guanine, and cytosine, which are strung together in sequences. There are two strands of DNA nucleotides, which bond together to form a double helix. The bond between these two strands is created by the pairing of adenine with thymine and guanine with cytosine.

Genes are composed of sequences of DNA that contain the "genetic instructions" for making proteins. There are two copies of each gene, called alleles, with one allele located on each member of the chromosome pair. The genes carry the data—the DNA sequences needed to make proteins that play important roles in the growth and development of the various structures and characteristics of the human body via the processes of transcription and translation. *Transcription* is the process by which a complementary ribonucleic acid (RNA) copy of a DNA sequence is created (commonly referred to as messenger RNA or mRNA). This differs from *translation,* where short strands of transfer RNA (tRNA) nucleotides (carrying amino acids) pair with the corresponding mRNA bases that have traveled from the cell nucleus to the cell's cytoplasm. The end result of these processes is the decoding of the genetic code and the assemblage of a protein with a specific amino acid sequence. Among the proteins that result from these processes are several hundred that are essential for the normal formation and function of the auditory system.

Changes may occur in the DNA material of the genes (called *mutations*) for a variety of reasons. If such changes occur, then alterations in the end products of the genes (i.e., their proteins) may result. In turn, abnormalities in the specific human growth or development processes in which these proteins are involved are likely to occur. Several types of gene mutations can occur, including nucleotide substitutions, deletions, and insertions. A comprehensive discussion of gene mutations is beyond the scope of this chapter. The reader interested in additional, but readily understandable, information on this topic is referred to Welch (2006).

The inheritance of a disorder can be caused by a single gene mutation or by more than one gene mutation, as in the case of digenic inheritance or modifier genes (see discussion below on nontraditional modes of inheritance for additional information on these types of gene interactions). There are two types of inheritance patterns: Mendelian inheritance and nontraditional inheritance. When discussing Mendelian inheritance patterns, there are three patterns of inheritance that are commonly discussed:

1. autosomal recessive
2. autosomal dominant
3. X-linked

The location of the gene (i.e., on either an autosome or the sex-linked X chromosome) and the number of mutated alleles (one or two) will determine the exact pattern of inheritance.

An important concept when one is discussing Mendelian inheritance patterns is that of zygosity. *Zygosity* refers to the similarity of the gene's two alleles. If the two alleles of a single gene are

---

[1]A nucleotide is a molecule that consists of a nitrogen-containing base (adenine, guanine, thymine, or cytosine in DNA and adenine, guanine, uracil, or cytosine in RNA), a phosphate group, and a sugar (deoxyribose in DNA and ribose in RNA).

identical they are said to be *homozygous*, whereas if one of the alleles is a wild-type (or normal) allele and the other is mutated they are referred to as being *heterozygous*. If both alleles of a gene are affected but by different mutations, then the term *compound heterozygous* is used. The term *hemizygous* is used to refer to the condition where only one allele is present, as would be the case in sex-linked genes where only one X chromosome is inherited (e.g., XY).

An additional inheritance pattern sometimes seen in families with hearing loss is the mitochondrial inheritance pattern. This inheritance pattern is not as common as the other inheritance patterns and is considered to be nontraditional. It is unique in that the inherited trait or characteristic can only be passed by a mother to her child through her mitochondrial DNA (mtDNA).

When an individual is seen for genetic evaluation, a geneticist or genetic counselor will draw a pictorial representation of the family, called a pedigree, which includes the history of the family and the occurrence of a specific disorder or syndrome within the family. The individual who first brought the disorder or syndrome to medical attention is called the *proband,* and this individual is typically indicated in the pedigree by the presence of an arrow. The various symbols used in drawing a pedigree are shown in Figure 9–1, and these will be used in the pedigrees included in this chapter.

Autosomal Recessive Inheritance Pattern

In the autosomal recessive inheritance pattern, both autosomal gene alleles must have a mutation in order for the individual to have the disorder or syndrome. In this pattern of inheritance, the individual

receives one allele from each parent. If both parents have an autosomal recessive disorder, then the offspring will necessarily inherit the disorder, as the offspring will receive a mutated allele from each parent; however, if both parents are heterozygotes (i.e., they each have one mutated allele and one nonmutated or wild-type allele), the offspring may or may not inherit the disorder depending on the specific allele received from each parent, as depicted in Figure 9–2. In the latter scenario, neither parent will manifest the disorder or condition, but both will be carriers of the trait, which they then can pass down to their offspring. In such a situation, each parent has a 50% chance of passing a mutated allele to their offspring, and as such, there is a 25% chance of having an offspring with the disorder or syndrome, a 50% chance of having an offspring who does not have the disorder or condition, but who would be a carrier (i.e., the offspring would have one mutated allele), and a 25% chance of having an offspring who would neither be a carrier nor have the disorder or syndrome. The same probability exists for every pregnancy and does not change as the number of pregnancies increases. Consanguinity (i.e., parents related by descent) significantly increases the chance that two parents will be carriers for the same mutated recessive gene that they inherited from their common ancestors. Figure 9–3 shows an example of a pedigree that might be observed when there is an autosomal recessive inheritance pattern.

Autosomal Dominant Inheritance Pattern

In the autosomal dominant inheritance pattern, the inheritance of one mutated allele is sufficient to cause a disorder or

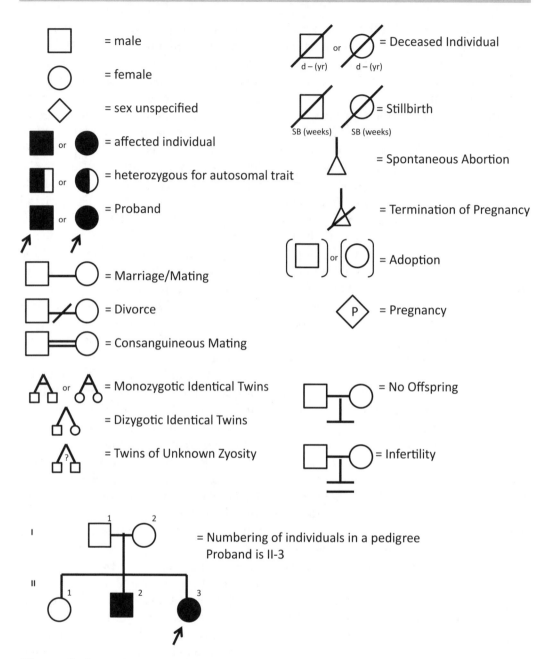

Figure 9–1. *The key to reading symbols of a pedigree.*

syndrome (Figure 9–4). With every pregnancy, there is a 50% chance for a parent with a specific disorder or condition to pass the mutated allele to his or her offspring. If the mutated allele is passed to the offspring, he or she will have the same

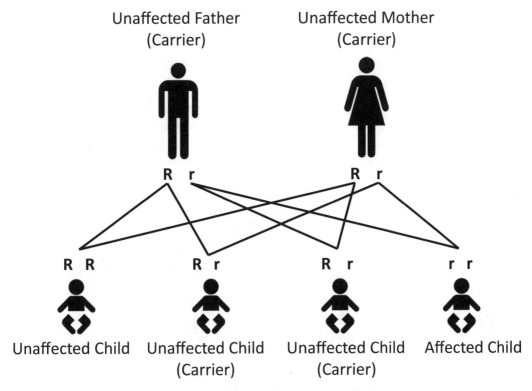

Figure 9–2. *Inheritance pattern for autosomal recessive conditions.*

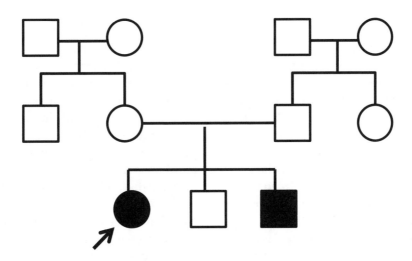

Figure 9–3. *Pedigree showing autosomal recessive inheritance.* Note: *the shaded symbols represent individuals in the family tree with the condition and the arrow indicates the proband.*

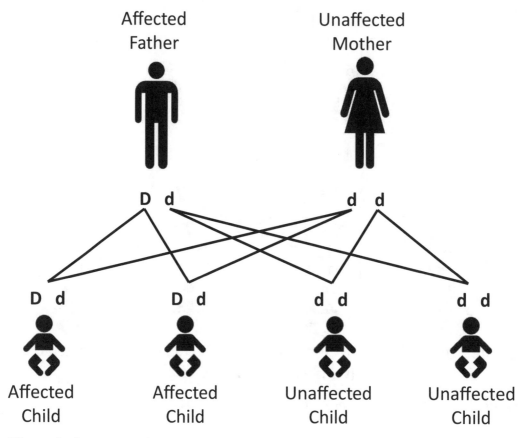

Figure 9–4. Inheritance pattern for autosomal dominant conditions.

condition or syndrome as the affected parent. Here, unlike in the case of autosomal recessive inheritance, many individuals in different generations of the family may have the disorder or syndrome, but the severity and the age of onset of the condition may vary among these individuals. This phenomenon is called variable expression and refers to the range in phenotype[2] that a particular genotype might cause (Welch, 2006). For example, the same gene mutation may result in varying degrees of hearing loss within a family, with some individuals having profound hearing loss while others experience milder forms of hearing loss. Another phenomenon that can be associated with autosomal dominant inheritance patterns is reduced penetrance. This refers to the likelihood that a particular genotype will be expressed as a phenotype less than 100% of the time. For example, if 75% of individuals with a particular mutation are deaf and the remainder have normal hearing, this mutation is said to have reduced penetrance. Figure 9–5 pro-

---

[2]The clinical presentation or observable characteristics that result from the expression of a particular genotype (i.e., the constitution of a set of alleles present at one or more sites).

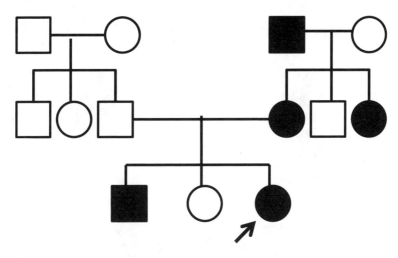

Figure 9–5. *Pedigree showing autosomal dominant inheritance.*
Note: *the shaded symbols represent individuals in the family tree with the condition and the arrow indicates the proband.*

vides an example of a pedigree that might be observed when there is an autosomal dominant inheritance pattern.

X-Linked Inheritance Pattern

This refers to the mode of transmission of genes on the X chromosome. This is a unique inheritance pattern, as females have two X chromosomes (XX) whereas males have one X and one Y chromosome (XY), and most of the X chromosome genes do not have corresponding alleles on the Y chromosome. As a result, if a male has a mutation in a gene on the X chromosome, he will have the condition or disorder associated with that mutation, because he has one mutated allele, but females will not typically have the condition or disorder, because they have one mutated allele and one wild-type allele. Figure 9–6 shows the inheritance pattern for a recessive X-linked disorder with a maternal carrier. In this inheritance pattern, there is a 25% chance that the couple will have a

male offspring with the disorder or syndrome, a 25% chance that the offspring will be an unaffected male, a 25% chance that the offspring will be an unaffected female, and a 25% chance that the offspring will be an unaffected female who is a carrier for the condition. Figure 9–7 depicts a representative pedigree for a family with this type of X-linked recessive trait. The above information discusses the mode of inheritance with a maternal carrier; however, if a male with the disorder or condition mates with a female with two wild-type (normal) alleles, then none of the male offspring will be affected, but all of the females will be carriers and may or may not show milder manifestations of the disorder.

Mitochondrial Inheritance

Although most of the DNA in humans is located in the nucleus, a small amount is located in the energy-producing organelles called mitochondria. Humans obtain their mitochondrial DNA from their mothers

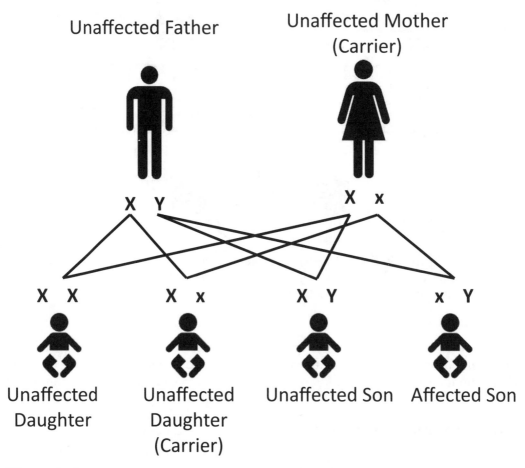

Figure 9–6. *Inheritance pattern for X-linked recessive conditions.*

because egg cells contain mitochondria and sperm cells do not. Hence, any mutations in the mtDNA are passed from the mother to all of her children, both males and females. Figure 9–8 shows an example of a pedigree that might be observed when there is a mitochondrial inheritance pattern.

Multifactorial Inheritance Patterns

For many disorders and conditions, the inheritance pattern can be multifactorial (i.e., there can be an intricate interaction between genes and the environment). In these cases, individuals may inherit a predisposition to develop a disorder, but the disorder does not necessarily manifest itself if the individual is not exposed to the environmental conditions that will trigger the response.

An inheritance pattern can also be digenic. In these cases, mutations in two genes interact to cause deafness or hearing loss. In other cases of inherited hearing loss, there are modifier genes that may determine if a genetic mutation will lead

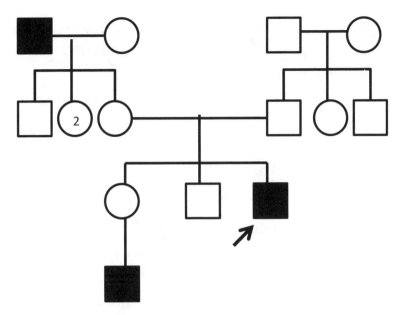

Figure 9–7. *Pedigree showing X-linked recessive inheritance. Note: the shaded symbols represent individuals in the family tree with the condition and the arrow indicates the proband.*

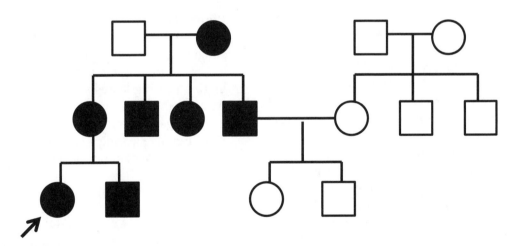

Figure 9–8. *Pedigree showing mitochondrial trait inheritance. Note: the shaded symbols represent individuals in the family tree with the condition and the arrow indicates the proband.*

to a condition or disorder or not. Modifier genes interact with other genes in a variety of ways. As discussed by Welch (2006), one gene may determine if a person has hearing loss (or not), and a second gene may determine the degree of hearing loss experienced (mild versus profound, etc.). It is also possible that a gene may determine if a person has a hearing loss or not, and an allele at a modifier locus may "save" the individual with the genotype from experiencing hearing loss. In this case, the individual presents phenotypically with normal hearing.

THE GENETICS OF HEARING LOSS

In humans, hearing loss comprises the most common sensory deficit. The prevalence of congenital hearing loss in newborns is 1 to 3 children per 1000 (Lalwani, 2008). The overall prevalence of hearing loss increases dramatically with age, due to the significant increase in the number of individuals with acquired hearing loss in older populations. It is estimated that 30 to 35% of individuals between the ages of 65 and 75 years of age have hearing loss, and the percentage rises to 40 to 50% for those over the age of 75 years (National Institute on Deafness and Other Communication Disorders, 1997).

This increase is due in part to the fact that genetic and environmental factors contribute to the development of hearing loss in many individuals (e.g., many individuals inherit a gene that increases their susceptibility to the damaging effects of noise exposure). Genetic etiologies account for the majority of hearing losses (50–60%) diagnosed in infancy (detected by newborn hearing screening) or in early childhood, and they also contribute to a significant proportion of hearing losses of later onset (Center for Disease Control and Prevention, 2011).

Genetic hearing losses (as well as hearing losses in general) are often classified by type and onset of the hearing loss. These classifications are described below.

CLASSIFICATION OF HEARING LOSS

Types of Hearing Loss

1. **Conductive:** Occurs due to abnormalities of the external auditory canal and/or middle ear.
2. **Sensorineural:** Occurs as a result of malfunction of inner ear (cochlea) and/or eighth cranial nerve.
3. **Mixed:** A combination of the previous two types.
4. **Central Auditory Dysfunction:** Due to a malfunction at the level of the auditory brainstem, cerebral cortex, and/or interhemispheric pathways.

Onset of Hearing Loss

1. **Prelingual:** Hearing loss develops before the acquisition of speech. All congenital (present at birth) hearing losses are prelingual, but not all prelingual hearing losses are congenital. Around 50% of this type of hearing loss is due to genetic causes (Figure 9–9).
2. **Postlingual:** Hearing loss occurs after the development of normal speech.

Perhaps the most common and useful classification of hereditary hearing loss is nonsyndromic versus syndromic hearing loss. These types of genetically based hearing losses are discussed below.

Nonsyndromic Hearing Loss

Hearing loss is one of the most common of the sensory disorders. Either at birth, during early childhood, or by adulthood significant hearing loss affects about 2 in

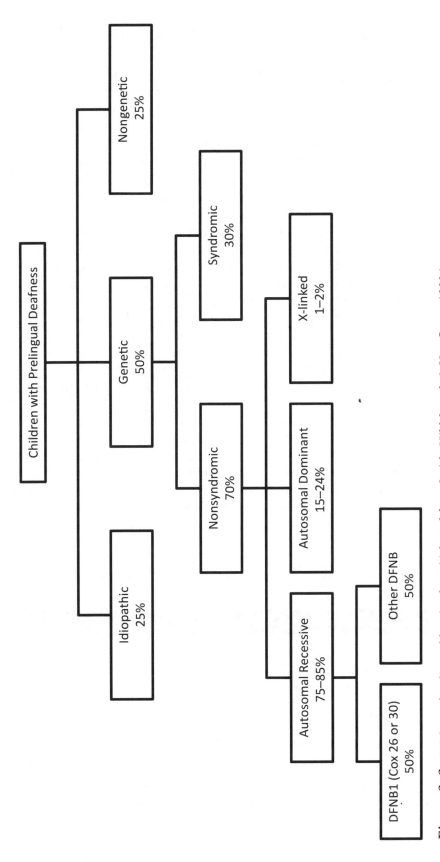

Figure 9–9. *Etiology of prelingual hearing loss. (Adapted from Smith, Hildebrand, & Van Camp, 1999.)*

1000 individuals and more than half of these are related to genetic causes (Li & Friedmann, 2002; Reardon, 1992). Interestingly, even in hearing loss related to aging in the elderly population (i.e., presbycusis), genetics (along with environmental cases) may likely play a role (Li & Friedmann, 2002). Genetic hearing losses can be segmented into two main categories—syndromic and nonsyndromic. Syndromic hearing loss, which will be discussed later, involves not only the auditory system but also other systems, making it a multifaceted disorder. Nonsyndromic hearing loss (NSHL) involves primarily the auditory system; however, in some situations more than the auditory system can be involved, but not nearly to the degree as is observed in syndromic hearing loss.

Nonsyndromic hearing losses are more common than syndromic hearing losses. Approximately 70% of genetic hearing loss is nonsyndromic, with syndromic hearing loss accounting for about 30% of the genetically based hearing losses (Li & Friedmann, 2002). Nonsyndromic hearing loss can be autosomal dominant or autosomal recessive, with the recessive form accounting for about 80% and the dominant form 18% of nonsyndromic hearing loss. Another 2% are reported to be X-linked (Li & Friedmann, 2002). Table 9–1 provides examples of genes associated with autosomal recessive nonsyndromic hearing loss. The designation of DFNA in this table indicates an autosomal dominant pattern of inheritance and DFNB refers to an autosomal recessive inheritance pattern, with the latter pattern of inheritance being more common in NSHL. Table 9–2 provides a list of some of the autosomal dominant genes along with their functions. In addition, the typical onset of the hearing loss (i.e., either prelingual or postlingual) associated with these gene mutations is provided for each of the genes listed.

Genes create proteins that play a critical role in the development, function, and dysfunction of structures throughout the various systems in the body. There are

Table 9–1. Examples of Genes Associated with Autosomal Recessive Nonsyndromic Hearing Loss

Gene Locus	Gene Symbol	Onset of HL	Function
DFNB1	GJB2 (Connexin 26) GJB6 (Connexin 30) GJB3 (Connexin 31)	Prelingual	Homeostasis
DFNB2	MY07A	Pre- or Postlingual	Cytoskeletal System
DFNB3	MY015	Prelingual	Cytoskeletal System
DFNB21	TECTA	Prelingual	Extracellular Matrix
DFNB36	ESPN	Prelingual	Cytoskeletal System

DFN = Deafness

Table 9–2. Examples of Genes Associated with Autosomal Dominant Nonsyndromic Hearing Loss

Gene Locus	Gene Symbol	Onset of HL	Function
DFNA1	DIAPH1	Postlingual	Cytoskeletal System
DFNA3	GJB2, GJB6	Prelingual	Homeostasis
DFNA10	EYA4	Postlingual	Transcription Factors
DFN17	MYH9	Postlingual	Cytoskeletal System
DFN36	TMC1	Postlingual	Cytoskeletal System
DFN48	MY01A	Postlingual	Unknown

DFN = Deafness

a variety of genes associated with the auditory system (Hood & Keats, 2011). The genes that have been identified at the molecular level encode proteins that have functions related to cytoskeleton, extracellular matrix, transcription factors, and ion channels (Kalatzis & Petit, 1998). According to Li and Friedmann (2002), more that 50 genes for NSHL have been identified, but a far smaller number have been characterized molecularly. These investigators relate that identifying genes is a challenging process, which includes defining the phenotype and finding families that have the genotype of interest, and then pursuing detailed family histories. The chromosomal location of the mutated or affected gene must be identified and a series of molecular-level processes (including gene cloning) are utilized to further learn about the affected area of the chromosome. Li and Friedmann (2002) provide an extensive review of gene mutations that can result in NSHL. A few of the better-known genes (especially to the audiology and otology community) are MYO7A, MYO15, and MYH9, which

are motor molecules that encode the myosin protein. Also notable are the GJB2, GJB6, and GJB3 genes, which are all categorized as gap junction proteins that encode the proteins connexin 26, 30, and 31, respectively. The myosin genes are associated with movement of actin filaments and the maintenance of the tip links of hair cells. These "movement" proteins make one think of the motile properties of the outer hair cells and the critical role they play in hearing. The GJB2 gene was one of the first identified genes associated with a high percentage of NSHL (autosomal recessive). The connexin 26 protein associated with GJB2 plays a key role in the development and maintenance of cochlear supporting cells, the stria vascularis, and electrolyte exchange across cells (Hood & Keats, 2011). There have been over 80 mutations of the GJB2 gene categorized, with some mutations yielding more hearing loss than others (Hood & Keats, 2011).

Mutations of genes such as the ones that have been mentioned above and/ or referred to in the tables can result in hearing loss. Although in some cases certain mutations can result in severe to profound hearing loss, a similar mutation may also result in minimal hearing loss. This kind of variability seems common (Hood & Keats, 2011). Having said this, some trends in regard to hearing loss have been reported. First, a very high percentage of NSHL is sensorineural in nature, as the various gene mutations affect proteins that influence structures and functions of the cochlea. There is also some evidence for gene mutations to yield a certain configuration of hearing loss, although the degree of loss may vary. A report by Wilcox and colleagues (2000) revealed that mutations of the GJB2 gene resulted in mostly high-frequency sensorineural hearing loss. Although the degree of loss varied from mild to profound, there was a trend toward the high frequencies (4000 to 8000 Hz) being more involved than the low and middle frequencies in individuals with mutations of this particular gene. The audiograms from individuals that had two connexin 26 mutations had a higher percentage of high-frequency hearing loss than those with one or no connexin 26 mutations. In this study, the second most common audiometric configuration was a flat audiogram, followed by a U-shaped audiogram.

Syndromic Hereditary Hearing Loss

A total of 427 syndromes (most of which are rare) with associated hearing losses have been identified (see Toriello, Readon, & Gorlin, 2004). These syndromes can be the result of chromosomal anomalies, a single gene mutation, or a combination of genetic and environmental factors. Most of these syndromes are inherited in the autosomal dominant fashion, but some are inherited in autosomal recessive and X-linked transmission patterns (see Tables 9–3 and 9–4 for information on some common syndromes, along with their modes of transmission, gene symbols, and clinical findings).

The following syndromes are relatively common ones that have been selected for discussion. The information that follows has been based on information provided by Northern and Downs (1978, 1991, 2002), unless other or additional references are noted.

Pendred Syndrome

The gene for this syndrome is referred to in shorthand as PDS, and the mode of inheritance is autosomal recessive. The incidence of PDS is 1 per 7500 (Hood & Keats, 2011). It is reported that Pendred syndrome makes up approximately 2% of syndrome hearing loss cases (Mozaria, Westerberg, & Kozak, 2004). Patients with this syndrome will usually have a U-shaped audiogram. The hearing loss is sensorineural in nature, and the high frequencies tend to be more involved than the low frequencies. The hearing loss is progressive, bilateral, often ranging from moderate to profound, and usually noted before 2 years of age. A characteristic of patients with Pendred syndrome is enlarged vestibular aqueducts (EVA), which cause an enlargement of the endolymphatic duct and sac (see discussion on vestibular aqueducts below). This genetic condition results in a defect in the ion transportation in endolymphatic fluid resorption, and patients have euthyroid goiter. The mutation of the SLC 26A4 gene may be responsible for up to 50% of this syndromic hearing loss (Hood & Keats, 2011).

Table 9–3. Syndromic Hearing Loss: Examples of Autosomal Recessive and X-Linked Genetic Syndromes

Syndrome	Mode of Transmission	Gene Symbol	Clinical Findings
Usher syndrome	Autosomal recessive (most common)	MYO7A, USH1C, CDH23, PCDH15, SANS, USH2A, VLGR1, USH3, GPR98, DFNB31	Retinitis pigmentosa, congenital sensorineural hearing loss
Pendred syndrome	Autosomal recessive (second most common)	PDS	Goiter, enlarged vestibular aqueduct, labyrinthine deformity (i.e., Mondini dysplasia), congenital sensorineural hearing loss
Jervell and Lange-Nielsen syndrome	Autosomal recessive (third most common)	KVLQT1, KCNE1	Syncopal episodes, prolonged QT interval on EKG, sudden death, congenital profound sensorineural hearing loss
Biotinidase deficiency	Autosomal recessive	BTD	Seizures, hypertonia, developmental delays, ataxia, visual impairment, sensorineural hearing loss (if biotin not administered)
Refsum disease	Autosomal recessive	PAHX	Retinitis pigmentosa, severe progressive sensorineural hearing loss
Alport syndrome	X-linked	CoL4A3, CoL4A4, CoL4A5	Progressive glomerulo nephritis leading to renal failure, ocular abnormalities (anterior lenticous and retinal flekes), conductive or progressive sensorineural hearing loss
Norrie disease	X-linked	Gene on XP11.3	Eye disorders (pseudotumor, retinal hyperplasia or necrosis, and cataracts), mental retardation, progressive sensorineural hearing loss

Table 9–4. Syndromic Hearing Loss: Examples of Autosomal Dominant Genetic Syndromes

Syndrome	Mode of Transmission	Gene Symbol	Clinical Findings
Waardenburg syndrome	Autosomal dominant (most common)	MITF, PAX3, SOX10, SLUG	Dystopia canthorum, pigmentary abnormalities of skin and hair (white forelock), heterochromia irises, sensorineural hearing loss
Branchiootorenal syndrome	Autosomal dominant (second most common)	EYA1, SIX1, SIX5	Branchial fistulas, cysts or clefts, preauricular pits, renal malformations, conductive, sensorineural, or mixed hearing loss
Stickler syndrome	Autosomal dominant	COL2A1, COL11A1, COL11A2	Cleft palate, spondyloepiphyseal dysplasia leading to osteoarthritis, eye abnormalities (severe myopia and cataracts) progressive sensorineural hearing loss
Neurofibromatosis type II	Autosomal dominant	NF2	Bilateral acoustic tumors (leading to sensorineural hearing loss), meningiomas, astrocytomas, ependymomas, juvenile cataracts
Treacher Collins syndrome	Autosomal dominant	TCOF1	Craniofacial deformity (mandibulofacial dysostosis), malformations in middle and inner ear structures causing conductive, sensorineural, or mixed hearing loss
Apert syndrome	Autosomal dominant	FGFR2	Premature fusion of skull bones and of fingers and toes, conductive hearing loss
CHARGE syndrome	Autosomal dominant	CHD7	Cranial nerve involvement, sensorineural or mixed hearing loss

Usher Syndrome

The prevalence of Usher syndrome has been reported to be in the 3 to 6% range of all individuals with severe to profound hearing loss (Boughman, Vernon, & Shaver, 1983). Several genes have been identified for this syndrome (see Table 9–3). It constitutes the most common cause of autosomal recessive syndromic hearing loss. These genes have a role in the structure and function of the cytoskeleton of stereocilia of the hair cells. Mutations in these genes are associated with retinitis pigmentosa, progressive visual loss and blindness, and vestibular dysfunction and ataxia in some cases. Usher syndrome is classified into 3 types (see Cohen, Bitner-Glindziez, & Luxon, 2007; Hood & Keats, 2011):

➤ Type I: 90% of cases. Onset of retinitis pigmentosa by 10 years of age. Profound congenital hearing loss and absent vestibular responses.
➤ Type II: 10% of cases. Onset of retinitis pigmentosa in the early 20s. Normal or decreased vestibular function and moderate progressive hearing loss.
➤ Type III: <1% of cases. Onset of retinitis pigmentosa at puberty. Progressive hearing loss and variable vestibular function.
➤ Types I, II, and III have autosomal recessive inheritance (subtypes have also been categorized; for additional information, see Cohen et al., 2007).

This syndrome is associated with bilateral cochlear hearing loss that usually manifests after the presentation of visual symptoms (visual field cuts and night blindness). Cataracts can also develop in individuals with Usher syndrome.

Apert Syndrome

This syndrome has an autosomal dominant transmission and has an incidence of about 1 in 65,000 cases (Genetics Home Reference, 2011). Skull and skeletal malformations may include syndactyly (fusion of fingers and toes). A flat conductive loss is often noted bilaterally, although sensorineural loss may be present in some cases. Congenital fixation of the stapes footplate is frequently noted in patients with Apert syndrome and is the cause of the flat conductive hearing loss often observed. There have also been reports of malformed cochlear aqueducts and large internal auditory meati in patients with Apert syndrome, which could play a role in the sensorineural hearing loss occasionally noted in this population. This sensorineural hearing loss is related to changes in the hydrodynamics of the cochlea. This may especially be the case in regard to what is commonly termed "enlarged cochlear aqueduct syndrome," which can yield sensorineural loss that is usually unilateral and not bilateral. Cognitive capabilities can be normal or mildly to moderately impaired (Genetics Home Reference, 2011).

Waardenburg Syndrome

The following discussion of Waardenburg syndrome (WS) draws on the excellent review of Schultz (2006). This syndrome has an autosomal dominant inheritance and occurs in about 1 in 10,000 to 20,000 individuals (Genetics Home Reference, 2011). There are four subtypes of WS, with the condition of dystonia canthorum key to distinguishing between types I and II. Dystopia canthorum is identified by lateral displacement of the inner canthi of the eyes without this displacement of the pupils. Dystopia canthorum is present in type I, but not in type II, WS. Types III and IV are less common than types I and II. Type III is a more severe form of type I, with musculoskeletal abnormalities of the arms, deafness, broad nasal root, dystonia canthorum, and blue irises. Type IV is similar to type II, but includes intestinal and pigmentary abnormalities. A hearing loss exists in 20 to 25% of individuals with type I, and vestibular dysfunction is present in 75%. Type II has a high penetrance of hearing loss—perhaps as great as 50% (Hageman, 1977). The hearing loss is often congenital, sensorineural, nonprogressive, and of a moderate to profound degree, and it presents with a variety of audiometric configurations. Asymmetric hearing loss as well as normal hearing can occur. Hearing loss can progress to be profound, but if less severe hearing loss is observed, the low and middle frequencies are often most involved. Unilateral or bilateral involvement is possible. Histopathic findings include severely defective or even absent organs of Corti and reduced populations of auditory nerve fibers. Patients have colored irises and a white forelock. Cleft lip and palate exist in 10% of the affected individuals, and severity of hearing loss may be related to the number of skin and hair pigmentation differences (Reynolds, Meyer, & Landa, 1995).

Alport Syndrome

Alport syndrome has an incidence of about 1 per 50,000 live births (Hood & Keats, 2011).

This syndrome has an autosomal dominant (5%), an autosomal recessive (15%), and also an X-linked inheritance pattern (80%) (Hood & Keats, 2011). There is progressive nephritis with hematuria and proteinuria in the first or second decade of life. Males are more severely affected than females in regard to the disease effects. Craniofacial dysostosis, brachiocephaly, bilateral proptosis, saddle nose, ankylosis, and spinal bifida have all been observed in Alport syndrome. Progressive sensorineural hearing loss and vestibular hypofunction can exist, but flat, conductive hearing loss affecting both ears is a common occurrence in this disorder. The severity of the hearing loss tends to be greater in men than women, and usually ranges from mild to severe. Age of onset of the hearing loss is usually in the preteen years.

Branchiootorenal Syndrome

Branchiootorenal (BOR) syndrome affects about 1 in 40,000 people. The term "branchio" in the name of this syndrome is related to the fact that there is maldevelopment of the second branchial arch in patients with this syndrome, which contributes to tissue on the lateral and front of the neck. There can be structural changes in the middle and inner ear. In approximately 90% of the cases, the syndrome is passed on from one affected parent to the offspring in an autosomal dominant inheritance pattern (Genetics Home Reference, 2011). There are three genes related to BOR. One is EYA1, which codes for transcription factor, another is SIX5, and the third is SIX1. Most of the gene mutations involve the EYA1 gene; however, there are many people with BOR who have none of these three gene mutations (Genetics Home Reference, 2011). Patients have conductive, sensorineural, or mixed hearing loss, branchial cleft cysts, auricular abnormalities, preauricular pits, preauricular skin tags, and renal abnormalities (dysplastic or polycystic kidneys).

Jervell and Lange-Nielsen Syndrome

Approximately 1% of infants with profound sensorineural hearing loss may have Jervell and Lange-Nielsen syndrome (JLNS), which is a recessive autosomal disorder (Hood & Keats, 2011). This is primarily a cardiovascular disorder caused by mutations in one of two genes (KVLQT1 and KCNE1) that are potassium channel genes, which lead to disturbances in endolymph homeostasis. The bilateral sensorineural hearing loss is congenital and is usually profound. There is elongation of QT intervals on EKGs, resulting in syncopal attacks and risk of sudden death related to functional heart disease. Carriers of this mutation (parents) may have no hearing difficulties, but should be screened for long QT intervals. A family history of sudden death should encourage consideration of this syndrome. Life expectancy is severely shortened if untreated.

Treacher Collins Syndrome

Treacher Collins syndrome has an incidence of about 1 in 10,000 to 50,000 births (Hood & Keats, 2011). It is caused by a mutation in the TCOF1 gene (autosomal dominant). This disorder is characterized by facial bone abnormalities such as depressed cheek bones, fishlike mouth, and dental deformities. Hearing loss can be mixed, conductive, or sensorineural. When present, the sensorineural hearing loss is usually in the high frequencies. There are auricular deformities and ossicular malformations. External ears are small and deformed and at times just nubs, and atresia of the external auditory meatus are observed. Additionally, the ossicular chain can be absent or malformed. The cochlea and vestibular end organ also can be malformed, but this is not as likely as malformations of the conductive mechanism are.

Stickler Syndrome

This syndrome is caused by mutation in collagen genes. Stickler syndrome is characterized by a flattened facial appearance and affected individuals have severe nearsightedness. They may also have cleft palate, and because of facial bone deformities they can have difficulty breathing and eating. It is estimated that 1 in 9000 births may have Stickler syndrome. This disorder is inherited in an autosomal dominant pattern. The degree of hearing loss can vary, but the hearing loss often affects the high frequencies and can be progressive. Because this is a collagen mutation, the epithelium of the inner ear is at risk; hence, sensorineural hearing loss is common (Genetics Home Reference, 2011). However, in cases with cleft palate and facial problems, it stands to reason that conductive hearing loss could also manifest.

Down Syndrome

In this genetic disorder, there is usually trisomy for chromosome 21 (i.e., an extra chromosome). The risk for having a child with this condition increases with maternal age. Translocation of chromosomes can be the basis for Down syndrome, but this etiology is relatively rare. The occurrence of Down syndrome is related to maternal age, with an occurrence of 1 case of the syndrome in 350 births for mothers who give birth at the age of 20 to an occurrence of 1 in 10 births for mothers who give birth at the age of 34 (National Down Syndrome Society, 2011).

Down syndrome manifests facial features such as epicanthal folds, open mouth, protruding tongue, flattened nose, and rectangular-shaped ears. Affected individuals can also suffer from severe cognitive compromise, hypotonia, congenital heart disease, shortened hands, and dermatologic problems.

Hearing loss is estimated to occur in about 50% of children with this syndrome, with bilateral conductive or mixed hearing loss being the most common. This is linked to a high incidence of upper respiratory and sinus infections in individuals with Down syndrome. Sensorineural loss by itself has been reported, but is rare. A curious finding in the early latency ABR waves is often observed when testing patients with this particular syndrome. This unique finding is that the interwave intervals of I–III and I–V are often shortened in their latencies. Even when compared to other populations with various types of developmental disabilities, the differences in interwave intervals remain significantly shorter for the Down syndrome population (Kittler et al., 2009). As reviewed by Kittler et al. (2009), there is no firm agreement as to why ABR interwave intervals are shorter in the Down syndrome population; however, smaller brain volume and faster development early in life (quicker myelination) have been considered.

Biotinidase Deficiency

Biotinidase deficiency is an inherited metabolic disorder defined by the lack of biotin, the B-complex vitamin (Wolf, Spencer, & Gleason, 2002). The lack of the enzyme biotinidase can affect certain kinds of protein synthesis, which in turn can result in abnormalities of the central nervous system, as well as other medical manifestations (seizures, hypertonia). In some cases, however, symptoms may not manifest until several years after birth.

The symptoms can be treated with biotin if early identification of the genetic condition is achieved, but once symptoms occur, they are difficult to reverse. Currently, however, screening for biotinidase deficiency is carried out in all states, so future occurrences of this condition can and should be managed effectively. Both hearing loss and vestibular problems have been reported in individuals with biotinidase deficiency. This disorder has also been shown to affect myelin in the central nervous system. Therefore, both central and peripheral auditory and vestibular involvement should be considered. Profound or partial biotinidase deficiency has an incidence of approximately 1 in 60,000 newborns (Genetics Home Reference, 2011).

Refsum Disease

Refsum disease is inherited as a recessive trait, and presents as a disorder of lipid metabolism. It has been associated with severe peripheral neuropathies (it is possible that the inefficient lipid metabolism could influence the development of myelin, resulting in poor nerve conduction, etc). Poor coordination, muscle weakness, retinitis pigmentosa, and hearing loss are among its symptoms. The hearing loss is progressive, bilateral, and sensorineural in nature. The gene for Refsum disease has been linked with chromosome 10 (National Center for Biotechnology Information, 2010), but the incidence of Refsum disease is unkown.

Norrie Disease

Norrie disease is a rare genetic disorder, and its incidence is unknown. It is an X-linked recessive disorder (Genetics Home Reference, 2011). Norrie disease primarily manifests as a progressive, severe eye disorder that results in blindness at birth or early in life. The retina does not develop normally. About one-third of those with Norrie disease will develop progressive, bilaterally symmetrical sensorineural hearing loss; however, the onset of the hearing loss can be late. Developmental motor delays are common, as is intellectual disability. Males are affected with this disorder much more often than females.

CHARGE Syndrome

The occurrence of CHARGE syndrome is somewhere in the range of 1 in 8500 to 10,000 persons (Genetics Home Reference, 2011). CHARGE syndrome is a result of a defect in the CHD7 gene, which was discovered in 2004 (see Hartshorne, Hefner, Davenport, & Thelin, 2011). Hartshorne and colleagues (2011) provide a current review of CHARGE syndrome, which is the basis for our discussion here. The CHD7 gene plays a key role in the development of the neural crest embryologically. The neural crest is responsible for the development of the 12 cranial nerves; hence, dysfunction related to these important structures is a main factor in understanding the problems related to CHARGE syndrome. CHARGE stands for the following:

C = Coloboma (missing segment or tear of the eye)

H = Heart (cardiac involvement)

A = Choanae (blocked nasal passages)

R = Retardation (of growth and development)

G = Genitourinary (genital, urinary problems)

E = Ear (otologic, audiologic problems)

It is useful to modestly elaborate on the dysfunctions related to CHARGE syndrome as listed above. Eye anomalies such as coloboma of the iris, optic discs, retina, and choroids have been shown to occur at a high frequency (80–90%). Blocked or maldeveloped nasal passages (choanal atresias) in the back of the nose are also present, but not as often as eye disorders. There can also be anomalies of cranial nerves I, VII, VIII, IX, and X. The pinnae are often short and wide, protrude, and are asymmetric, with reduced amounts of cartilage being observed. Although in CHARGE the pinnae are often malformed in some way, this seldom leads to any hearing loss. In the middle ear, ossicular malformations can result in maximal conductive losses. Dysfunction of the Eustachian tube is the second most common cause of conductive hearing loss in CHARGE. Mondini defects in the cochlea results in various degrees of hearing loss, and, when combined with conductive loss, can yield a considerable degree of mixed hearing loss. Like the cochlea, the peripheral vestibular apparatus can be maldeveloped or incompletely developed. Auditory and vestibular nerves in CHARGE syndrome can be absent or reduced in size. Maldevelopment of the central auditory system can also exist in CHARGE syndrome, but it is difficult to assess because the peripheral system often is compromised to the degree that testing of the central auditory nervous system is not possible (Thelin, 2011).

The incidence and degree of hearing loss in CHARGE has been reviewed by Thelin (2011), who reports that 15% have normal hearing, 38% have mild to moderate loss, and 47% have severe to profound loss. Given these findings, it is clear that hearing loss is a major factor in the overall well-being of individuals with this syndrome.

There are other physical anomalies associated with CHARGE, such as genital hypoplasia and delayed puberty. Cardiovascular problems as well as growth deficiency and cleft lip and/or palate are seen in CHARGE syndrome. Tracheal and esophageal fistulas and renal anomalies are also relatively common in this syndrome (see Hartshorne et al., 2011).

Eighth Nerve

Special mention of neurofibromatosis type I (NF1), also known as von Recklinghausen disease, and neurofibromatosis type II (NF2) is in order when discussing hereditary hearing loss. These disorders can result in acoustic tumors and have a strong hereditary link. NF1 is an autosomal dominant problem characterized by heterozygous mutations in the NF1 gene. More than 500 different gene mutations have been identified for the NF1 gene. The mutations are thought to be "loss of function" mutations due to truncation. Other mutations such as deletion, nonsense mutations, amino acid substitutions, insertions, intronic changes, and gross chromosomal rearrangements can also occur (Jett & Friedman, 2010). About half of the mutations are inherited; the other half are spontaneous (Boyd, Korf, & Theos, 2009).

Neurofibromas occur in the peripheral nerves and can be cutaneous or subcutaneous. They often develop during puberty. The number of neurofibromas vary from a few to thousands. Fifty percent of patients with NF1 have plexiform neurofibromas, which are often discrete and missed clinically. Most plexiform neurofibromas usually grow slowly throughout the lifetime, but can grow rapidly during childhood. Gliomas of the brain, brainstem, or cerebellum are also seen in patients with NF1 and often follow a less aggressive course than in other patients presenting with brain tumors (Jett & Friedman, 2010).

The first symptom to originate is the café au lait spots, which are often seen at birth. Estimates are 90% of patients with NF1 will have these spots by the age of 7 years (Jett & Friedman, 2010).

NF2 is an autosomal dominant disease that can result in bilateral acoustic neuromas, meningiomas, and ependymomas. However, bilateral tumors are not necessary for the diagnosis of NF2. Interestingly, 50 to 60% of individuals with NF2 do not have a family history of the disease, which is due to the "de novo" (new) gene mutation of the NF2 gene. In addition, 25 to 33% of the cases are specifically due to truncating gene mutations. About 70% of individuals with this disease have skin tumors and a large proportion of patients may develop visual problems secondary to cataracts. By the age of 60 years practically all individuals with the disease have manifested symptoms (Gareth & Evans, 2009).

The hearing loss associated with NF1 and NF2 is consistent with what is usually observed with acoustic tumors. This was covered in Chapter 6, Auditory Nerve Disorders. Tumors that appear in the brainstem and/or cerebrum often demonstrate the same kind of hearing difficulties as other central auditory disorders, which are discussed in Chapter 7, Disorders Affecting the Central Auditory Nervous System.

Auditory Neuropathy/Auditory Dyssynchrony (Auditory Neuropathy Spectrum Disorder)

Auditory neuropathy/auditory dyssynchrony (AN/AD) has recently received attention for a possible genetic basis.

Studies on the genetic link to AN/AD are difficult because many etiologies can contribute to the manifestation of the disorder. For example, Charcot-Marie-Tooth disease often manifests as AN/AD and this disease has long been known to be inherited. However, in other cases where otoacoustic emissions have been present, but hearing loss and abnormal ABRs have been demonstrated, no identifiable genetic syndrome or disease was observed (Varga et al., 2003). These results indicate that AN/AD may be a result of both syndromic and nonsyndromic autosomal dominant, autosomal recessive, X-linked, and mitochondrial mutations. Autosomal dominant mutation of the HMSN gene and autosomal recessive mutation of the NDRG1 gene have been reported, as have X-linked recessive syndromic AN/AD associated with Mohr-Tranebjaerg syndrome and mitochondrial mutations associated with Leber hereditary optic neuropathy. However, the majority of nonsyndromic AN/AD are autosomal recessive, with many of the individuals presenting with mutations of the OTOF gene that codes for the protein otoferlin (Hood & Keats, 1991) (see Chapter 6, Auditory Nerve Disorders, for additional information on AN/AD).

Central Auditory Disorders

Although there are a number of inherited disorders of the central nervous system, there is a paucity of information on these kinds of disorders that are linked to central auditory dysfunction. However, the recent work of Bamiou and colleagues (2007) yields new information in this regard. The PAX6 gene mutation has been associated with panocular maldevelopment with anaridia (absence of the iris) and structural brain abnormalities. These structural brain abnormalities often seem to manifest in the region of the corpus callosum. This could indicate that interhemispheric auditory transfer may be affected in patients with PAX6 mutations. Bamiou et al. (2007) tested patients with PAX6 gene mutations and demonstrated interhemispheric auditory processing problems in this group. Specifically, left ear deficits in dichotic listening were demonstrated in this patient population—a finding consistent with interhemispheric transfer problems. Anaridia has an incidence of about 1 in 60,000 (Vincent, Pujo, Olivier, & Calvas, 2003).

CONGENITAL MALFORMATIONS

Congenital malformations can exist for the external, middle, and/or inner ear. These malformations may have a hereditary link in that they may be part of an inherited syndrome or they can be associated with embryonic maldevelopment (which may or may not be genetically linked). Definitive information in regard to a genetic or embryologic cause is difficult to determine in many cases with congenital ear malformations. The information that follows on ear malformations has mostly been obtained from Northern and Downs (1978, 1991, 2002).

External and Middle Ear Malformations

External ear malformations are usually related to abnormal embryologic development of the first branchial groove. External and middle ear malformations can be viewed as aplasias or atresias.

Aplasia usually indicates that the pinna is deformed, but that an ear canal opening remains that allows an acoustic pathway to the middle ear. Atresia usually means this opening is not complete. One of the best-known conditions that can be an aplasia or atresia is the microtic ear. The severity of this problem ranges from mild abnormalities of only the pinna to total absence of the pinna and complete atresia of the external ear canal. This condition can be bilateral, but it is common to observe a unilateral problem, and the condition is more common in males than females. If the middle and inner ears are intact, surgical intervention in these severe cases can provide a pathway for sound to the middle ear. Surgical reconstruction of the pinna is extremely challenging, and what is deemed a "successful" surgery is debatable.

Middle ear malformations are usually related to problems with the embryologic development of the branchial arches (usually the first and second). Absence of the ossicles, either partial or complete, is possible. In addition, fusion of the ossicles may be observed and an absence of the oval and/or round windows may occur.

External and middle ear problems require teamwork from the surgeon and the audiologist as well as other professionals depending on the nature of the deficits. Proper audiologic diagnosis as to the degree of conductive loss or sensorineural loss is essential. Utilization of both air- and bone-conducted ABR is an important consideration in these diagnoses. In some cases, surgical intervention may correct most of the hearing deficit; in other cases, little can be done surgically to improve hearing. Because conductive loss is usually the primary deficit, bone conduction hearing aids may be a useful approach. Careful, long-term monitoring of hearing status in both aided and unaided conditions is required for good audiologic management. Counseling as to audiologic expectations, educational implications, and social challenges that may be experienced, as well as the coordination of necessary referrals, is the responsibility of the audiologist (Northern & Downs, 2002).

Inner Ear Malformations

Aplasias

Inner ear malformations that will be included in our review are Michel-Type, Mondini, Scheibe, and Bing-Siebenmann aplasias (Omerod, 1960). *Michel-Type* is an aplasia of the inner ear that is characterized by complete absence of the inner ear and auditory nerve. The outer and middle ear may be normal; however, the stapes may be malformed or absent in some cases. ABR and radiologic work-ups are critical to the diagnosis of this congenital disorder.

Mondini aplasia of the inner ear often manifests as a partially developed cochlea that has a flattened appearance. Both the membranous and bony cochlear structures are typically involved, with only part of the cochlea (often the basal turn) intact. The auditory nerve and vestibular canal may also be compromised. Involvement may be unilateral or bilateral and residual hearing can be present. Mondini malformations are among the most common inner ear aplasias (Jackler, 1998).

Scheibe malformations are generally limited to the membranous cochlea and the saccule and are the most frequently occurring of membranous inner ear aplasias. Membranous cochlear structures, such as the stria vascularis, basilar membrane, and tectorial membrane are often damaged; however, in many cases, there is residual hearing. This condition can be unilateral or bilateral, and it has been shown to be present in a number of syndromes (Waardenburg, Usher, etc.).

Bing-Siebenmann malformation is one that reveals a normal inner ear bony capsule but abnormally developed membranous cochlea and vestibular structures. Hearing loss is usually profound and sensorineural in nature (Rodriguez, Shah, & Kenna, 2007).

Vestibular and Cochlear Aqueduct Malformations

Vestibular and cochlear aqueduct malformations have become diagnostically popular in recent history. Jackler's review (1998) highlights key points of interest, which are discussed here. In many cases, the enlarged vestibular aqueduct accompanies other congenital abnormalities of the cochlear or vestibular apparatus. It also can exist alone as a probable cause of sensorineural hearing loss. Arrested embryologic development is believed to result in a shortened but broad-shaped vestibular aqueduct. The common term for this condition is large vestibular aqueduct syndrome, defined as when the width of the vestibular aqueduct is larger than 2 mm (measured halfway between the common crus and its external aperture). Hearing loss is sensorineural in nature and present at birth. It often progresses into the teenage years, but it can be highly variable in its degree and progression. Head trauma can result in marked decreases in hearing when this condition is present. Estimates are that approximately 40% of individuals with this condition will eventually develop profound hearing loss.

The diagnosis of an enlarged cochlear aqueduct is somewhat questionable although it can be absent or not patent, most commonly in malformed ears. A fibrous mesh in the lumen of the cochlear aqueduct prohibits rapid cerebrospinal fluid (CSF) exchange from the brain and likely protects the cochlea.

Auditory Nerve and Internal Auditory Meatus

There are also congenital abnormalities of the internal auditory meatus (IAM). There have been reports of both narrow and wide internal auditory canals (Jackler, 1998). These anomalies were brought to light by cochlear implantation investigations. As Jackler (1998) relates in his review, a narrow IAM could indicate an abnormal or absent auditory nerve. For example, if there is abnormal facial function and the IAM is less than 3 mm, it is possible that the auditory nerve is absent. Narrow IAMs may accompany anomalies of the inner ear or they can exist alone and are often considered a contraindication to cochlear implantation. An enlarged IAM may be related to inner ear anomalies but, by itself, is usually an incidental finding in normal individuals. A large IAM is considered one that is larger than 10 mm in diameter. The presence of a large IAM could be a factor in stapes surgery in that it could be a potential route for CSF leak during the surgery.

GENETIC EVALUATION AND COUNSELING FOR HEARING LOSS

Genetic evaluation and counseling is a critical component in the identification and management of individuals with hearing loss. According to the American College of Medical Genetics (ACMG), every individual identified with congenital hearing loss should undergo a genetic evaluation (ACMG, 2002). It is important to delineate the difference between a genetic evaluation and genetic counseling, as they each have separate functions. A genetic evaluation is a medical evaluation performed by a trained clinical geneticist/ physician, which may or may not result in a diagnosis of a genetic condition. The diagnosis would depend on the outcome of the evaluation conducted. Only a geneticist/physician is qualified to make the clinical diagnosis of a genetic disorder.

The genetic counselor is a professional with specialized training in counseling individuals about genetic disorders, but these professionals do not make genetic diagnoses. The genetic counselor, like the geneticist, has many key roles in patient care. These professionals provide education, guide decision making, provide support to the patient and/or the family, and make appropriate referrals when necessary. They are also often involved in counseling families with respect to the probability that a genetic trait was inherited and what is the probability that the individual may pass an inherited genetic trait to offspring (Ciarleglio, Bennett, Williamson, Mandell, & Marks, 2003).

Genetic Evaluation

The genetic evaluation requires a multitiered approach that typically includes obtaining the patient's history, completing a comprehensive diagnostic evaluation, counseling the patient, and recommending interventions and referrals to other specialists when necessary. The initial genetic evaluation begins with a detailed history that has a special focus on the occurrence of genetic conditions in the patient's family, the patient's risk factors

for a genetic condition, and a comprehensive physical examination (ACMG, 2002). This is particularly important because early detection can decrease the chance of morbidities and mortalities that may be associated with some genetic conditions (Cooke-Hubley & Maddalena, 2011).

A detailed medical history is the foundation for all genetic evaluations. The evaluation should specifically include a review of the patient's pedigree to determine the likelihood of an inherited syndromic or nonsyndromic condition, a consideration of the patient's ethnicity and country of origin, and a review of any audiometric evidence of hearing loss, as well as of any evidence or documentation of vestibular involvement and/or other associated syndromic features. Also, medical evaluation for comorbid conditions such as cardiac, vision, and renal impairments should be pursued (ACMG, 2002). The pedigree is a component of the evaluation that deserves special attention. The pedigree can be defined as a chart or diagram which demonstrates the occurrence of the particular trait of interest (i.e., hearing loss). The geneticist or the genetic counselor will draw a family pedigree that covers three or more generations of the family, showing relatives with hearing loss along the lineage. In addition, they will also note any history or other significant findings that may suggest disorders, traits, or conditions that are associated with a syndromic disorder (e.g., the presence of heart conditions along with hearing loss, which may suggest CHARGE syndrome). The pedigree is carefully examined to find evidence that suggests the presence of an inherited trait and the probable inheritance pattern if a family pedigree is consistent with a genetic etiology.

In addition to careful analysis of the patient's pedigree, the geneticist will evaluate the patient in order to determine if the hearing loss may be associated with a specific syndrome. This is accomplished through either physical examination and/or a detailed history of the various systems (visual, endocrine, cardiac, renal), and they will also be evaluated for dysmorphic features. Patients are examined for visual involvement such as retinitis pigmentosa, which is associated with Usher syndrome. Additionally, the patient and family members may be examined for dysmorphic features such as preauricular pits or aural atresia. Patients are also examined for signs and symptoms that may include the endocrine, cardiac, and renal systems. Finally, careful attention should be paid to other integumentary changes (e.g., abnormal pigmentation, white forelocks, etc.), as such findings during the physical examination of the patient could point to certain syndromes or diseases (e.g., a white forelock in Waardenburg syndrome or preauricular pits in branchiootorenal syndrome).

There are several important elements that should be taken into consideration with respect to the physical examination of the patient. Patients should undergo audiologic and neurologic examinations. In addition, they should have an otologic examination with emphasis on the evaluation of the airway and documentation of any dysmorphic features. Additional risk factors for hearing loss should be considered, including meningitis, hypoxia, ototoxic exposure, prenatal alcohol exposure, extracorporeal membrane oxygenation (use of an artificial lung machine), and intrauterine infections (cytomegalovirus, rubella, etc.), as such findings in the medical history and/or evaluation may help to establish a nongenetic basis for the hearing loss (e.g., meningitis or cytomegalovirus infection, injury, or prenatal maternal infection).

As outlined by the ACMG (2002), the following triage/testing paradigm is recommended when evaluating a patient who is at risk for a genetic hearing loss:

I. If syndromic deafness is suspected:
   ➤ Gene-specific mutation screening
II. If nonsyndromic deafness is suspected and the patient is a simplex case (i.e., one that presents with a single disorder):
   ➤ CMV testing
   ➤ Connexin 26 (GJB2) screening
III. If nonsyndromic deafness is suspected and the patient is multiplex (i.e., presenting with a multifactorial disorder) with first-degree hearing-impaired relatives, proceed to connexin 26 screening
IV. If nonsyndromic deafness is suspected and the pedigree suggests dominant inheritance, connexin-related deafness is not excluded and gene-specific mutation screening for other loci may be available on a research or clinical investigation basis
V. If nonsyndromic deafness is suspected and the pedigree suggests mitochondrial DNA inheritance:
   ➤ Testing for the A1555G mutation (associated with aminoglycoside-induced hearing loss) and the A7445G mutation, both of which are associated with some rare familial cases of hearing loss, may be appropriate after common GJB2 mutations are excluded
VI. If nonsyndromic deafness is suspected and both parents are deaf:
   ➤ Connexin-related deafness will be strongly suspected
   ➤ After triage/testing, it will be possible to ascribe a genetic

etiology to the hearing loss in many persons

➤ Alternatively, mutation screenings may be negative. A negative mutation screening must NOT be taken to mean that deafness is not genetic

To be able to answer questions about the presence of a syndromic or nonsyndromic hearing loss, a geneticist needs to determine the cause of hearing loss (Willems, 2000). The geneticist will determine if the hearing loss is genetic (50% of severe to profound hearing loss cases) or whether it is a result of other causes like infections, head trauma, etc. If the hearing loss is found to be genetic, the geneticist will also be able to identify whether it is due to a syndromic or nonsyndromic etiology. Once that is determined, then the mode of inheritance (autosomal dominant, autosomal recessive, X-linked, mitochondrial, or multifactorial) is studied. Depending on the findings, the patient's spouse, parents, and siblings are frequently encouraged to have hearing testing and may also be asked to undergo genetic testing. The geneticist will often work in conjunction with the genetic counselor to provide a multitiered approach to evaluation and management of these patients.

Genetic Counseling

Genetic counselors are health professionals with degrees in medical genetics and counseling. As outlined by the 2006 National Society of Genetic Counselors' Definition Task Force (Resta et al., 2006), they are trained to assist families to understand the "medical, psychological, and familial implications of genetic contributions of a disease." Genetic counsel-

ing is an important resource for patients and their families throughout the genetic evaluation process. Once reserved for high-risk patients, genetic counseling has become a routine part of many aspects of medicine. The goal of genetic counselors is to assist with interpretation of family medical histories and assess the likelihood of disease occurrence (or reoccurrence). In addition, they provide the educational framework for education regarding inheritance, testing, prevention, and management of genetic disorders (Resta et al., 2006).

At the outset, it must be stressed that genetic counseling should be "nondirective." In other words, it is recommended that it be supportive and informative, but it should not prescribe the steps that the individual and/or family should take. The purpose of genetic evaluation and counseling is to answer the various questions that may arise about how genetic factors could cause hearing loss and other conditions (e.g., in the case of syndromic hearing losses) and the risk of the hearing loss (and other conditions, if they exist) to worsen or progress with time. It is also to ensure that the family understands the results of the genetic evaluations. A common question addressed during genetic counseling is, "What is the probability that the genetic condition could be passed down to offspring if a couple mates?"

After completion of the genetic evaluation, a meeting is held with the proband and other family members (at the proband's request) to explain the findings. The findings may reveal whether the hearing loss is genetic in nature and, if so, what its mode of inheritance is. If a syndrome is detected, then the physical and medical features are described. In other cases, the cause of the hearing loss may not be found; however, it may still be genetic.

The most common genetic cause in such a case is an autosomal recessive etiology where each normally hearing parent has one mutation in a gene, and the affected person has inherited these two mutations, which results in hearing loss. The probability of this occurring is 25% with each pregnancy. The chance for these persons to have children with hearing loss is small (i.e., unless they marry someone with the same recessive gene for hearing loss or who has a dominant form of hearing loss).

Another possible pattern that may be observed is that the person with hearing loss may have a dominant gene that is new to him or her (or modified by a new mutation). In this case, the chance that this person will have a child with the same hearing loss is 50%. If the hearing loss is in a male, then it is possible that this hearing loss is due to a recessive X-linked mode of inheritance. In this case, the son would have inherited this gene from his mother. If the cause of hearing loss remains unknown, an estimated risk is calculated based on studies involving families with similar histories. Therefore, if a couple presents with normal hearing and has one child with profound deafness, then their chance of having another deaf child is 10%. If both parents are deaf, then the chance of having a deaf first child is 10%.

The above analysis of inheritance patterns are only a few examples of the counseling issues that genetic counselors encounter and about which they educate patients and their families on a daily basis. The information and support they provide to patients and their families with hearing loss are critical to the care and well-being of the patient. As a result, they play a critical role in the overall management of patients with hearing loss, making them an integral part of the health care team.

SUMMARY

Genetics, heredity, and congenital hearing loss are complex topics that are difficult to overview. Genetic evaluation and counseling have become an important part of the identification, treatment, and management of individuals with hearing impairment. As genetic testing becomes even more highly integrated into audiologic and otologic practices, so will the need for the support of geneticists and genetic counselors. The role of genetics in the identification, treatment, and management of hearing loss is one that has become highly important to patients and their families, and also to their fellow health care professionals.

Acknowledgment. The authors gratefully acknowledge the contributions of Kathleen S. Arnos, PhD, Professor and Chair, Department of Biology, Gallaudet University, and Abbas Younes, MD, Assistant Professor, Department of Otolaryngology, University of Kentucky, to this chapter.

REFERENCES

American College of Medical Genetics (ACMG). (2002). Genetic evaluation guidelines for the etiologic diagnosis of congenital hearing loss. *Genetics in Medicine, 4*(3), 162–171.

Bamiou, D. E., Free, S. L., Sisodiya, S. M., Chong, W. K., Musiek, F., Williamson, K. A., . . . Luxon, L. M. (2007). Auditory interhemispheric transfer deficits, hearing difficulties, and brain magnetic resonance imaging abnormalities in children with congenital aniridia due to PAX6 mutations. *Archives of Pediatric and Adolescent Medicine, 161*(5), 463–469.

Bayazit, Y. A., & Yilmaz, M. (2006). An overview of hereditary hearing loss. *ORL: Journal for Oto-rhino-laryngology and Its Related Specialties, 68*(2), 57–63.

Boyd, K. P., Korf, B. R., & Theos, A. (2009). Neurofibromatosis type 1. *Journal of American Academy of Dermatology, 61*(1), 1–14.

Boughman, J. A., Vernon, M., & Shaver, K. A. (1983). Usher syndrome: Definition and estimate of prevalence from two high-risk populations. *Journal of Chronic Diseases, 36*(3), 595–603.

Center for Disease Control and Prevention. (2011). *Genetics of hearing loss.* Retrieved 6/15/11 from http://www.cdc.gov/ncbddd/hearingloss/genetics.html

Ciarleglio, L. J., Bennett, R. L., Williamson, J., Mandell, J. B., & Marks, J. H. (2003). Genetic counseling throughout the life cycle. *Journal of Clinical Investigation, 112*(9), 1280–1286.

Cohen, M., Bitner-Glindziez, M., & Luxon, L. (2007). The changing face of Usher syndrome: Clinical implications. *International Journal of Audiology, 46*(2), 82–93.

Cooke-Hubley, S., & Maddalena, V. (2011). Access to genetic testing and genetic counseling in vulnerable populations: The d/Deaf and hard of hearing population. *Journal of Community Genetics, 2*(3), 117–125.

Gareth, D., & Evans, R. (2009). Neurofibromatosis type 2 (NF2): A clinical and molecular review. *Orphanet Journal of Rare Diseases, 4,* 16–32.

Genetics Home Reference. 2011. *Your guide to understanding genetic conditions.* Retrieved 6/15/11 from http://www.ghr.hlm.hih.gov

Hageman, M. J. (1977). Audiometric findings in 34 patients with Waardenburg's syndrome. *Journal of Laryngology and Otology, 91*(7), 575–584.

Hartshorne, T. S., Hefner, M. A., Davenport, S. L. H., & Thelin, J. W. (Eds.). (2011). *CHARGE syndrome.* San Diego, CA: Plural.

Hood, L. J., & Keats, B. J. (2011). Genetics of childhood hearing loss. In R. Seewald & A. M. Tharpe (Eds.), *Comprehensive handbook of pediatric audiology* (pp. 113–123). San Diego, CA: Plural.

Jackler, R. (1998). Congenital malformations of the inner ear. In C. W. Cummings, J. M. Fredickson, L. A. Harker, C. J. Krause, M. A. Richardson, & D. E. Schuller (Eds.), *Otolaryngology—head and neck surgery* (3rd ed.) (pp. 418–438). New York, NY: Mosby.

Jett, K., & Friedman, J. M. (2010). Clinical and genetic aspects of neurofibromatosis 1. *Genetics in Medicine, 12*(1), 1–11.

Kalatzis, V., & Petit, C. (1998). The fundamental and medical impact of recent on research on hereditary hearing loss. *Human Molecular Genetics, 7*(10), 1589–1597.

Kittler, P. M., Phan, H. T., Gardner, J. M., Miroshnichenko, I., Gordon, A., & Karmel, B. Z. (2009). Auditory brainstem evoked responses in newborns with Down syndrome. *American Journal on Intellectual and Developmental Disabilities, 114*(6), 393–400.

Lalwani, A. K. (Ed.). (2008). *Current diagnosis and treatment in otolaryngology—head and neck surgery.* New York, NY: McGraw-Hill.

Li, X. C., & Friedmann, R. (2002). Nonsyndromic hereditary hearing loss. *Otolaryngologic Clinics of North America, 35*(2), 275–285.

Mozaria, S., Westerberg, B. D., & Kozak, F. K. (2004). Systematic review of bilateral sensorineural hearing loss in children. *International Journal of Pediatric Otorhinolaryngology, 68*(9), 1193–1198.

National Center for Biotechnology Information (NCBI). (2010). *The bookshelf.* Retrieved 6/15/11 from http://www.ncbi.nlm.nih.gov/books/NBK22208/

National Center for Biotechnology Information (NCBI). 2011. *Gene tests.* Retrieved 6/15/11 from http://www.ncbi.nlm.nih.gov/sites/GeneTests/

National Down Syndrome Society (NDSS). (2011). http://www.ndss.org

National Institute for Deafness and Other Communication Disorders. (1997). *Presbycusis.* Retrieved 6/15/11 from http://www.nidcd.nih.gov/health/hearing/presbycusis.htm

Northern, J. L., & Downs, M. P. (1978). *Hearing in children* (2nd ed.). Baltimore, MD: Williams & Wilkins.

Northern, J. L., & Downs, M. P. (1991). *Hearing in children* (4th ed.). Baltimore, MD: Williams & Wilkins.

Northern, J. L., & Downs, M. P. (2002). *Hearing in children* (5th ed.). Baltimore, MD: Williams & Wilkins.

Omerod, F. C. (1960). The pathology of congenital deafness. *Journal of Laryngology and Otology, 74,* 919–950.

Reardon, W. (1992). Genetic deafness. *Journal of Medical Genetics, 29*(8), 521–526.

Resta, R., Biesecker, B. B., Bennett, R. L., Blum, S., Hahn, S. E., Strecker, M. N., . . . Williams, J. L. (2006). A new definition of genetic counseling: National Society of Genetic Counselors' Task Force report. *Journal of Genetic Counseling, 15*(2), 77–83.

Reynolds, J. E., Meyer, J. M., Landa, B., Stevens, C. A., Arnos, K. S., Israel, J., . . . Diehl, S.R. (1995). Analysis of variability of clinical manifestations in Waardenburg syndrome. *American Journal of Medical Genetics, 57*(4), 540–547.

Robin, N. H. (2008). *Medical genetics: Its application to speech, hearing, and craniofacial disorders.* San Diego, CA: Plural.

Rodriguez, K., Shah, R. K., & Kenna, M. (2007). Anomalies of the middle and inner ear. *Otolaryngologic Clinics of North America, 40*(1), 81–96.

Schultz, J. (2006). Waardenberg syndrome. *Seminars in Hearing, 27*(3), 171–181.

Smith, R. J. H., & Van Camp, G. (2009). *Deafness and hereditary hearing loss.* GeneReview-NCBI Bookshelf. Retrieved 6/15/11 from http://hereditaryhearingloss.org/

Smith, R. J., Hildebrand, M. S., & Van Camp, G. (1999). Deafness and hereditary hearing loss overview. GeneReview-NCBI Bookshelf. Retrieved 6/15/11 from http://www.ncbi.nlm.nih.gov/books/NBK1434/

Thelin, J. W. (2011). Hearing. In T. Hartshorne, M. Hefner, S. Davenport, & J. Thelin (Eds.), *CHARGE syndrome* (pp. 25–42). San Diego, CA: Plural.

Toriello, H. V., Readon, W., & Gorlin, R. J. (Eds.). (2004). *Hereditary hearing loss and its syndromes* (2nd ed.). New York, NY: Oxford University Press.

Varga, R., Kelley, P. M., Keats, B. J., Starr, A., Leal, S. M., Cohn, E., & Kimberling, W. J. (2003). Non-syndromic recessive auditory neuropathy is the result of mutations in the otoferin (OTOF) gene. *Journal of Medical Genetics, 40*(1), 45–50.

Vincent, M. C., Pujo, A. L., Olivier, D. & Calvas, P. (2003). Screening for PAX6 gene mutations is consistent with haploinsufficiency as the main mechanism leading to various ocular defects. *European Journal of Human Genetics, 11*(2), 163–169.

Welch, K. O. (2006). Fundamentals of human genetics. *Seminars in Hearing, 27*(3), 127–135.

Willems, P. J. (2000). Genetic causes of hearing loss. *New England Journal of Medicine, 342*(15), 1101–1109.

Wilcox, S. A., Saunders, K., Osborn, A. H., Arnold, A., Wunderlich, J., Kelly, T., . . . Dahl, H. H. (2000). High frequency hearing loss correlated with mutations in the GJB2 gene. *Human Genetics, 106*(4), 399–405.

Wolf, B., Spencer, R., & Gleason, A. (2002). Hearing loss is common in symptomatic children with profound biotinidase deficiency. *Journal of Pediatrics, 140*(2), 242–246.

Glossary

Acceptable Masking: The level at which the patient can tolerate the masking sound as a substitute for the tinnitus

Acetylcholine: A common, usually excitatory neurotransmitter.

Acute Otitis Media (AOM): A condition of otitis media with rapid development of purulent effusion.

Alleles: A form of a DNA sequence of a gene.

Ankylosis: Rigidity, stiffness, at a joint (such as the knee).

Anoxia: An overall decrease in oxygen level.

Anterior Inferior Cerebellar Artery (AICA): A branch of the basilar artery in the pons.

Anticonvulsants: Class of medications used to treat epileptic seizures that act to suppress the rapid firing of neurons.

Antioxidants: A molecule capable of inhibiting the oxidation of other molecules in turn protecting the health of the cell.

Anxiolytics: A class of drugs used to treat anxiety and its related disorders.

Aplasia: Defective development or congenital absence of an organ or tissue.

Ataxia: Symptoms of lack of coordination of muscle movements, often related to cerebellar dysfunction.

Audiogram: A graphical representation of hearing thresholds plotting frequency as a function of intensity.

Auditory Hallucinations: The perception of hearing sounds, typically voices or music, when no sounds are present.

Aural Atresia: A condition in which the external auditory canal fails to develop resulting in an abnormally closed or absent canal.

Auricle: The outer most structure of the ear that is comprised of elastic cartilage; also known as the pinna.

Autoinsufflation: The process by which an individual equalizes the pressure between their outer and middle ear space.

Autophony: Excessive loudness of one's own breath and speech due to a patulous Eustachian tube.

Autosome: A non–sex chromosome with an equal number in males and females (22 pairs).

Autosomal Dominant: A pattern of inheritance whereby an individual requires only one abnormal gene from a parent to inherit the disease.

Autosomal Recessive: A pattern of inheritance whereby two copies of an abnormal gene are needed in order for the trait to develop.

Avulsion: A tearing away.

Axial: Situated around a central location or plane.

Barotrauma: Development of negative middle ear pressure due to rapid descent from high altitudes or ascension during diving.

Battle's Sign: Bruising around the eyes; also known as raccoon sign.

Branchial Arches: Structures in the pharynx which lead to the formation of the outer and middle ears during embryonic development.

Brachycephaly: Improper fusion of (cranial) coronal sutures resulting in a "flat head" appearance.

Burst and Taper: A term treating patients with corticosteroids. Initially a large dose is given early to control the inflammatory process, then the dosage is reduced to minimize the adverse effects of steroids.

Carhart Notch: An audiometric phenomenon where at times a notch is observed at 2000 Hz by bone conduction in otosclerotic patients.

Cerebellopontine Angle (CPA): An anatomical recess where the eighth nerve projects to the brainstem.

Cerebral Vasospasm: The contraction of a blood vessel, narrowing its lumen.

Charcot-Marie-Tooth Disease: A peripheral degenerative nerve disorder that often affects the auditory nerve.

Chelation Therapy: Administration of agents, usually to remove heavy metals from the blood.

Cholesteatoma: Collection of epithelial skin cells resulting in a benign, yet potentially destructive, mass within the middle ear space.

Chromosomes: A threadlike structure that is made up of DNA, located in the nucleus of a cell.

Chronic Otitis Media with Effusion (COME): The presence of serious effusion for more than 30 days.

Chronic Suppurative Otitis Media (CSOM): Persistent inflammation and disease of the middle ear.

Cisterns (outer hair cell): Tubular structures along the walls of the OHC which aid in expansion and contraction of the cell.

Cleft Palate: Craniofacial anomaly in which both sides of the palate fail to fuse together during development.

Click Stimulus: Traditional stimulus (a short broadband noise) used to elicit an evoked response.

Comminuted: This refers to a fracture in which bone is broken, splintered or crushed into a number of pieces. This is different than a compound fracture in which the bone is protrudes through the skin.

Commissure: To a bundle of nerve fibers that cross the midline at their level of origin or entry joining separate structures.

Conductive Hearing Loss: Type of hearing loss resulting in impairment of sound transmission from the outer and/or middle ear.

Connexin 26: Genetic disorder that results in flawed copies of the GJB2 gene.

Consanguinity: Parents related by descent.

Contralateral: Relating to the opposite side.

Coronal: This in anatomy or radiology is a frontal plane dividing into anterior-posterior segments.

Cyclophosphamide: An alkylating agent used in the treatment of cancer and some autoimmune disorders.

Depolarization: Process by which the electrical potential within a neural cell changes from a large negative value to a less negative value through an increase in sodium flow into the cell.

Demyelinization: The loss of myelin along the axon of a neuron.

Deoxyribonucleic Acid (DNA): Nucleic acid that contains the genetic blueprint for all living organisms.

Digenic: Induced by two genes.

Effective Masking: Refers to the ability to successfully cover the tinnitus so that the patient can no longer hear it; also refers to sufficiently masking a sound at a given level.

Ehlers-Danlos Syndrome: An inherited connective tissue disorder resulting from poor synthesis of collagen.

Endochondral: Typically referring to development and ossification that takes place from centers arising in cartilage.

Ependymoma: A central nervous system tumor from the ependyma tissue.

Epileptic Foci: The locus of seizure activity in the brain, determined by EEG methods.

Epitympanum: Portion of the middle ear space above the tympanic membrane which contains the head of the malleus and the short process of the incus.

Eustachian Tube: Organ which connects the middle ear space to the nasopharynx.

Eustachian Tube Dysfunction: Occurs when the Eustachian tube does not equalize the air pressure between the outer and middle ear space.

Extra-axial: Outside but usually impinging on the brainstem, usually referring to the locus of lesions.

Fasciculation: Small involuntary muscle contraction in a particular area.

Fissula Ante Fenestrum: Area just anterior to the stapes footplate, which is a common origin for otoslcerosis to occur.

Fistula: An abnormal hole within the body.

Fistulae of the Labyrinth: A hole in the labyrinth, often in the oval or round window.

FM System: An assistive listening device often used with school aged children in which the sound is transmitted directly from the sound source to the receiver via frequency modulated (FM) waves.

Free Radicals: A molecule that has a single unpaired electron which can be damaged by oxidative stress.

Friedrich's Ataxia: An inherited disorder that results in progressive degeneration of the nervous system, in particular the sensory nerves.

Fundus: Opposite of the opening; for example. the fundus of the internal auditory meatus would be the end opposite of its opening into the posterior fossa.

Gamma Knife Surgery: Stereotactic radiologic surgery (utilized in acoustic neuromas).

Globus Pallidus: One of the three nuclei making up the basal ganglion.

Glomus Jugulare: Initial term used to describe glomus tumors.

Glomus Tumor: Benign, slow-growing, high, vascularized tumor at the base of the skull.

Glossopharyngeal Nerve: Ninth cranial nerve whose primary function is to receive sensory input from the tonsils, pharynx, middle ear, and tongue.

Hematoma: Localized collection of blood, secondary to bleeding, such as subdural hematoma.

Hemotympanum: Blood behind the eardrum.

Heterozygote: A person possessing two different forms of a particular gene.

Homozygote: A person possessing two of the same forms of a particular gene.

Hyperacusis: Consistently exaggerated or inappropriate responses to sounds that are neither threatening nor uncomfortably loud to a typical person.

Ipsilateral: Relating to the same side.

Hyperbilirubinemia: A condition that is a result of high bilirubin levels in the blood that can affect the health of nuclei within the central nervous system.

Hypopneumatic Atresia: Atresia in which there is total stenosis along with poorly pneumatized mastoid and the facial nerve has an aberrant course.

Hypotympanum: The portion of the middle ear space that is the location of the bony covering of the jugular bulb.

Hypoxia: Deprivation of oxygen supply.

Immittance: A term used to represent energy flow by measuring admittance and impedance of the middle ear system.

Interaural Time Differences (ITD): The difference between the time information arriving at the right and left ears.

Interaural Intensity Differences (IID): The difference between the intensity information arriving at the right and left ears.

Intra-axial: Within the brainstem, usually referring to the locus of lesions.

Intronic: RNA splicing that removes a nucleotide sequence within a gene.

Iodinated Contrast Agents: These compounds work by altering the magnetic properties of nearby hydrogen nuclei, thereby enhancing visual resolution of the image.

Ischemia: Lack of blood supply that can lead to damaged tissue.

Jahrsdoerfer Scale: A 10-point grading scale based on temporal bone anatomy commonly used in determining candidacy for surgical intervention.

Kinocilium: The tallest cilia in the vestibular end organ.

Levator Veli Palatini: An elevator muscle of the soft palate.

Longitudinal Fracture: The most common type of temporal bone fracture.

Mastoid Antrum: Cavity in the middle ear space that communicates with the mastoid air cells and the epitympanic recess.

Mastoidectomy: Surgical procedure which involves removal of infected mastoid cells.

Meatal Atresia: Atresia that involves the lateral cartilaginous portion of the canal; also known as Type A atresia.

Mendelian Inheritance: A set of laws related to the transmission of hereditary characteristics from parent to offspring.

Meningioma: A relatively common, usually benign brain tumor arising from the meninges.

Methotrexate: An antimetabolite and antifolate drug used in treatment of cancer.

Mesotympanum: A portion of the middle ear space which contains the handle of the malleus, the long process of the incus, the stapes, oval and round windows, and a portion of the facial nerve.

Microtia: Malformation or absence of the pinna.

Misophonia: Dislike of a particular sound.

Mitochondria: An energy-producing organelle in the cell.

Mixed Hearing Loss: A type of hearing loss resulting from both conductive and sensorineural involvement.

MR Angiogram: MRI procedures that serve to elucidate the views of blood vessels.

Magnetic Resonance Imaging (MRI): A medical imaging technique used to visualize detailed internal structures.

Multiplanar Reconstruction (MPR): Permits CT images to be developed from the original axial plane in either the coronal, sagittal, or oblique plane.

Myringotomy: Surgical procedure by which a small incision is made in the tympanic membrane in order to allow fluid to drain and/or be suctioned.

Nasopharyngoscope: Scope used to examine the nose and throat.

Neurofibroma: A nerve sheath tumor in the peripheral nerves.

Neuropathy: Damage to nerves of the peripheral nervous system.

Neuroepithelium: Highly specialized cells of a sensory organ (visual, auditory. etc.).

Oblique: An angle of view, usually between vertical and horizontal planes in imaging or anatomy.

Odd-Ball Paradigm: A manner of presenting a signal that varies in relation to other signals in the paradigm. Often used in P300 evoked potentials and fMRI.

Ossicles: Chain of small bones within the middle ear space responsible for transmitting sound vibrations from the outer ear to the inner ear.

Ossiculoplasty: Surgical reconstruction of the ossicles.

Otalgia: Ear pain.

Otic Capsule: The bony cochlear shell.

Otitis Media: Inflammation of the middle ear.

Otomicroscopy: Otoscopy using a binocular microscope.

Ototopical: Surface application to the ear.

Otorhea: Discharge from the ear.

Otosclerosis: A metabolic bone-remodeling disease of the temporal bone which primarily affects the otic capsule and ossicles.

P50 Response: An evoked potential occurring at approximately 50 msec after the onset of the stimulus.

Paragangliomas: Rare neuroendocrine tumor.

Partial Atresia: Atresia that involves narrowing of the cartilaginous and bony portions of the canal; also known as Type B atresia.

Patulous Eustachian Tube: A Eustachian tube which fails to close.

Perilymph Fistula: A perforation resulting in abnormal communication between the middle and inner ear spaces.

Phonophobia: Fear of sounds.

Pontomedullary Junction: An anatomical demarcation between the medulla and pons.

Pressure Equalization (PE) Tube: Small ventilation tube surgical placed in the ear drum to compensate for a malfunctioning Eustachian tube; also known as tympanostomy tube.

Proband: Relating to the particular person being examined.

Prussak's Space: Posterior epitympanic space.

Pinna: Outer most structure of the ear that is comprised of elastic cartilage; also know as auricle.

Pneumatic Insufflation: Process by which mobility of the tympanic membrane is evaluated by delivering air manually.

Politzer Test: Inspection of the tympanic membrane while air is injected into the nasopharynx as the patient swallows.

Polypoid: Resembling a polyp.

Protympanum: The anterior-most space of the middle ear that contains the opening of the Eustachian tube.

Putamen: A structure in the basal ganglia.

QT Interval: A defined part of the heart's electrical cycle.

Recurrent Acute Otitis Media (RAOM): Three or more bouts of AOM within six months or four or more episodes in one year.

Residual Inhibition: The phenomenon by which there is a decrease or elimination of the perception of tinnitus following the delivery of masking.

Retinitis Pigmentosa: A genetic eye disorder eventually leading to blindness.

Rhinorrhea: Discharge from the nose.

Rhinoscopy: Examination of the inside of the nose.

Ribonucleic Acid: Similar to DNA is composed of nucleotides. It controls gene expression and the synthesis of proteins.

Sagittal: In anatomy or radiology the vertical plane passing anterior to posterior dividing into left and right sides.

Schwartze's Sign: A reddish hue at the promontory that can be visualized on otoscopic exam in otosclerotic patients.

Scutum: Sharp spur formed by the lateral wall of the tympanic cavity.

Sensorineural Hearing Loss: Type of hearing loss resulting from impairment to the inner ear, auditory nerve or retrocochlear auditory structures.

Sigmoid Sinus: A large vein posterior and slightly inferior to posterior temporal bone.

Speech Awareness Threshold: The softest level at which an individual is aware of speech 50% of the time.

Speech Recognition Threshold: The softest level at which an individual can recognize speech 50% of the time.

Stapedectomy: Surgical intervention which involves removal of a portion of the entire stapes footplate and replacing with a prosthesis.

Sternocleidomastoid: Muscle which acts to rotate the head.

Tensor Veli Palatini: A ribbonlike muscle that tenses the soft palate.

Temporalis Fascia: Covering of the temporalis muscle.

Tinnitus: The internal perception of sound with the absence of acoustic stimulus.

Torus Tubarius: The base of the cartilaginous portion of the Eustachian tube.

Total Atresia: Atresia that involves complete stenosis of the cartilaginous and bony portions of the canal; also known as Type C atresia.

Transient Ischemic Attack (TIA): Temporary lack of blood supply to a particular area of the brain.

Transverse Temporal Bone Fracture: A fracture occurring as a result of blunt force trauma to the skull.

Trigeminal Neuralgia: Dysfunction of the fifth cranial nerve (trigeminal), often resulting in facial pain.

Tuning Curves: A measurement of frequency selectivity.

Tympanic Membrane: The membrane that separates the outer and middle ears; also known as eardrum.

Tympanometry: Clinical measure used to measure the pressure, volume, and compliance of the middle ear system.

Tympanoplasty: Surgery in which disease is removed from the middle ear and a weakened or perforated eardrum is repaired.

Vagus Nerve: The tenth cranial nerve responsible for many instinctive responses from the body.

Valsalva Test: Forced expiration with closed mouth and occluded nose while the tympanic membrane is inspected.

Vasculitis: Inflammation of blood vessels.

Vasodilators: Agents that increase the lumen of blood vessels and increasing blood supply.

Vertebrobasilar Blood Supply: From the vertebral arteries which course on each side of the medulla and form the basilar artery on the ventral side of the pons.

Voxels: A volume element, representing a value on a regular grid in three-dimensional space. This is analogous to a pixel, which represents 2-D image data used in various types of imaging (radiology, television).

Wallerian Degeneration: Degeneration of the nerve fiber due to trauma. Specifically, the axon separates from the nerve body.

X-linked: Mode of transmission of genes on the X-chromosome.

We acknowledge the use of:

Menda, L. Danhauer, F., & Singh S. (1999). *Pocket Dictionary of Audiology.* San Diego, CA: Singular Publishing.

Stach, B. (1998). *Clinical Audiology: An Introduction* (1st ed.). San Diego, CA: Singular Publishing.

Wikipedia.com

Index